T0075136

Spirituality and Mental Health Across Cultures

Spirituality and Mental Health Across Cultures

Edited by

Alexander Moreira-Almeida
Research Center in Spirituality and Health (NUPES)
School of Medicine
Universidade Federal de Juiz de Fora (UFJF)
Brazil

Bruno Paz Mosqueiro
Psychiatrist
Federal University of Rio Grande do Sul (UFRGS)
Porto Alegre

and

Dinesh Bhugra
Institute of Psychiatry, Psychology and Neuroscience (IoPPN)
King's College
UK

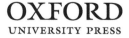

OXFORD
UNIVERSITY PRESS

OXFORD
UNIVERSITY PRESS

Great Clarendon Street, Oxford, OX2 6DP,
United Kingdom

Oxford University Press is a department of the University of Oxford.
It furthers the University's objective of excellence in research, scholarship,
and education by publishing worldwide. Oxford is a registered trade mark of
Oxford University Press in the UK and in certain other countries

© Oxford University Press 2021

The moral rights of the authors have been asserted

First Edition published in 2021

All rights reserved. No part of this publication may be reproduced, stored in
a retrieval system, or transmitted, in any form or by any means, without the
prior permission in writing of Oxford University Press, or as expressly permitted
by law, by licence or under terms agreed with the appropriate reprographics
rights organization. Enquiries concerning reproduction outside the scope of the
above should be sent to the Rights Department, Oxford University Press, at the
address above

You must not circulate this work in any other form
and you must impose this same condition on any acquirer

Published in the United States of America by Oxford University Press
198 Madison Avenue, New York, NY 10016, United States of America

British Library Cataloguing in Publication Data

Data available

Library of Congress Control Number: 2020952930

ISBN 978–0–19–884683–3

DOI: 10.1093/med/9780198846833.001.0001

Printed and bound by
CPI Group (UK) Ltd, Croydon, CR0 4YY

Oxford University Press makes no representation, express or implied, that the
drug dosages in this book are correct. Readers must therefore always check
the product information and clinical procedures with the most up-to-date
published product information and data sheets provided by the manufacturers
and the most recent codes of conduct and safety regulations. The authors and
the publishers do not accept responsibility or legal liability for any errors in the
text or for the misuse or misapplication of material in this work. Except where
otherwise stated, drug dosages and recommendations are for the non-pregnant
adult who is not breast-feeding

Links to third party websites are provided by Oxford in good faith and
for information only. Oxford disclaims any responsibility for the materials
contained in any third party website referenced in this work.

Foreword

This book *Spirituality and Mental Health Across Cultures*, highlights a very important domain for most individuals across different cultures and context. It is estimated that 80% of the world population are religiously affiliated. Research evidence shows that religiosity and spirituality are related to lower frequency of depression, suicide, overall mortality, and substance use/abuse, and positively correlated with well-being, meaning, and quality of life. The World Psychiatric Association recently released the 'Position Statement on Spirituality and Religion in Psychiatry', recommending the integration of religiosity and spirituality in clinical practice.

Research in different countries has demonstrated that most mental health professionals report some obstacles in integrating religiosity and spirituality in clinical practice. The most common reported barriers are fear of trespassing ethical barriers, lack of training, and lack of time. This book aims to help fill this gap by providing ethically sound, evidence-based guidelines, which will be directly useful to clinicians' daily practice.

In the first section, the reader will find a thorough discussion of the principles and fundamental questions in the relationship between science, history, philosophy, religion, and spirituality, and their importance for mental health. The second section explores the main beliefs and practices related to major world religions (including 'spiritual but not religious', agnosticism, and atheism) and their implications for individuals' mental health. The final section is strongly clinical oriented, where readers will find straightforward and practical guidelines to be implemented by clinicians in their daily practice.

This book will be of special interest to clinicians and students in the field of mental health, including psychiatry, psychology, nursing, and social work. It will also be of interest to researchers, public health professionals, physicians, as well as intelligent laypersons interested in the relationship between religiosity and spirituality.

Pedro Ruiz, MD
President, American College of Psychiatrists (2000–01)
President, American Association for Social Psychiatry (2000–02)
President, American Board of Psychiatry and Neurology (2002–03)
President, American Psychiatric Association (2006–07)
President, World Psychiatric Association (2011–14)
President, World Association on Dual Disorders (2015–21)

Foreword

Contents

Section II **General principles of religions and relationship with mental health**

Section III **Clinical practice**

Abbreviations

AA	Alcoholics Anonymous		mPFC	medial prefrontal cortex
ACT	Acceptance and commitment therapy		MRI	magnetic resonance imaging
APA	American Psychiatric Association		MTG	middle temporal gyrus
			NDE	near-death experience
AYUSH	Ayurveda, Yoga, Unani, Siddha and Homeopathy		NHS	National Health Service
			OCD	obsessive compulsive disorder
BDNF	brain-derived neurotropic factor		OFC	orbitofrontal cortex
			PCC	posterior cingulate cortex
CBT	cognitive behavioural therapy		PCMH	President's Commission on Mental Health
CFI	cultural formulation interview		PE	psychotic experience
CofE	Church of England		PFC	prefrontal cortex
CPC	Children's Pastoral Care		PNES	psychogenic non-epileptic seizures
DBT	dialectical behaviour therapy		PTSD	post-traumatic stress disorder
DID	dissociative identity disorder		RC	Roman Catholic
DMN	default mode network		RCP	Royal College of Psychiatrists
DMT	N, N-Dimethyltryptamine		RERF	Rajyoga Education and Research Foundation
EEG	electroencephalography			
EMDR	eye movement desensitization and reprocessing		R/S	religiosity and spirituality/ religion and spirituality
ELE	end-of-life experience		RSNs	resting state networks
fMRI	functional magnetic resonance imaging		SERT	serotonin transporter
			SIP	spiritually integrated psychotherapy
IPL	Inferior parietal lobe			
LGBT	lesbian, gay, bisexual, and transgender		SSRI	selective serotonin re-uptake inhibitor
LOC	lateral occipital cortex		TCI	Temperament and Character Inventory
LSD	lysergic acid diethylamide			
MBI	mindfulness-based intervention		TFH	traditional and faith healer
			TP	temporal pole
MBSR	mindfulness-based stress reduction		TPN	task positive network
			UHR	ultra-high-risk
MCT	metacognitive therapy		UK	United Kingdom
MD	mental disorder		VIA-IS	Virtues in Action Inventory of Strengths
MDD	major depressive disorder			
ME	mystical experience		WHO	World Health Organization
MEG	magnetoencephalography		WPA	World Psychiatric Association

Contributors

Olatunde Ayinde
Lecturer,
Department of Psychiatry,
College of Medicine, University of
Ibadan
Honorary Consultant Psychiatrist,
Department of Psychiatry,
University College Hospital,
Ibadan,
Nigeria.

Haim Belmaker
Professor Emeritus of Psychiatry
Ben Gurion University of the Negev
Israel

German E. Berrios
Emeritus Professor of the
Epistemology of Psychiatry
Emeritus Consultant & Head of
Neuropsychiatry
Life Fellow, Robinson College
University of Cambridge, UK

Dinesh Bhugra
Institute of Psychiatry, Psychology
and Neuroscience (IoPPN)
King's College
UK

Arjan W. Braam
Professor
Department of Humanist Chaplaincy
Studies for a Plural Society
University of Humanistic Studies
Utrecht
The Netherlands

Etzel Cardeña
Thorsen Professor of Psychology
Center for the Research on
Consciousness and Anomalous
Psychology (CERCAP)
Lund University
Sweden

King Yee Agatha Chong
Honorary Clinical Assistant
Professor
Department of Psychiatry
Li Ka Shing Faculty of Medicine
University of Hong Kong
Hong Kong SAR, China

C. Robert Cloninger
Department of Psychiatry
Wallace Renard Professor of
Psychiatry and Director of Center for
Well-being
Washington University in St. Louis
USA

Thomas J. Coleman III
Brain, Belief, and Behaviour Lab
Centre for Trust, Peace and Social
Relations (CTPSR)
Coventry University
UK
Society and Cognition Unit
University of Bialystok
Poland

Christopher C.H. Cook
Professor of Spirituality, Theology
and Health
Department of Theology and
Religion
Durham University
UK

Marianna de Abreu Costa
Anxiety Disorders Outpatient
Program, Hospital de Clínicas de
Porto Alegre, Federal University of
Rio Grande do Sul, Porto Alegre,
Brazil

Rodolfo Furlan Damiano
Institute of Psychiatry
University of São Paulo
São Paulo
Brazil

Julie J. Exline
Professor
Department of Psychological
Sciences
Case Western Reserve University
Cleveland
Ohio
USA

Miguel Farias
Brain, Belief, and Behaviour Lab
Centre for Trust, Peace and Social
Relations (CTPSR)
Coventry University
UK

Peter Fenwick
Senior Lecturer
King's College
London
UK

Wai Lun Alan Fung
Co-Chair, World Psychiatric
Association Section on Religion,
Spirituality, and Psychiatry
Vice-Chair, American Psychiatric
Association Caucus on Spirituality,
Religion and Psychiatry
Research Professor
Tyndale University
Medical Director, Mount Sinai
Hospital Wellness Centre
University of Toronto Faculty of
Medicine
Toronto, Ontario
Canada

Bangalore N. Gangadhar
Former Professor of Psychiatry and
Director
National Institute of Mental Health
and Neurosciences
Bangalore
India

Alison J. Gray
Institute of Clinical Sciences
University of Birmingham
UK
Priest Associate
The Church of the Ascension
Munich
Germany

Susham Gupta
East London Foundation NHS Trust
London

Oye Gureje
Professor
Department of Psychiatry
University of Ibadan
Nigeria

Simone Hauck
Professor
Department of Psychiatry
Universidade Federal do Rio Grande
do Sul
Hospital de Clínicas de Porto Alegre
Porto Alegre
Brazil

Malcolm Huxter
Clinical Psychologist
Compassionate Mind Research
Group
School of Psychology
The University of Queensland
St Lucia
Queensland
Australia

Larkin Kao
Assistant Professor of Psychiatry
Boston University School of
Medicine
Consultation-Liaison Psychiatrist
VA Boston Healthcare System
USA

Matcheri S. Keshavan
Stanley Cobb Professor and
Academic Head of Psychiatry
Department of Psychiatry
Beth Israel Deaconess Medical
Center and Massachusetts Mental
Health Center
Harvard Medical School
USA

Harold G. Koenig
Director, Center for Spirituality,
Theology and Health
Professor of Psychiatry and
Behavioral Sciences
Associate Professor of Medicine
Duke University Medical Center/
King Abdulaziz University
Durham/Jeddah
USA/Saudi Arabia

Pesach Lichtenberg
Professor of Psychiatry
School of Medicine
Hebrew University in Jerusalem
Israel

Lena Lindström
Center for the Research on
Consciousness and Anomalous
Psychology (CERCAP)
Lund University
Sweden

**Alessandra Lamas Granero
Lucchetti**
School of Medicine
Federal University of Juiz de Fora
Juiz de Fora—MG
Brazil

Giancarlo Lucchetti
School of Medicine
Federal University of Juiz de Fora
Juiz de Fora—MG
Brazil

Leonardo Machado
Postgraduate Program in
Neuropsychiatry and Behavioral
Sciences (POSNEURO)
Medical Sciences Center (CCM)
Universidade Federal de
Pernambuco (UFPE)
Brazil

Victor Makanjuola
Senior Lecturer/Consultant
Psychiatrist
Department of Psychiatry
University of Ibadan
Nigeria

Ivana S. Marková
Hull York Medical School
University of Hull
Hull
UK

Alexander Moreira-Almeida
Research Center in Spirituality and
Health (NUPES)
School of Medicine
Universidade Federal de Juiz de Fora
(UFJF)
Brazil

Akin Ojagbemi
Senior Lecturer
Department of Psychiatry
University of Ibadan
Nigeria

Ahmed Okasha
Professor of Psychiatry
Founder Okasha
Institute of Psychiatry
Faculty of Medicine
Ain Shams University
Cairo
Egypt

Tarek A. Okasha
Professor of Psychiatry
Director of the World Psychiatric
Association Collaborating Centre for
Training and Research in Psychiatry
Okasha Institute of Psychiatry
Faculty of Medicine
Ain Shams University
Cairo
Egypt

Ananda K. Pandurangi
Distinguished Career Professor of
Psychiatry
Virginia Commonwealth University
Richmond
Virginia

Kenneth I. Pargament
Professor Emeritus
Department of Psychology
Bowling Green State University
Ohio
USA

Bruno Paz Mosqueiro
Universidade Federal do Rio Grande
do Sul (UFRGS)
Psychiatrist at Grupo Hospitalar
Conceição Brazil (GHC)
Scientific Director of Spirituality and
Psychiatry
Department of Psychiatric
Association of Rio Grande do Sul
(APRS)
Chair of Brazilian Psychiatry
Association Commission on
Spirituality and Mental Health (ABP)
Secretary of World Psychiatry
Association Section on Religion,
Spirituality and Psychiatry (WPA)

John Peteet
Dana-Farber Cancer Institute and
Brigham and Women's Hospital
Harvard Medical School
Boston
USA

Leandro Pizutti
Psychiatrist
Department of Psychiatry and
Spirituality
Associação de Psiquiatria do Rio
Grande do Sul (APRS)
Porto Alegre
Brazil

Mario Fernando Prieto Peres
Institute of Psychiatry
University of São Paulo, São
Paulo—SP
Hospital Israelita Albert Einstein
São Paulo
Brazil

David H. Rosmarin
Director
Spirituality and Mental Health
Program
McLean Hospital
Assistant Professor
Harvard Medical School
USA

Sujatha D. Sharma
Consultant Clinical Psychologist,
Parivartan Center for Mental Health
Founder-Director, MindSpecialists &
Better Minds
Chairperson, RAHAT Charitable &
Medical Research Trust
Visiting Faculty, National Institute
of Public Cooperation & Child
Development
India

Avdesh Sharma
Consultant Wellbeing Psychiatrist,
Parivartan Center for Mental Health
Founder-Director, Better Minds &
MindSpecialists
Managing Trustee, RAHAT
Charitable & Medical Research Trust
Chair, Section on Religion,
Spirituality, and Psychiatry, World
Psychiatric Association
India

Victor A. Shepherd
Professorial Fellow
Wycliffe College, University of Toronto
Professor Emeritus
Tyndale University
Toronto, Ontario, Canada

Andreas Sommer
Independent Scholar
UK

Rael Strous
Professor of Psychiatry
Sackler Faculty of Medicine
Tel Aviv University
Israel

Harald Walach
Department of Pediatric
Gastroenterology
University of Medical Sciences
Poznan
Poland
University Witten-Herdecke
Department of Psychology
Witten
Change Health Science Institute
Berlin
Germany

Cameron Watson
Academic Foundation Doctor—Barts
Health NHS Trust
London
UK

Introduction

Dinesh Bhugra, Bruno Paz Mosqueiro, and
Alexander Moreira-Almeida

Both religion and spirituality (R/S) have played a major role in lives of human beings since the dawn of mankind and that remains the case in many cultures. In times of stress, individuals look towards internal or external sources for help, succour, and support. Looking outwards towards a transcendental realm of life and/or a greater being, organized religions rely on belief systems, moral codes, rituals, prayers, taboos, and support. Attendance in places of worship often provides a sense of belonging and purpose with real and perceived social support, and contributes to social and cognitive development of individuals and the community. Spirituality is an individual internal matter and provides succour and feelings of betterment. Considering that, the World Psychiatric Association (WPA)'s 'Position Statement on Spirituality and Religion in Psychiatry' recommends the integration of R/S in psychiatry research, training, and clinical practice. Sections on R/S have been created at the World Psychiatric Association, Latin American Psychiatric Association, American Psychological Association, and in national psychiatric associations such as in Brazil, Germany, South Africa, the UK, and the USA.

R/S, indeed, represent an important domain for most individuals across different cultures and contexts. Furthermore, there has been a growing academic recognition of the implications of R/S for health, with an increasing number of studies on this relationship. Scientific literature shows a remarkable increase in high-quality research publications in the past decades providing insights and evidence-based information into the relationship between R/S and mental health. Generally, measures of R/S are inversely associated with depression, suicide, overall mortality, and substance use/abuse, and are positively associated with quality of life and well-being. On the contrary, religious conflicts, struggles, or fundamentalisms are recognized sources of mental health suffering that must be acknowledged and addressed in psychiatry.

Most patients agree that it is very, or extremely, important to receive health care that is respectful and compassionate. Many of them wish to share their beliefs and for their spiritual, religious, and cultural needs to be met in health care. The assessment of R/S in mental health care represents a key feature in a qualified and effective clinical approach, also with large implications for mental health promotion and prevention. However, despite most mental health professionals acknowledging the importance of R/S issues in clinical practice, there has a been a large gap in translating this knowledge to clinical practice and professional training in mental health. Research in different countries has shown that most mental health professionals report some obstacles in integrating R/S in clinical practice. The most common reported barriers are fear of trespassing ethical barriers, lack of training, and lack of time.

Based on these unmet needs and on the robust available evidence, the present volume, *Spirituality and Mental Health Across Cultures* presents a comprehensive and sensitive review and summary of evidence and recommendations regarding R/S and mental health to inform clinical practice. This book will be of especial interest to clinicians and students in the mental health field, including psychiatry, psychology, nursing, occupational therapy, and social work, and to all other mental health professionals. It may also be of interest to researchers, public health professionals, physicians, policymakers and individuals personally interested in the relationship between R/S and mental health.

Section I: Theory

The handbook is divided into three complementary sections. In this first section, the reader will find a thorough discussion of the principles and fundamental questions in the relationship between science, history, philosophy, religion, and spirituality with implications for mental health.

Moreira-Almeida and Bhugra (Chapter 1) set the scene for the discussion of the relationships between R/S and mental health, dealing with the question, 'What are religion and spirituality and why are they important in mental health?' The chapter starts with the definitions of religion and spirituality, and the implications of various definitions. Based on the literature, the authors propose defining spirituality as referring to a transcendent realm of reality that is considered sacred, and religion as the institutional or communal aspect of spirituality. They look at the roles of spirituality and religion in the context of a modern and yet changing contemporary and highly secularized world. They explore the challenge as to whether it is indeed possible for science to get into a dialogue with R/S, whether R/S has any impact on mental health, and whether it can be researched. These authors propose a bio-psycho-socio-spiritual evidence-based approach as the best one to inform mental health research, training, prevention, and clinical practice.

Berrios and Marková, in their (Chapter 2), provide a scholarly analysis of the history of the concept of spirituality. In addition, they provide historically informed insights on other key concepts for the field such as religion, sacred, spirit, soul, and spiritual experience. They highlight the complexities and the need to understand the origin and manifold meanings assumed by these words throughout history. They conclude by discussing more recent forms of secular spirituality, not necessarily linked to religious institutions.

Taking up the challenge from Chapter 1, Sommer (Chapter 3) points out that the ongoing debate between science and religion ignores the complex nature of both subjects as well as the complicated relationship between the two topics. There appears to be a clear tension between the Western 'scientific' materialism dating from the nineteenth century, and naturalistic notions of empirical approaches emanating from existing theological and political anxieties. Spirit visions from the Enlightenment to the increasing current preoccupation with professionalization of modern psychology indicate a shift in focus and that in itself is an important challenge. Recent re-emergence of spiritually integrated approaches for treating various psychiatric disorders that had fallen to the wayside for about a century indicates that the pendulum is swinging back, and clinicians need to be aware of ongoing repercussions on scientific and medical practice and research.

Walach (Chapter 4) argues about the philosophical distinctions between religion and spirituality and raises interesting questions about religion as a conceptual, ethical, ritual, and at times also political framework. The distinction of spirituality as the experiential core of all religions is worth noting. Spirituality, through a theoretical framework, can also provide important theoretical insights. In an interesting observation, Walach points out that, because religion has been left behind by the new scientific narrative of a self-evolving world, driven by random accidents and natural laws, there seems to be no place for spirituality either, thereby creating a sense of alienation and isolation.

Taking this one step further, in their overview, Machado and Moreira-Almeida (Chapter 5) provide a comprehensive review of the distinction between religious, spiritual, or cultural experiences and psychopathology. It is not uncommon that, in many cultures, patients with mental disorders have symptoms with religious or spiritual contents, and, on the other hand, spiritual experiences often involve dissociative and psychotic-like phenomena. Clinical differentiation and assessment are thus critical to avoid delaying proper treatment. The overview provided by these authors can help clinicians to reach appropriate diagnoses based on the best current scientific evidence and clinical guidelines to help the distinction between R/S experiences and mental disorders with R/S content.

Building on this theme, Cardeña and Lindström (Chapter 6) present a perspective of self-transcendence and mystical experiences. They develop this theme with brain-imaging research, and ontological implications. It is well recognised that people have described alterations of consciousness during which they experienced a sense of transcendence. These experiences have been foundational for many religious or spiritual practices, although there have been occasions when they have been treated as suspect or outright pathological, thereby pathologizing normal human experiences.

Lucchetti et al. (Chapter 7) review the growing impact of R/S on health, quality of life, wellness, and common mental disorders such as depression, anxiety, and substance use disorders. They observe that a large number of studies have shown that R/S beliefs and practices have a clear impact on mental health, both in a positive and a negative manner, and present potential strategies to spiritually integrated interventions to mental health care.

Koenig (Chapter 8) brings together the genetic, psychological, social, behavioural, environmental, individual-level, and biological pathways in the R/S research highlighting that these connections may contribute to our understanding of the relationship between religion and mental health both in positive and negative ways.

Bhugra et al. (Chapter 9), in their chapter on sexual variation and religion. offer brief descriptions of religious attitudes to alternative sexualities, and suggest the ways that these can be linked with identity formation and coming out. They observe that, in many cultures, religion plays a major role in attitudes towards homosexuality and other sexual variations. The authors highlight the benefits of spirituality to those individuals with R/S beliefs as a source of meaning, self-acceptance, strength and well-being.

Section II: General principles of religions and relationship with mental health

The second section explores the main beliefs and practices related to the major world's religions (including 'spiritual but not religious', agnosticism, and atheism) and their implications to mental health. It provides key information to help clinicians and researchers to better understand the mindset and practices of the main religious traditions, a crucial step for cultural competence.

Gray and Cook (Chapter 10) summarize the impact of the Christian faith on mental health and illness. Through a broad and careful overview of the history of the Christian church founded in the teachings of Jesus Christ, they also highlight the variations between the key beliefs and distinctions from other monotheistic religions and between different forms of Christianity in beliefs and practices of various churches, as well as their long and ongoing history of involvement in health care. It is worth recalling that churches are often at their best healing communities offering community, prayer, and rituals such as Baptism and the Eucharist. These authors observe that elements of Christian faith and practice can benefit those with psychotic disorders and depression, increasing happiness and resilience, and decreasing the risk of substance abuse or suicide. These observations are worth recalling because, in many settings, churches can play a significant role in developing community based healthcare services.

Okasha and Okasha (Chapter 11) describe the concepts of madness, or 'majnoon', in Islam and basic perspectives of Islam as a religion. Using clinical and research observations, they illustrate the attitude of Islam to many psychiatric conditions including the act of suicide, which has been confirmed in very many studies. Practical advice on how Muslim patients can be treated successfully can combine R/S and psychiatric interventions.

Keshavan et al. (Chapter 12) present a dialogue between mental health and Hinduism. They highlight that Hinduism is not only a polytheistic religion: it is much more of a philosophy. They note that ancient Hindu scriptures such as the Upanishads and the Bhagavad-Gita (the Gita) offer important insights to the mind and mental health in ways that can be seen as complementary to those derived from Western psychology. Unlike Descartes philosophy, in the Gita, the mind and body are viewed in non-dualistic terms. Psychopathology is often a result of too much or misplaced attachment and a faulty concept of self. Parallels can be drawn between the Gita and the principles of Western psychotherapeutic models such as cognitive and metacognitive therapies.

Buddhism developed from Hinduism. Huxter and Pizutti (Chapter 13) describe principles and practices of Buddhism in relation to mental health. They suggest that the Buddhist framework can assist clinicians in treating mental health suffering. Buddha's 'four noble truths' and the 'eightfold path' as frameworks for clinical applications can help in suitable cases. Meditation and mindfulness from a Buddhist perspective can help manage some common mental disorders especially through managing anxiety.

Belmaker et al. (Chapter 14) provide a perspective about mental health and Judaism, which is also a monotheist religion. After providing a historical perspective, they point out that, while most Jews today are secular participants in Western democratic liberal cultures, orthodox and especially ultra-orthodox Jews are a rapidly growing minority with vulnerabilities to certain psychiatric disorders, and also requiring culturally appropriate and culturally sensitive interventions.

Increasingly in many countries, notions of atheism and agnosticism are becoming more prominent. In a review, Farias and Coleman (Chapter 15) discuss the relationships between mental health, atheism, and agnosticism. After careful definitions, these authors suggest that, with non-religious experience and a lack of a belief in God, patients do not lack psychological health. Again, it is crucial that clinicians respect their attitudes and feelings.

Ayinde et al. (Chapter 16) provide an unusual perspective regarding African religions and mental health. There is no doubt that, in much of the African continent, religion plays a prominent role in most areas of life. Traditional African religions are many and diverse with their own rituals and symbolisms, often confined to a specific ethnic and language group. Even though most subscribe to the notion of a supreme deity, the common feature of these religions is their polytheistic philosophy in which there are many layers of deities, spirits, and ancestors. Thus, often patients and their families will use these approaches in a complementary way and professional medicine may be acceptable only if it is provided in a respectful manner.

Mosqueiro (Chapter 17) highlights the substantial degree of increased interest in scientific publications about the impact of religiosity and spirituality on mental health and well-being of patients. A growing attention has been devoted to the emergence of people often describing themselves as 'spiritual but not religious', which differentiates their beliefs and faiths from those proposed by religious organizations and from those people without religious beliefs. Mosqueiro discusses the clinical implications of this form of expressing R/S.

Section III: Clinical practice

The final section is strongly clinically oriented, with straightforward and practical guidelines to be implemented by clinicians. It offers, for instance, practical suggestions and guidelines for assessing and integrating R/S in personal history anamnesis and psychotherapy, additionally reviews the relationship with positive psychology and psychiatry, and gives an overview of implications of R/S issues in face of specific clinical situations.

Cook and Moreira-Almeida (Chapter 18) discuss the implications for clinical practice, teaching, research, and public health using the WPA's position statement on religion and psychiatry. Research findings on the topic influence clinical care and the professional boundaries that need to be taken into account.

In (Chapter 19), Kao and Peteet present the evidence-based approaches in order to explain how to take a spiritual history. The first, most basic step to informing this decision is to ascertain a spiritual history that can help the clinician to understand not only the patient's R/S but also whether they or their family would like R/S included in their clinical care.

Taking on the agenda for mental health promotion and prevention of mental illnesses, Braam (Chapter 20) provides an overview on using aspects of R/S as epidemiological factors linked with better or poorer mental health. Three main targets of prevention are suggested. These include contributions R/S can make and how to educate accordingly; secondly to address religious struggle and positive elements of R/S in people with mental illnessess and lastly to prevent associated disabilities.

Hauck and Cloninger (Chapter 21), after a review of evidence, offer contributions to the fields of positive psychology and positive psychiatry. Both disciplines take the focus away from illnesses and aim to study what is 'right' about people—their positive attributes, psychological assets, and strengths—thereby facilitating individuals, communities, and societies to thrive.

In their chapter, Costa and Rosmarin (Chapter 22) recognize that it is important to understand how spirituality is related to mental health and distress, and propose how it can be integrated into psychotherapy. Spiritually integrated psychotherapy involves the adaptation of secular psychotherapies in order to be more culturally sensitive and client-centered to spiritually and religiously inclined clients. Research evidence suggests that these integrated therapies, including cognitive behaviour therapies, are as effective as conventional psychotherapy for treating different mental disorders.

Similarly Pargament and Exline (Chapter 23) review the growing literature on religious and spiritual struggles and their implications for clinical practice, with a focus on people with psychiatric problems. A variety of forms can be used to improve lives of people with psychiatric disorders. This chapter offers practical recommendations to help patients name and normalize their struggles, as well as potential resolutions to their struggles.

Fenwick and Mosqueiro (Chapter 24) state that providing spiritual care to people approaching the end of life can be an important task for mental health professionals. The authors suggests that, under these circumstances, understanding their mental and spiritual experiences constitutes a key aspect to providing a more effective treatment and improving their quality of life.

Fung et al. (Chapter 25) present an overview of evidences, experiences, and implications to foster fruitful collaborations between mental health professionals and religious and spiritual communities to foster mental health in general society.

We hope readers find in this book an inspiring and dedicated review, built upon the contribution of worldwide experts in the field of R/S and mental health, to bring insights, knowledge, and resources to improve the mental health care regarding R/S, to ensure that it is sensitive and open to different cultures' perspectives.

Section I

Theory

Chapter 1

Religion, spirituality, and mental health: Setting the scene

Alexander Moreira-Almeida and
Dinesh Bhugra

Introduction

Several questions emerge whenever anyone talks about religion and spirituality (R/S) and their relationship with mental health. The first key question is about what is meant by R/S. Then other crucial questions follow: is R/S relevant in the contemporary and highly secularized world? Is it possible for science to have a dialogue with R/S? Is it possible, or indeed advisable, for science to investigate R/S? If so, does R/S have any impact on mental health? Would this impact be mostly positive or negative? Do we need to deny or neglect scientific knowledge about bio-psycho-social aspects of mental health and mental disorders to incorporate R/S in our approaches? Even if R/S has an impact on mental health, is it appropriate to approach it in clinical care and public health? Would it not configure the trespassing of ethical boundaries? Naturally, these are complex and challenging questions impossible to fully address in a single chapter, but we wish to start the debate. In this chapter, we will discuss these topics because our main aim is to provide a brief, but as comprehensive as possible, answer to the question, 'What are religion and spirituality and why are they important in mental health?'. In this chapter, we will use the term 'R/S'.

What do religion and spirituality mean?

We propose working definitions for R/S although, in the past century, dozens of definitions have been described. In addition, we will formulate descriptions for spirituality and religion that make sense of the core of what humanity has experienced as R/S and what else has been proposed by many prominent scholars of R/S.

In the past, the word 'religion' tended to be used more frequently than spirituality, and in a broader sense than used today. More recently, the use of the term 'spirituality' has become more common. However, two major dangers have emerged in the academic discourse regarding these definitions. One is the polarization of spirituality as individual, open, and good; and religion as institutionalized, dogmatic, and bad. The second danger is losing the *sacred and transcendent* core of spirituality, usually defining it as just a search for meaning or as positive mental health constructs such as well-being, sense of purpose, or peacefulness. In doing this, one cannot distinguish spirituality from other human experiences that may also bring purpose and/or well-being, such as politics and sports (1–3). Several scholars (4–6) see in this move 'vested interests of an ideological character ... *interest in quasiscientific legitimation of the avoidance of transcendence* ... to provide quasiscientific legitimations of a secularized world view' (p. 128) as put by the sociologist Peter Berger (4).

There have been many definitions for these terms with wide variations of inclusiveness and specificity. In order to be precise, useful, and to do justice to R/S in the real world (outside the academic environment), it is important to avoid extremes. A too-specific and limited definition would not include many varieties of what have been considered throughout history and cultures as expression of R/S. On the other hand, a too inclusive definition may lack specificity and the ability to discriminate R/S from other human experiences, beliefs, and behaviours. In this sense, in line with a long tradition of prominent scholars on R/S, we propose that the distinctive aspect of spirituality *is the relationship or contact with a* **transcendent** *realm of reality that is considered* **sacred***, the ultimate truth or reality*. As support and further clarification of this definition that focuses on the *transcendent* and the *sacred*, the following definitions provided by key authors in the R/S field, and coming from different intellectual backgrounds, are worth noting:

> A minimum definition of Religion[1] [is] the belief in Spiritual Beings. (Tylor, p. 383)(7)
>
> Religion ... consists of the belief that there is an unseen order. (James, p. 46)(8)
>
> Religion is the definition of man's relationship to the origin of everything [usually called God], and the purpose acquired as a result of this relationship, and of the rules of conduct that follow from this purpose. (Tolstoy, p. 120)(9)
>
> The word 'holy' ... includes ... a clear overplus of meaning ... without it no religion would be worthy of the name.... These terms, 'supernatural' and 'transcendent' (literally, supramundane) ... become forthwith designations for a unique 'wholly other' reality and quality, something of whose special character we can feel. (Otto, pp. 5–6, 30)(10)

---

[1] As stated previously, the term 'religion' used to have a broader meaning, basically referring to what it is currently called 'spirituality'. This is why definitions of religion provided by some authors (especially the ancient ones) were listed to illustrate the meaning of spirituality.

Spirituality can be defined as belief in an absolute reality that is also sacred and transcending (Eliade, p. 202)(11). Such transcendental reality is about a "a feeling that 'Something Other' than the self can be sensed'" (Hardy, p. 131) (12) or "transcendent entities in the conventional sense—God, gods, supernatural beings and worlds" (Berger, p. 128)(4). Spirituality has also been defined as a search for the sacred, and the sacred understood as encopassing "God, the divine, and the transcendent" (Pagament, p. 12)(2). Hufford (p. 10)(5) sees spirituality as reffering "to the domain of spirit(s): God or gods, souls, angels, djinni, demons" whereas Armstrong (p. 5)(13) too sees it as " a transcendent dimension of life". Also seeing it as different from humanism, values, morals, etc., Koenig et al. (p. 46)(14) state that what distinguish spirituality is " its connection to which is sacred, the transcendent". Walach (p. 18)(15) sees it as "related to the reality that transcends the ego" and spiritual experiences as "a direct, unmediated experience of an absolute reality. Stark (pp. 25–26)(6) sees religion as fundamentally "concerned with the supernatural", beyond the physical aspects of the universe. This transcendent and non-physical power is also key to Holloway's concept of religion (p. 8)(16).

In line with contemporary distinctions between religion and spirituality, we propose defining religion *as the institutional or communal aspect of spirituality, as a shared set of beliefs, experiences, and practices related to the transcendent and the sacred.* Below are some definitions of religion that support and expand the proposed definition of religion: it has an institutional structure of its own but, as Hufford (p. 11)(12) notes, it is " the institutional aspect of spirituality". Like culture, religion is an organized and shared system of beliefs, practices, and symbols (Koenig et al. p. 4 5)(14). These rituals and symbols often enable an individual to experience the transcendent. Thus, as Walach (p. 18)(15) argues, religion can be seen as "the vessel for spiritual experience".

Naturally, it is possible to present diverse distinctions between religion and spirituality. However, we think the proposed definitions have the advantage of keeping the currently prevalent academic approach of considering spirituality as something broader and more personal, with religion being more institutional and communal. And, at the same time, preserving the core that is central and unique to R/S: the sacred transcendent. Thus, religion is a community-based spirituality that also allows rites, rituals, and communal worship, whereas spirituality is very much an individualistic thought and practice which, in turn, may be well-placed in egocentric societies.

Are religion and spirituality still relevant in the contemporary world?

Since the mid-1800s in the academic environment, there has been a widespread acknowledgement of variations in what has been called 'secularization thesis'. In general, this states that R/S are vestiges of superstition, pathology, or primitive thought that would disappear with modernization, reason, and scientific knowledge. The thesis is usually coupled with materialist/physicalist scientism, an ideology that states that only natural scientific research can provide knowledge, and that science has proved that matter and physical forces are the only constituents of reality (16–19). Some seminal authors for this thesis were Feuerbach, Marx, and Freud; Dawkins is a contemporary proponent of it. This creed has led much of academia to neglect R/S and even to deny their relevance to the contemporary world. However, at the end of the twentieth century, the sociologist Rodney Stark (20) had already stated in his paper 'Secularization R.I.P.': 'once and for all, let us declare an end to social scientific faith in the theory of secularization, recognizing that it was the product of wishful thinking' (p. 269). However, rather than dying out in many countries and especially those with cultures in transition, religion and its practice have become much more prominent as people are trying to hand on to what they are familiar with in the face of an onslaught of change in cultural values. Traditional societies are likely to be socio-centric. Therefore, organized religion and its practice may take on an important role. With the advent of the practice of mindfulness, the spiritual practice in an egocentric society is much more likely to be individual even when it is being practised in public or in a group.

Nowadays, it is widely recognized that R/S have been important features in virtually all societies and cultures throughout human history, since the dawn of *Homo sapiens*. Historians and archaeologists have proposed that Palaeolithic cave paintings probably had mainly ritualistic or spiritual purposes (21–23). Some famous illustrative examples are the French cave paintings from Chauvet-Pont-d'Arc (34,000 BC) and Lascaux (12,000 BC). It is worth noting that the two oldest figurative artworks (from around 40,000 BC), the sculpture Lion Man (24, 25) from Germany and the rock art panel from the cave of Leang Bulu' Sipong in Indonesia (21), represent beings that do not exist in physical reality, possibly refer to transcendental beings and are related to religious rituals.

Since dawn of Homo sapiens, R/S have been seminal in many of the highest and best human achievements. Just to list a few: pyramids in Egypt, Parthenon in Greece, Notre Dame Cathedral, Michelangelo's Pietà, Taj Mahal, Universities (26), anti-slavery movement (27), and Beethoven's 9th symphony around Schiller's Ode to Joy (28). On the other hand, many wars, violence, and intolerance have happened under actual or alleged R/S motivations (29, 30) and indeed continue to do so.

The Soviet Union put to test several hypotheses related to the secularization thesis. Among them: R/S would depend on low educational level, social coercion, supportive cultural environment, and lack of access to basic human needs (health care, food, and housing). Soon after the Bolshevik Revolution in 1917, all forms of R/S started to be violently opposed. Religious leaders were assassinated or sent to Gulags, churches were closed or destroyed, and religious teachings or talks were forbidden. In addition, basic human needs were attended to by the government, and there was a huge educational effort that also included mandatory classes of 'scientific atheism' (31, 32). Despite more than 70 years of systematic and violent suppression of R/S, in 1991, just after the fall of Berlin Wall, 31% of Russians still persisted in declaring themselves Orthodox Christians. Fewer than two decades later, in 2008, only 18% of Russians declared themselves to be religious unaffiliated (33), similar to the highly religious United States (34). This is a striking example of the resilience of R/S and puts to question several assumptions related to the secularization thesis. However, there is no doubt that, as societies become less traditional and more modern, the practice of religious rituals does change.

The most recent data regarding the global religious landscape, provided by the Pew Research Center, shows that 84% of humanity declares some religious affiliations: 31.2% Christians, 24.1% Muslims, 15.1% Hindus, and 6.9% Buddhists (33). Although 16% have reported being unaffiliated, it does not necessarily mean they have no R/S: many may simply not belong to any organized religion. Half of them are from China, where religions face severe state restrictions, so there may be under-reporting of R/S (35). In addition, many of those declaring non-affiliation to a religion may still have some form of spirituality. For example, in China, where more than 90% of the population declare having no religion, 78% endorse the doctrine of karma, 27% pray to Buddhas or Bodhisattvas, and about half believe that their families and friends are the consequence of their behaviour in previous lives (36). The projections to 2060 are of even higher religiosity within the world's population, with non-affiliation declining to 13% (37).

Somewhat similar data was provided by Gallup polls in 163 nations involving more than 1 million individuals participating in interviews. In the world population, 81% report religious affiliation and 74% acknowledge that religion plays an important part in their daily lives. Only in Vietnam, China, and South Korea did more than 20% report being atheist (35). The World Values Survey has shown that at least two-thirds of the world's population hold one of the core beliefs of most R/S traditions: the belief in life after death (38). There is also evidence that this belief is not usually related to lower educational level (contrary to another common assumption of the secularization thesis) (39).

In addition to religious affiliation and beliefs, religious experiences are also very prevalent in the contemporary world. In 2009, 49% of the US population reported having had 'a religious or mystical experience—that is, a moment of religious or spiritual awakening'. This rate has more than doubled since 1962, when 22% reported such experiences (40). Most Latin American Catholics and Protestants say they have witnessed speaking in tongues, praying for a miraculous healing, and prophesying at church, at least occasionally (41).

In summary, there is overwhelming and robust evidence that R/S are still relevant in the contemporary (and not so secularized) world, and will probably remain so for at least several decades.

Science, religion and spirituality, and mental health

It is often argued that science and R/S have always lived in a perennial conflict, that it is not possible that science investigates R/S, and that R/S usually have a detrimental impact on mental health. Ronald Numbers (26), one of the most prominent contemporary historians of science, edited a book that lists 25 myths about science and religion and he opens the introduction stating: 'The greatest myth in the history of science and religion holds that they have been in a state of constant conflict' (p. 1). A few pages later, he presents another impressive conclusion of high-quality historical studies: 'No scientist, to our knowledge, ever lost his life because of his scientific views' (p. 6)—in other words, there is no single science martyr killed because of religious opposition to their science. Two examples of martyrs of modern science who usually come to mind are of Giordano Bruno and Galileo Galilei. However, Galileo was condemned to house arrest and not death. Bruno was indeed killed by the Inquisition, but he was condemned because of his religious, not scientific, views. Among other myths exposed are that the medieval Christian Church suppressed the growth of science, taught that the Earth was flat, and prohibited human dissection; that scientific revolution liberated science from religion; that Isaac Newton's mechanistic cosmology eliminated the need for God; and that evolution destroyed Darwin's faith in Christianity. In the past decades, a large and high-level scholarship in the history of science and religion has shown that their relationship has been much more complex, interesting, and often fruitful than usually has been assumed by academics in the past 150 years (30).

When we consider the impact of R/S on mental health, we conclude that, between the ends of nineteenth century and of the twentieth century, psychiatry and psychology tended to ignore or to pathologize R/S. R/S beliefs, practices, and experiences were often considered related to immature personality, or symptoms or causes of mental disorders (42). This is further discussed in detail in Chapter 3. However, these views were not based on well-designed epidemiological studies that only started to investigate R/S and mental health mainly in the last decades of the twentieth century. Usually, considering some expression of R/S (e.g. frequency of prayer or church attendance; use of religious coping strategies or religious commitment) as a predictor and health measures (e.g. depression score, suicide mortality, substance use) as outcomes, the epidemiology of religion flourished. A systematic review of more than 3,300 empirical studies on R/S and health have found some robust and consistent findings (14, 43). To summarize the main evidence regarding R/S and mental health (14, 43–45) (discussed further in Chapter 7):

- R/S is a common coping strategy used worldwide to deal with stressors and illness.

- Higher levels of religious involvement (especially religious service attendance, positive religious coping, and intrinsic religiosity) are usually related to less depression, suicidal behaviour (suicide attempts or deaths), use or abuse of alcohol and other substances, and lower general mortality. It is also usually related to higher levels of quality of life, well-being and human flourishing. Many religions proscribe suicide so the role of religion in understanding epidemiology becomes very important.

- Negative religious coping and extrinsic religiosity are related to more depression and mortality, and a worse quality of life.

- Taking patients' spiritual history does not take much time, is well accepted by patients, and may indeed improve therapeutic alliance and rapport, as well as and patients' satisfaction with treatment (46). (See Chapter 19.)

- Spiritually integrated psychotherapies are at least as effective as conventional psychotherapies in symptoms reduction and perhaps more effective in increasing spiritual well-being (47–49). See Chapter 23 for further details.

- Most patients would like physicians to address R/S in medical consultations (50).

- There is a 'religiosity gap' between mental health professionals (especially psychiatrists and psychologists) and the patients they see. Despite most clinicians having some R/S, they tend to have lower rates of religious affiliation or involvement and lower levels of belief in God than general population (51).

- Lack of training and of the necessary skills are the most common reasons cited for psychologists and psychiatrists not addressing R/S in clinical practice. This lack of training may also be expressed as fear of trespassing professional boundaries, as well as lack of time (51–54).

In summary, the idea of an inevitable and perennial conflict between science and R/S is a historical myth and their relationship is much more complex, nuanced, and often fruitful. It is possible for science to investigate R/S, because there are thousands of empirical studies that have shown that R/S has a significant impact (usually positive, but also negative) on mental health.

Bio-psycho-social-spiritual approach

Some people fear that emphasizing R/S would imply disfavouring scientific and medical knowledge. So, the question is: Do we need to deny or neglect scientific knowledge about bio-psycho-social aspects of mental health and mental disorders in order to incorporate R/S into our clinical or scientific practices?

First, let's briefly discuss the many factors that interact to promote health or disease. It is very important always to keep in mind that the health–disease continuum is a delicate, complex, and extremely dynamic balance of pathogenic and salutogenic factors (55, 56). In addition to the conventional biological, psychological, and social factors, the importance of religious and spiritual factors is now well established for this balance. This is why we propose a *bio-psycho-social-spiritual* approach to health. Taking R/S into consideration is not denying biology or other factors in causing or managing distress: we are just adding another crucial factor. It is essential to avoid an 'either/or' approach and develop a genuine 'and' approach. Unfortunately, psychiatry and psychology's history is plagued with exclusivist approaches, usually with detrimental effects to both patients and the general population. One example is the psychoanalysts' denial of biological factors for schizophrenia and the creation of the concept of 'schizophrenogenic mother' (57). On the other extreme, it is the evidence that believing in biogenetic models for mental disorders, and viewing them basically as brain disorders, actually increases stigma (58). This is why we must work with all dimensions of human beings to provide a comprehensive and integral approach that is more evidence-based and effective (59) (see also Chapter 22 in this volume). Not acknowledging this multidimensional approach by neglecting R/S does not mean being rational and science- oriented: it actually means holding a dogmatic and anti-scientific approach by ignoring a strong body of scientific evidence. All the bio-psycho-social-spiritual dimensions are deeply interlinked.

A recent study, the largest study ever conducted on R/S and suicide, illustrates this very well. The genetic, social, and psychological factors related to suicide are well known but what about R/S? Almost 90,000 American women were followed up for 14 years. Even after adjusting for a wide range of covariates (demographic, lifestyle, depressive symptoms, social interaction, and medical history), those who attended religious services at least once a week had a suicidal death rate fivefold lower than those who never attended. Although regular religious service attendance was related to biological (less alcohol use), social (higher social integration), and psychological (lower depressive symptoms) factors that have an impact on suicidal behaviour, these factors did not mediate the impact of religious attendance on suicide (60).

The bio-psycho-social-spiritual approach recognizes that we all have pathogenic and salutogenic aspects in all four domains, for example:

- Biological: genetic vulnerabilities or protections, patterns of substance use, sleep, exercise, and diet habits, etc.
- Psychological: cognitive framework, central beliefs, etc.
- Social: childhood adversity, role models, support, poverty, marriage, work environment, etc.
- Spiritual: beliefs about God, meaning of life, church attendance, prayer, meditation, religious coping styles, etc.

The health–disease continuum is similar to an old scale with two arms. Diseases develop when the pathogenic factors as a whole (from all the four dimensions) weigh more than the salutogenic ones. On the other hand, promoting prevention or treatment is a matter of decreasing the weight of pathogenic factors and increasing the salutogenic ones.

In summary, acknowledging the evidence for the impact of R/S on mental health and integrating it into theory and practice does not mean being antiscientific or neglecting the bio-psycho-social determinants of health. Given the amount of robust evidence of R/S on health, neglecting it would be antiscientific. We claim for a truly bio-psycho-socio-spiritual approach that is evidence based and acknowledges the contributions of each of these as pathogenic and salutogenic factors in the delicate and dynamic health–disease balance.

Is it appropriate to integrate religion and spirituality into clinical care and public health?

While acknowledging that R/S has an impact on mental health, there still remains the question as to whether it is appropriate to approach R/S in clinical care and public health. Would it not configure the trespass of ethical boundaries or imposition of one's own values? Some wonder if R/S is a too private a topic, that touching the subject would be offensive to patients, that it should not be part of health care. Indeed, ethical and boundary issues are very important when dealing with R/S and health. The key aspect here is that any approach must be *patient centred*, neither prescribing, nor imposing spiritual or anti-spiritual perspectives. The point is to address (to assess, respect, and integrate) what matters to patients and not necessarily to clinicians. Neither approach is proper: a religious clinician imposing R/S beliefs or practices on an atheist patient or a secular humanist psychiatrist choosing to neglect or depreciate R/S beliefs or practices of a religiously committed patient. If R/S matters to the patient and there is plenty of evidence that it has an impact on health, it is our ethical duty to address it in a sensible and respectful manner (46), as was recommended in the World Psychiatric Association (WPA)'s 'Position statement on spirituality and religion in psychiatry' (61) (see also Chapter 18 in this volume).

Regarding public health, there has been an increasing awareness of the key role of R/S and faith communities in this area (62, 63). Some examples are special issues published in recent years by *The Lancet* (a series on faith-based health care www.thelancet.com/series/faith-based-health-care) (64) and the *American Journal of Public Health* ('Faith-based organizations and public health') (65). From an institutional perspective, it is worth noting the American Psychiatric Association's Mental Health and Faith Community Partnership (www.psychiaty.org/faith). These promising collaborations come after decades of, in the words of Doug Oman (62), 'intellectual blindness' within public health teaching and research that refused to see the 'proverbial elephant in the room: An enormous body of empirical evidence that now links religious and spiritual (R/S) factors to health—and very commonly to *better health*' (p. 2). More recently, it has been recognized that faith-based organizations deliver a substantial volume of world health care, because they have for centuries founded hospitals, provided health professional training and been involved in public health campaigns. A benchmark for fruitful partnership between faith communities and public health is, for example, the Children's Pastoral Care (CPC) developed by the Catholic Church in Brazil. Around 260,000 volunteers track (and provide basic paediatric health education) monthly to 1.8 million children and 95,000 pregnant women in deprived areas of 3,300 towns. Compared with control areas, those with CPC's activity have shown higher birth weight and duration of breast-feeding as well as lower child mortality and criminality (66). This successful experience of partnership could be adapted and implemented in pressing public mental health issues where R/S has a relevant role, such as in substance abuse and suicide prevention.

As noted by Summerskill and Horton (64) in their introductory article in *The Lancet's* series on faith-based health care: 'Appreciation of spiritual, social, and cultural dimensions of health are crucial to care and public health. Better understanding of the reasons for different practices provides opportunities to reframe faith as part of the solution, rather than the problem, in complex consultations' (p. 1709). However, as recently noted by a group of leading public health researchers, a major barrier for this integration is that public health training usually neglects current scholarship on R/S (63). In order to overcome the barriers to effective integration, they provide four recommendations to public health scholars and practitioners: '(1) academic and intellectual humility; (2) engagement with a wider range of literature; (3) building relationships with people and communities of faith; (4) considering the goals and ends of communities served by the public health' (p. 4).

In summary, with respect to the evidence available and to the R/S beliefs, behaviours, and values of most of the world's population, it is not only appropriate but a scientific and ethical responsibility to integrate R/S into clinical care and public health.

Why are religion and spirituality important in mental health?

After all, why are R/S important in mental health and needing to be integrated in research, teaching, prevention, and treatment? We end this introductory chapter answering that question by listing the main reasons underlying the rationale for integrating R/S into mental health, and which will be discussed in the following chapters:

- Most of the world's population has some R/S, more than four-fifths have a religious affiliation, and even the non-religious usually have some spirituality (understood as some relationship with the transcendent and sacred).
- R/S is a prevalent, often the most used, coping strategy to deal with stressors and illness.
- Thousands of empirical studies have consistently shown that R/S has an impact on health, usually in a positive way, but may also (although less frequently) have a negative impact.
- Addressing patients' R/S (e.g. by taking a spiritual history or providing spiritually integrated treatments) affects prognosis positively.
- Most patients would like their clinicians to address their R/S in the clinical encounter.
- It is a scientific and ethical duty to address and consider seriously what matters to patients and affects their health and well-being, no matter our (professionals') personal R/S beliefs.

◆ R/S is a key component of an evidence-based and integral patient's assessment that needs to consider the main bio-psycho-socio-spiritual pathogenic and salutogenic factors.

◆ For the above reasons, the integration of R/S into mental health research, teaching, and practice has been recommended by many leading medical and health organizations, such as the World Psychiatric Association (which published the Position Statement on Spirituality and Religion in Psychiatry) (61) in 2016 and the World Health Organization (which integrated R/S in the concept of quality of life) (67).

References

1. **Moreira-Almeida A, Koenig HG.** Retaining the meaning of the words religiousness and spirituality: a commentary on the WHOQOL SRPB group's 'a cross-cultural study of spirituality, religion, and personal beliefs as components of quality of life' (62: 6, 2005, 1486–1497). *Social Science & Medicine.* 2006;**63**(4):843–5.

2. **Pargament KI.** The psychology of religion and spirituality? Yes and no. The *International Journal for the Psychology of Religion.* 1999;**9**(1):3–16.

3. **Koenig HG.** Concerns about measuring 'spirituality' in research. *Journal of Nervous and Mental Disease.* 2008;**196**(5):349–55.

4. **Berger PL.** Some second thoughts on substantive versus functional definitions of religion. *Journal for the Scientific Study of Religion.* 1974;**13**(2):125–33.

5. **Hufford DJ.** An analysis of the field of spirituality, religion, and health. **Metanexus** 2005. Available from: https://metanexus.net/analysis-field-spirituality-religion-and-health-david-j-hufford

6. **Stark R.** *Why God? Explaining religious phenomena.* First edition. West Conshohocken, PA: Templeton Press; 2017.

7. **Tylor EB.** *Primitive culture: researches into the development of mythology, philosophy, religion, art, and custom.* London: J. Murray; 1871.

8. **James W.** *Varieties of religious experience: a study in human nature.* Centenary edition. London and New York: Routledge; 2002. lxiii, 415 pp.

9. **Tolstoy L, Kentish J.** *A confession and other religious writings.* Harmondsworth, UK, and New York: Penguin; Viking Penguin; 1987. 238 pp.

10. **Otto R.** *The idea of the holy.* 2nd edition. Oxford: Oxford University Press; 1958. 256 pp.

11. **Eliade M.** *Myths, dreams, and mysteries; the encounter between contemporary faiths and archaic realities.* London: Harvill Press; 1960. 256 pp.

12. **Hardy A.** *The spiritual nature of man: a study of contemporary religious experience.* Oxford: Clarendon Press; 1979.

13. **Armstrong K.** *The case for God.* First edition. New York: Knopf; 2009. xviii, 406 pp.

14. **Koenig HG, King DE, Carson VB.** *Handbook of religion and health.* Second edition. Oxford and New York: Oxford University Press; 2012. xv, 1169 pp.

15. **Walach H.** *Secular spirituality: the next step towards enlightenment.* New York: Springer; 2014.

16. Holloway R. *A little history of religion.* New Haven: Yale University Press; 2016.

17. Haught JF. Science and scientism: the importance of a distinction. *Zygon.* 2005;40(2):363–8.

18. Kelly EF, Kelly EW, Crabtree A. *Irreducible mind: toward a psychology for the 21st century.* Lanham, MD; Rowman & Littlefield; 2007.

19. Gabriel M. *I am not a brain: philosophy of mind for the 21st century.* Malden, MA: Polity; 2017.

20. Stark R. Secularization, R.I.P. *Sociology of Religion.* 1999;60(3):249–73.

21. Aubert M, Lebe R, Oktaviana AA, Tang M, Burhan B, Hamrullah AJ, et al. Earliest hunting scene in prehistoric art. *Nature.* 2019;576(7787):442–5.

22. González A. El misterio rupestre. *Pensamiento.* 2019;75:1039–59.

23. Rickert T. Rhetorical prehistory and the Paleolithic. *Review of Communication.* 2016;16(4):352–73.

24. Cook J. The Lion Man: an Ice Age masterpiece. The British Museum blog, 10 October 2017. Available from: https://blog.britishmuseum.org/the-lion-man-an-ice-age-masterpiece

25. Kind C-J, Ebinger-Rist N, Wolf S, Beutelspacher T, Wehrberger K. The smile of the Lion Man. Recent excavations in Stadel Cave (Baden-Württemberg, south-western Germany) and the restoration of the famous Upper Palaeolithic figurine. *Quartär.* 2014;61:129–45.

26. Numbers RL. *Galileo goes to jail: and other myths about science and religion.* Cambridge, MA: Harvard University Press; 2009.

27. Stark R. *For the glory of God: how monotheism led to reformations, science, witch-hunts, and the end of slavery.* Princeton, NJ: Princeton University Press; 2003.

28. Feld M. Beethoven's Symphony #9 (1824). **Columbia Center—Music Humanities.** Available from: http://www.columbia.edu/itc/music/modules/summa3/summa3_print.html

29. Cavanaugh WT. *The myth of religious violence: secular ideology and the roots of modern conflict.* New York and Oxford: Oxford University Press; 2009.

30. Harrison P. *The territories of science and religion.* Chicago, IL: University of Chicago Press; 2015.

31. Solzhenitsyn AI. *The Gulag archipelago, 1918–1956: an experiment in literary investigation.* First edition. New York: Harper & Row; 1974.

32. Fraser G. Why the Soviet attempt to stamp out religion failed. *The Guardian.* 26 October 2017.

33. Pew Research Center. *The changing global religious landscape.* Pew Research Center; 5 April 2017.

34. Pew Research Center. *The global religious landscape.* Pew Research Center; 2012.

35. Stark R. *The triumph of faith: why the world is more religious than ever.* First edition. Wilmington, DE: ISI Books; 2015.

36. Yao X, Badham P. *Religious experience in contemporary China.* Cardiff: University of Wales Press; 2007.

37. Pew Research Center. *The changing global religious landscape.* Pew Research Center; 5 April 2017.

38. **World Values Survey:** Wave 6 (2010–2914) [cited 8 March 2018]. Available from: www. worldvaluessurvey.org/WVSDocumentationWV6.jsp

39. **Curcio CSS, Moreira-Almeida A**. Who does believe in life after death? Brazilian data from clinical and non-clinical samples. *Journal of Religion & Health.* 2019;**58**(4):1217–34.

40. **Pew Research Center.** *Many Americans mix multiple faiths.* Pew Research Center; 9 December 2009.

41. **Pew Research Center.** *Religion in Latin America.* Pew Research Center; 13 November 2014.

42. **Moreira-Almeida A, Silva de Almeida AA, Neto FL.** History of 'Spiritist madness' in Brazil. *History of Psychiatry.* 2005;**16**(61 Pt 1):5–25.

43. **Koenig HG, McCullough ME, Larson DB.** *Handbook of religion and health.* Oxford and New York: Oxford University Press; 2001.

44. **Moreira-Almeida A, Neto FL, Koenig HG.** Religiousness and mental health: a review. *Brazilian Journal of Psychiatry.* 2006;**28**(3):242–50.

45. **VanderWeele, TJ.** Religion and health: a synthesis. In: **MJ Balboni & JR Peteet,** (eds), *Spirituality and religion within the culture of medicine: from evidence to practice.* New York: Oxford University Press; 2017. pp. 357–401.

46. **Moreira-Almeida A, Koenig HG, Lucchetti G.** Clinical implications of spirituality to mental health: review of evidence and practical guidelines. *Brazilian Journal of Psychiatry.* 2014;**36**(2):176–82.

47. **Anderson N, Heywood-Everett S, Siddiqi N, Wright J, Meredith J, McMillan D.** Faith-adapted psychological therapies for depression and anxiety: systematic review and meta-analysis. *Journal of Affective Disorders.* 2015;**176**:183–96.

48. **Captari LE, Hook JN, Hoyt W, Davis DE, McElroy-Heltzel SE, Worthington EL.** Integrating clients' religion and spirituality within psychotherapy: a comprehensive meta-analysis. *Journal of Clinical Psychology.* 2018;**74**(11):1938–51.

49. **Gonçalves JP, Lucchetti G, Menezes PR, Vallada H.** Religious and spiritual interventions in mental health care: a systematic review and meta-analysis of randomized controlled clinical trials. *Psychological Medicine.* 2015;**45**(14):2937–49.

50. **Best M, Butow P, Olver I.** Do patients want doctors to talk about spirituality? A systematic literature review. *Patient Education and Counseling.* 2015;**98**(11):1320–8.

51. **Paulino PRV, Pargament KI, Moreira-Almeida A.** Religiosity/Spirituality of Psychiatrists and Psychologists: a review. Submitted.

52. **Curlin FA, Lawrence RE, Odell S, Chin MH, Lantos JD, Koenig HG,** et al. Religion, spirituality, and medicine: psychiatrists' and other physicians' differing observations, interpretations, and clinical approaches. *American Journal of Psychiatry.* 2007;**164**(12):1825–31.

53. **Delaney HD, Miller WR, Bisonó AM.** Religiosity and spirituality among psychologists: a survey of clinician members of the American Psychological Association. *Professional Psychology: Research and Practice.* 2007;**38**(5):538–46.

54. **Menegatti-Chequini MC, Gonçalves JP, Leão FC, Peres MF, Vallada H.** A preliminary survey on the religious profile of Brazilian psychiatrists and their approach to patients' religiosity in clinical practice. *BJPsych Open.* 2016;**2**(6):346–52.

55. Lindström B, Eriksson M. Salutogenesis. *Journal of Epidemiology and Community Health*. 2005;**59**(6):440–2.

56. Patel V, Saxena S, Lund C, Thornicroft G, Baingana F, Bolton P, et al. The Lancet Commission on global mental health and sustainable development. *Lancet*. 2018;**392**(10157):1553–98.

57. Harrington A. The fall of the schizophrenogenic mother. *Lancet*. 2012;**379**(9823):1292–3.

58. Kvaale EP, Gottdiener WH, Haslam N. Biogenetic explanations and stigma: a meta-analytic review of associations among laypeople. *Social Science & Medicine*. 2013;**96**:95–103.

59. Cloninger CR. The importance of ternary awareness for overcoming the inadequacies of contemporary psychiatry. *Archives of Clinical Psychiatry*. 2013;**40**:110–3.

60. VanderWeele TJ, Li S, Tsai AC, Kawachi I. Association Between Religious Service Attendance and Lower Suicide Rates Among US Women. *JAMA Psychiatry*. 2016;**73**(8):845–51.

61. Moreira-Almeida A, Sharma A, van Rensburg BJ, Verhagen PJ, Cook CC. WPA position statement on spirituality and religion in psychiatry. *World Psychiatry*. 2016;**15**(1):87–8.

62. Oman D. *Why religion and spirituality matter for public health: evidence, implications, and resources*. New York: Springer Berlin Heidelberg; 2018.

63. Long KNG, Gregg RJ, VanderWeele TJ, Oman D, Laird LD. Boundary crossing: meaningfully engaging religious traditions and religious institutions in public health. *Religions*. 2019;**10**(7):412.

64. Summerskill W, Horton R. Faith-based delivery of science-based care. *Lancet*. 2015;**386**(10005):1709–10.

65. Morabia A. Faith-based organizations and public health: another facet of the public health dialogue. *American Journal of Public Health*. 2019;**109**(3):341.

66. Schumann C, Stroppa A, Moreira-Almeida A. The contribution of faith-based health organisations to public health. *BJPsych International*. 2011;**8**(3):62–4.

67. World Health Organization. *WHOQOL and spirituality, religiousness and personal beliefs (SRPB)*. Geneva: World Health Organization; 1998.

Chapter 2

Western spirituality: A historical epistemology

German E. Berrios and Ivana S. Marková

Introduction

To understand the concept of 'spirituality', the following are required: a) a recognizable object of inquiry; b) a manageable database; and c) methodology of study. The first two requirements are hard to meet: 'spirituality' remains opaque and poorly defined[1] (1–6);[2] and publications on the subject are often marred by bias, repetition, and triteness.[3] Regarding the third requirement, the kaleidoscopic nature of spirituality suggests an approach called 'historical

---

[1] No satisfactory general definition of 'spirituality' seems available.

[2] Furthermore, the concept is understood differently across history (Kirby J. Varieties of spirituality: a Western philosophical analysis. In: *Oxford Research Encyclopedia of Religion.* Oxford: Oxford University Press; 2019); cultures (Kim-Prieto C. *Religion and spirituality across cultures.* Switzerland: Springer; 2014); human disciplines (Souza M, Bone, J and Watson J. *Spirituality across disciplines.* Switzerland: Springer; 2016); religious denominations (Hinson EG. *Spirituality in ecumenic perspective.* Louisville: John Knox Press; 1993); Bartolini N, MacKian S, Pile S. *Spaces of spirituality.* London: Routledge; 2018); workplaces (Roberts GE, Cross JE. *Palgrave handbook of workplace spirituality and fulfilment.* Switzerland: Palgrave; 2018).

[3] During the past 20 years, the literature on spirituality has grown to the point of becoming unmanageable. One has the feeling that it has also become polarized. On the one hand, there are publications highly critical of secular spirituality, whether written or not from a religious perspective (Palmisano S, Pannofino, N. Spirituality. *Sociology Notebooks.* 2018;77:35–54). On the other hand, some of the literature on non-religious spirituality can be equally critical of religion's attempts to monopolize spirituality (Del Rio C, White LJ. Separating Spirituality from Religiosity: a hylomorphic attitudinal perspective. *Psychology of Religion and Spirituality* 2012;4(2):123–142).Work in between the two is also available and it is from this corpus that one expects the most illumination (Fuller RC. *Spiritual but not religious.* Oxford: Oxford University Press; 2001; Comte-Sponville A. *The Book of Atheistic Spirituality.* London: Bantam Press; 2007; Harris S. *Waking up: a guide to spirituality without religion.* New York: Simon & Schuster; 2014).

epistemology'.[4] This method of study is excellent at avoiding anachronism, but it demands detailed information not only on the protagonist notion but also on its conceptual retinue and general cultural background.

Despite the above, and the fact that in this field 'objectivity' of analysis is difficult to achieve, efforts to explore 'spirituality' should not be abandoned. Its unpacking should contribute to the understanding of religion and of philosophical anthropology[5]—that is, the discipline that deals with the definition of man (and of his emotional, ethical, and aesthetical yearnings).

The historical epistemology of spirituality purports to map the changes in meaning and function that this concept has undergone in response to cultural shifts. Its main focus is not on ontology[6] and hence it has little interest in whether 'spirituality' or 'spiritual need' a) are objects to be located in the brain of man; b) have emerged at some point in human evolution; c) represent a 'gift'

---

[4] Historiography names the discipline that studies the various methods and ideologies involved in the writing of history (Tucker A. *A companion to the philosophy of history and historiography*. Oxford: Blackwell; 2009; Bentley M. *Companion to historiography*. London: Routledge; 2006). 'Historical epistemology' (Rheinberger HJ. *On historicizing epistemology*. Stanford: Stanford University Press; 2010) can be considered as an offshoot of the history of ideas (Tobey JL. *The history of ideas* (vols I and 2). Santa Barbara: Clio Books; 1975) and of conceptual history (Koselleck R. *The practice of conceptual history*. Stanford: Stanford University Press; 2002), both important approaches to the historical study of ideas, concepts, and systems of thought in relation to their respective cultural background.

[5] Philosophical anthropology names a conceptual approach that seeks to develop a general theory of man based on the contribution of both the natural and social sciences (Groethuysen B: *Antropología filosófica*. Buenos Aires: Losada; 1951; Ladmann M. *Philosophical anthropology*. Philadelphia: Westminster Press; 1974; Plessner H. *Levels of organic life and the human. An introduction to philosophical anthropology*. New York: Fordham; 2019; Gosselin M. Homo Sapiens, *a problematic species. An essay in philosophical anthropology*. New York: University Press of America; 2015; Cassirer E. *Essay on man*. New York: Doubleday; 1944; Agassi J. *Towards a rational philosophical anthropology*. The Hague: Martinus Nijhoff; 1977). Differences can be noticed between the classical continental philosophical anthropology of Scheler, Plessner, Groethuysen, Cassirer, and Landmann, and the approach developed within Anglo-American philosophy. Biological, psychological, cultural, phenomenological, and theological varieties of philosophical anthropology can be identified (Pappé HO. On philosophical anthropology. *Australasian Journal of Philosophy*. 1961;39:47–64).

[6] Although the term was only coined during the seventeenth century by Glocenius, the questions it asks date to the earliest history of philosophical activity (Mohanty JN. *Phenomenology and ontology*. Den Haag: Martinus Nijhoff; 1970; Lowe EJ. *The four category ontology*. Oxford: Clarendon Press; 2006; Hartmann N. *Ontology: laying the foundations*. Berlin: Walter der Gruyer; 2019; Effingham N. *An introduction to ontology*. Cambridge: Polity Press; 2013).

from an external agency (e.g. God); and d) can be subject to manipulation, deviation, deformation, or disease.

Instead, historical epistemology is concerned to know whether certain phenomena: a) can be consistently recognized as 'spiritual'; b) have a common denominator; c) change in time; d) constitute a composite concept; e) relate to the cultural *Lebenswelt*; f) co-vary with other concepts such as mind, personality, self, health, disease, etc.

For reasons of space not all these questions will be tackled in this chapter.

Historical epistemology

Historical epistemology explores 'the biography of concepts', maps their life, and evaluates their functionality, relevance, rate of change, and capacity to cohere with one another. These tasks are made difficult by the ontological levity of many concepts—that is, by the fact that they are just ideal constructs rather than durable and independent things (i.e. heavy cores surrounded by hanging properties).

Historical epistemology posits that all disciplines (e.g. the natural and human sciences), in order to organize their chosen region of interest, construct concepts. On account of their specific and tailor-made functionality, to be imported into a different historical period, concepts need to be adapted (by changing their cognitive, rhetorical, emotional, and agential structure). This explains why concepts with the same name may have different meanings in different historical periods. Constructivist assumptions of this type run counter to the heavy ontological narrative of Divine Creation according to which a stable Platonic world underlies the surface ephemerality of things.

Soul, spirit, psyche, nous, mind, pneuma, experience, etc. constitute a family of concepts whose co-varying meanings have undergone a marked change. Their epistemological exploration is difficult because change may affect some concepts more than others. This explains the periodic search for common denominators for all these concepts, and indeed for 'spirit' and 'spirituality', the hope being that, despite any surface difference, there is still a deep unchangeable human attribute called 'spirituality'. Positing such an attribute has been the long-term solution proposed by organized religion: man has been created by God and equipped with a specific capacity to experience the divine.

Unfortunately, mapping the historical biography of 'spirituality' suggests otherwise. At least since the seventeenth century, a concept with that name has certainly been around, but its meaning has changed, most likely in response to new cultural demands.

Concepts in general

Concepts are cognitive, emotional, and rhetorical gadgets, constructed to create working pictures of reality.[7] Usually acting in clusters, they organize, date, and give meaning to information accruing to the mind. Concepts can fit together in ever-larger arrays, thereby capturing ever-larger regions of reality. In this sense, they can be considered as the building bricks of what in each historical period is accepted as 'legitimate knowledge'.

Concepts can be classified according to their history, form, intension, extension, duration, content, etc. For example, some have a narrow compass, work closer to reality, and are stable (simple, basic, primary concepts). Others cover larger regions of reality and consist in clusters of basic concepts (composite, superordinate, higher-level concepts). The basic concepts feed meaning into composite ones, render them stable, and form with them conceptual families. Scientific research can be described as an activity dedicated to improving the semantic and mathematical coherence of conceptual families.

In general, it is possible to date the construction of concepts and, on this basis, trace their migration and distinguish between short- and long-lived ones. Longevous concepts often create the illusion of having captured something eternal and immutable (e.g. nature, environment, planet, man, god, time, space).

Supporting concepts

If spirituality is a composite concept, then several basic concepts need to be briefly explored.

Religion

Of rather confused and disputed etymology (*religio, religare, relegere*) (7), the term 'religion', coined in the wake of the construction of Christianity (8), has since been generalized to refer to any 'unified system of beliefs and practices relative to sacred things: that is to say, things set apart and forbidden—beliefs and practices which unite into one single moral community called a Church, all those who adhere to them' (9, p. 47).

Once considered as intimately related, spirituality and religion have since gone their separate ways and their divergence causes controversy. Resolving

---

[7] The literature on what concepts are, how they function, and how they relate to reality has grown dramatically during the past three decades (Weitz M. *Theories of concepts*. London: Routledge; 1988; Loocke P. *The nature of concepts*. London: Routledge; 1999; Peacocke C. *A study of concepts*. Cambridge, Mass: MIT Press; 1992; Murphy GL. *The big book on concepts*. Cambridge, Mass: MIT Press; 2002).

this issue is of importance. For example, in the context of this book, it is important to decide whether spirituality or religion is the crucial concept in: a) the management of sufferers of mental disorder; b) the training of therapists; and c) the organization of the venues of care (10–12).

If the literature on spirituality is vast, that on religion is enormous.[8] Every cultural movement in the West has occurred within the ideological frame of Christianity. The very history of spirituality up to the eighteenth century cannot be understood unless it is sought in the religious literature. No doubt religion will be covered in depth in other chapters in this book.

The sacred

Holy and sacred belong to a family of concepts constructed early in the cultural history of man to: a) name objects and properties of objects recognized as special in a particular way; and b) to keep such objects separated from profane, daily ones.

Before the nineteenth century, 'sacred' (*Heilige, sagrado, sacré*, etc.), used to translate Biblical Greek terms such as *hieros, hagios* and *hosios*, were considered as adjectives rather than as nouns (13).

The Biblical Greek terms *hieros, hagios* and *hosios* formed a family of words used to refer to properties of objects and to the manner in which these properties relate to man. *Hieros* referred to the divine and to everything consecrated by it; *hagios* and *hosios* characterized the nature of the relationship between the sacred and man, and emphasized the moral duty of the latter to worship the former.

The reification of the 'sacred' (14) started at the turn of the century in the work of Windelband (15), Durkheim (16), Otto (17), and Jung (18, 19), and soon enough it acquired a substantival form. By the time Otto published his great book, *Das Heilige* (20) had become both ontologized and endowed with causal powers of its own.

Spirit

The historical etymology of the Greek 'psyche' and 'pneuma', the Latin 'spirit', and of their stem derivations in the European vernaculars are well known (21).

---

[8] The literature on the history, nature, and meaning of religion is enormous and there is little point in providing a long list of references apart from the following: (Ellwood RS, Alles GD (eds). *The encyclopedia of world religions*. New York: Infobase Publishing; 2007; Woodhead L. (ed.). *Religions in the modern world*. London: Routledge; 2002; Stuckrad K. (ed.). *The Brill dictionary of religion* (3 vols). Leiden: Brill; 2006; Yandell KE. *The philosophy of religion*. London: Routledge; 1999; Mesiter C, Copan P. *Routledge companion to the philosophy of religion*. London: Routledge; 2013).

Psyche and pneuma originally named physical events such as flow of air, breathing sounds, etc. (22). Associated as they were with biological functions, agony, etc., the sounds started to be considered as symbols of life and eventually became ontologized—that is, viewed as objects existing in space and time. Psyche thus starts to name a 'something' that abandons the body when a person dies, but this 'something' has nothing to do with anachronistic concepts such as mind and soul (23).

Psyche was translated as 'Spirit', the Latin term, which had meanings over and above those present in the Greek term 'psyche'; so, the terms were not semantically coterminous. This fact is important to understand the adventitious referents that psyche was to acquire in back translation. The meanings of *Spiritus* (24) are:

1) 'the action of breathing; respiration (also) a single breath; one's last breath; deep breathing; aspiration)';

2) 'a concomitant of life or consciousness';

3) 'the non-corporeal part of a person; the vital principle animating the world as a whole according to some philosophical systems';

4) 'divine afflatus or inspiration'; 'essential or pervading quality';

5) 'any disposition that causes a person to act in a particular way'; and

6) 'exhalation, scent, perfume, odour', etc.

The historian is confronted by the problem of meaning selection. Since usage frequencies are not available for all meanings, later derivations and choice of one meaning over the other tend to be governed by ideological convenience. The core meaning of trends and themes such as spiritual experience, spiritualism, spirituality are therefore shaped by contemporary bias rather than original usage.

Meanings can often be sharpened by creating contrasts and polarities (25, 26). In the case of spirit, the most common polarities have been body, matter, and physical world. Thus constructed, spirit appears as abstract, fleeting, transparent, shadowy, unsubstantial, gaseous, light, etc., all of which relate to its metaphorical origins of 'exhalation, wind breath', etc.

Soul

The relationship between 'spirit' and 'soul' has changed since Classical times (27, 28). Originally, body, soul and spirit were not necessarily polar notions. The soul named the final exhalation in agony and was responsible both for: a) life (vegetative role); and b) the conscious, spiritual, experiential attributes of the individual (29–31).

A dualist view of man starts to be discernible in Plato who conceived of psyche and body as essentially different: the psyche is immortal and imprisoned in a succession of perishable bodies. Augustine developed the Platonic view defining the soul as a substance endowed with reason whose main function is to govern the body (32, 33).

Although etymologically and metaphorically spirit, anima, and alma (soul) have the same origin, their later historical usage has differed. Soul has remained firmly embedded in the Christian definition of man, but spirit has been given at least two meanings. On the one hand, its Christian meaning as a central element in the complex concept of the Trinity (34, 35); and, on the other, a more material one, as illustrated by the physiological role that it was made to play by Descartes, Hartley, etc., whereby animal spirits were conceived of as circulating fluids carrying both information and agential force (36). It can be sensibly concluded that spirituality as a property of humans is directly related to the non-physiological usage of the term. In addition to historical and epistemological studies, spirit and spirituality have been the subject of psychology (37), anthropology (38), and other disciplines.

Lifeworld (*Lebenswelt*)(39)

Lifeworld is a term of art used by philosophers to refer to the quotidian experience (40), to the background that pre-conceptual daily life offers human beings, before they start applying scientific concepts to it. The term was redefined by Husserl late in his philosophical career (41, 42) and has since been worked upon by writers such as Heidegger, Gadamer, Merleau-Ponty, and Habermas (43, 44). Aspects of the lifeworld overlap with what in the English-speaking world is referred to as 'folk psychology' (45).

The concept of lifeworld can help with the analysis of the spiritual experience. However personal, subjective, and unobtrusive the feeling of the lifeworld may be, it already carries meaning about the world. Because this cannot be provided by mere sensory information (visual, auditory, tactile, etc.), it is likely to originate in the cultural envelope. If thus, it could be asked whether the spiritual experience is also present in the contents of the *Lebenswelt*. Interestingly, it has also been suggested that faith may also be required by the package of expectations built into the *Lebenswelt*: 'Faith in a far wider sense is necessary for human life and knowledge outside religion, since it is the basic acceptance that the universe is reliable, albeit unpredictable in many respects ... '(46).

The object of inquiry

'Spirituality' is meant to capture or outline a composite psychological attribute (including cognitive, emotional, aesthetic, rhetorical, and agential components). The agential component refers to the fact that, beyond mere musing or contemplation, the person is driven to search for answers to questions of a general type, of the type that the regionalized languages of the sciences do not tackle. These questions may be about the absolute origin and meaning of the universe, of life, of personal purpose, of ethical norms, etc. (47–49). Until the nineteenth century, it was the job of religion to answer these questions. As spirituality started to be thought of as a concept or space independent of religion, the answers began to be sought elsewhere.

Many still considered religion and spirituality as synonyms; and religion as the only legitimate response to spiritual needs and questions. Indeed, the very need to search for a transcendental explanation is considered by many as a natural response to needs for the divine that has been placed in man by God himself. Thus, man is spiritual because he is religious, rather than the other way around (50–52).

So, the very idea of dealing with spirituality independently from religion, or the claim that the spiritual need is primary, and that religion is just one among various answers to such a need is bound to appear as controversial. Those holding a separatist position have named their ideological stance as secular (53), non-religious (54), atheistic, (55) humanistic (56) spirituality.

Extension and applicability of concepts

The issue of whether it makes sense to ask general questions of the type listed above needs to be touched upon. The functionality, extension, and meaning of concepts such as causality, creation, origin, being, totality, universe, container, emptiness, etc. can be conceived of as being general (unlimited) or restricted (regionalized). If the former, then it is legitimate to apply explanatory concepts of this type to both individual objects and the universe at large. In other words, the question, 'Who has made this table?', and the question, 'Who has made the universe' should both be considered as valid and equivalent.

However, the option must be considered that usage validity depends upon the semantic functionality of each concept. This is determined by how extensive its original explanatory power was meant to be. For example, in the case of 'causality', we must decide first whether its power to explain the origin of things was limited to specific terrestrial objects or was unlimited (57–60). Theories of causality are not clear in this regard but what we know suggests that it is unlikely that the concept was constructed to be legitimately used in all possible worlds. So, it would be a category mistake, in the Rylean sense (61–63), to conceive of the entire universe or of the whole of reality as another specific object (like a table), which hence should also have a maker, a beginning in time, etc.

Given that spirituality can be considered as a part of the psychological make-up of persons, the first step should be to approach it from the perspective of the subject—that is, to focus on the 'spiritual experience'.

The spiritual experience

Efforts to 'explain' the nature of spiritual experience have been made by psychology, sociology, comparative anthropology, the neurosciences, and other disciplines (64–69). The legitimacy of these efforts has generated yet another debate—namely, whether spirituality (and religion) should be considered as *sui generis* in the sense that their essence, meaning, and nature cannot be reduced to anything else (e.g. mere social or neuroscientific objects) (70–73). It is not within the remit of this chapter to contribute to this debate.

Finding a description of how it feels to have a spiritual need is not easy for at least four reasons:

1) The said 'need' may not have been 'felt the same' throughout the centuries, on account of changes in both the feeling itself and in the semantics of the concept used to name it.

2) The verbal articulation of the need—that is, the speech act in which such need is conveyed—may also have changed in response to culture pressure: for example, up to the nineteenth century, such need was mostly expressed in terms of the organized religion to which the individual was supposed to belong.

3) The construction of psychology as a discipline during the nineteenth century created a pre- and post-psychology view of the mind (74). In practice, this means that concepts such as mental function, perception, sensation, emotion, passion, volition, etc., although still using the same name as before 1800, have now actually a different meaning.

4) Views on the structure of the mind and its relationship to the brain changed once again with the development of psychoanalysis, which added new layers of description and interpretation to the earlier structures (75–80).

Are these reasons deflationary enough to give up on any attempt to search for a definition of the (*Ur*) experience on which the concept of spirituality may be based? Within organized religions, this issue is not a problem for the creation of man in the image of God endowed him with need for the divine.

For example, Otto's 'numinous': '[includes] the sense of the sacred, the consciousness of creatureliness, nothingness, sin, and guilt, the assurance of redemption and salvation. Such effects are permeated by the apprehension of a meaning and value that is uniquely and irreducibly religious' (81).

Interestingly, Otto himself warned:

> The reader is invited to direct his mind to a moment of deeply felt religious experience, as little as possible qualified by other forms of consciousness. Whoever cannot do this, whoever knows no such moments in his experience, is requested to read no further; for it is not easy to discuss questions of religious psychology with one who ... cannot recall an intrinsically religious feelings (82).

It would seem as if Otto believed that at least some persons may not have the ability to entertain a religious (spiritual) experience.

Outside the realm of Creationism (83–85), explanations for the origins, nature, and persistence of a 'spiritual need or experience' need to be governed by: a) the conventional epistemology of experience, feeling, sensation, need, drive, etc. and related contents of consciousness; and b) the way in which these are configured into speech acts (86–89).

In this sense, 'experience' offers two conventional meanings: 1) accumulative dexterity after repeated task exposure, and 2) feeling, qualia, or personal sensation (90). The second meaning is relevant to our inquiries.

Experience and its types

Before it is decided whether there are experiences that can be identified as specifically 'spiritual', the general concept of experience must be explored.

Since antiquity, the term/concept of 'experience' has undergone transformation. In Classical Greece, 'experience' (a derivation of *empireia*) referred to the repeated exposure of someone to a given knowledge, task, or operation that in time led to an accumulation of memories, reinforcement of knowledge, and development of a skill. Indeed, *Empeiros* meant 'practised in' or 'acquainted with'(91) and referred to someone who had become an expert or perite (*peritus*) (92) in a task (e.g. smith, cobbler, 'practical' physician).

This reference to a given praxis was not accompanied by a conceptual abstraction or theoretical speculation as to how the skill might have developed. Nor there was any speculation as to how the practice might relate to the individual's subjectivity or contribute to general knowledge. Indeed, *empireia* referred only to knowledge of the particular (93). This is the reason why, in Classical times, medical practitioners were divided into those dealing with particulars, pejoratively called '*empeirikoi*' (94), and those who, on account of being equipped with a theory, were able to generalize their knowledge and experience.

Experience as feeling

The current definition of 'experience' as feeling is: 'The fact of being consciously the subject of a state or condition, or of being consciously affected by an event. Also an instance of this; a state or condition viewed subjectively; an event by which one is affected (95).'

In this definition, the concept of experience is linked to subjectivity, awareness, and related to a sensation/feeling rather than to a praxis or learning consequential to an external event. This is different from the Classical view of *empireia*.

The question here is whether a 'spiritual experience' can be distinguished from other types of experience, and on what bases (quality, intensity, content, etc.). Ideally, this detection should be performed before the official narratives designed to describe/satisfy the experience (e.g. religion, secular spirituality, aesthetics, etc.) can cloud the analysis. Whether this analysis is possible depends upon what is known of the historical epistemology of 'experience'.

In relation to the meaning of experience as feeling (as in 'I experienced severe pain'), the German and Spanish languages differentiate between a generic, informational notion of experience (*Erfahrung* (96), *experiencia* (97)) and a form of experience defined as unique, personalized, and specific to time and space (*Erlebnis* (98), *vivencia* (99)).

The spiritual experience can be studied from the two perspectives. Standard psychology is likely to consider the spiritual experience as an *Erfahrung*—that is, as a generic capacity shared by most persons. However, when Otto defined the numinous as the personal experience of a '*mysterium tremendum fascinans et augustum*' (100), he was thinking of it as an *Erlebnis*. Similar differentiation can be applied to the 'mystical experience' which can be treated as both a generic event and a very personal and unique experience (101).

While the German language uses two words to differentiate two different types of experience, French philosophy classifies experience in a different way. For example, in a classical publication on the concept, Alquié lists regional forms of experience in relation to the theoretical and social sciences, biology, mysticism, aesthetic, morality, and metaphysics (102).

The sublime

It is of some interest that, outside the realm of religion, an experience similar to the numinous was in fashion during the eighteenth century (103, 104). Developed within aesthetic theory, and out of an old Classical concept (105), 'the sublime' referred to the emotions (fear and terror) elicited by certain visual stimuli, especially those related to the majesty and roughness of nature (106).

Different from the beautiful, the sublime soon started a fashion in art, with painters trying to capture nature at its most violent. The concept was important in the development of the views on nature entertained by the Romantic movement and its influence is still found during the early nineteenth century—for example, in the work of Turner (107, 108).

The sublime also influenced Otto's idea of *das Heilige*. Indeed, he wrote: 'In the category and feeling of the sublime we have a counterpart to it, though it is true it is but a pale reflexion ... The analogies between the consciousness of the sublime and of the numinous may be easily grasped ... ' (109)

Introspecting, intuiting, etc.

Identifying a methodology that may allow for the identification of the spiritual experience in its pure form is not easy. Before 1900, it might have been possible to trust in 'introspection' (110–112); but, since then, its epistemological power has been seriously challenged (113, 114).

Husserl's eidetic intuition is another candidate (115, 116). Although opaque and much criticized, this method was used by this philosopher to capture the 'essence' of objects, qualities, relationships, etc. He observed various presentations of the object under study (in our case, this would be the various ways in which the spiritual experience may present itself) (117), abstracting from this variation some essential (eidetic) commonality. The obtained idea was not an object. Thus, Husserl rejected the accusation that he was searching for an ontologized Platonic idea (118). As far as it is known, no determined effort has been made to apply Husserl's eidetic intuition method to the spiritual experience itself, although there is a great deal of work on the phenomenology of the religious experience.

Origins and type of experience

Further to understanding the spiritual experience, it would be useful to know whether it is innate or acquired—that is, whether it is a mental function that has emerged as a result of evolution or whether it is part of a package of cultural configurators. Once again, the religious experience has from the start been considered as a divine gift but, if the spiritual experience is to be explored independently, then these questions stand.

Towards the end of the nineteenth century, the consciousness-centred model of the mind was challenged by writers who proposed a layered model according to which strata beyond the reach of consciousness nonetheless played a central agential role in human behaviour (119). A member of this group, C.G. Jung, suggested that a spiritual need could be part of an archetypal notion embedded in the collective unconscious (120). These concepts, endowed with descriptive, prescriptive, and explanatory function, have since received much attention (121). Whether they can resolve the nature–nurture debate remains to be seen.

Given the recognizable and consistent content of the spiritual experience (and the replicative questioning it engenders), the question remains as to its origins. This question is likely to demand both a conceptual and empirical answer. Recent work suggests that, at least in some cases, cultural configurators[9] may provide an explanation for both the origin and functionality of the spiritual experience (122).

Lastly, there is the issue of whether the primary nature of the spiritual experience is cognitive, emotional, ethical, or aesthetic. If cognitive, it must be asked whether its function is mostly epistemological, and its expression is exhausted by the application (whether legitimately or not) of concepts of limited semantic extension to totalities. On the other hand, if the primary engine of the spiritual experience is a search for the satisfaction of emotional, ethical, or aesthetic needs, then the cognitive questioning becomes secondary and societies must have at the ready repertoires of pre-conceptual, raw, experiential answers for their members to lead satisfactory lives.

For completion's sake, a final option must be mentioned. It could be argued that, as has been predicated of fideist forms of religion,[10] the spiritual experience is also unique (i.e. of one kind, sui generis, a thing apart, etc.) and hence it should not be reduced to any other cultural concept (cognition, emotion, ethics, aesthetics, etc.) but dealt with using proprietary categories and methods of analysis. It remains unclear whether these tools are already available.

Spirituality since the eighteenth century

As mentioned above, currently spirituality seems to refer to a set of needs that human beings are believed to possess. The existence/function/activity of such an attribute is primarily ascertainable from the perspective of the experiencer who may be driven by a 'need' to question and search for emotions, states of mind, and accounts relating to the origin and meaning of life, and the universe

---

[9] The concept of cultural configurator is explored in Berrios GE. The role of cultural configurators in the formation of mental symptoms. In: KS Kendler, J Parnas, (eds), *Philosophical issues in psychiatry III: the nature and source of historical change*. Oxford: Oxford University Press; 2015, pp.107–115.

[10] This refers to forms of religion in which 'all (or some) knowledge depends upon faith or revelation, and reason or the intellect is to be disregarded ... ' (Oxford English Dictionary, 1992). Faith itself is considered as an irreducible form of experience/behaviour which needs to be studied in its own right and by means of its own categories (Sessions WL. *The concept of faith: a philosophical investigation*. Ithaca : Cornell University Press ; 1994).

at large. Searching for evidence that this need was experienced in earlier centuries is complicated because of the omnipresence of religious talk.

Towards the end of the seventeenth century, Furetiere (123) defined *Spiritualité* as: '*Detachement des choses temporelles, application a la meditation des celestes.*[11] *Tous les livres de devotion s'appellent livres de spiritualité . . .*'

The French encyclopedia offers two definitions:

> on dit la spiritualité de l'âme, pour désigner cette qualité qui nous est inconnue, & qui la distingue essentiellement de la matière … le même mot se prend aussi pour une dévotion honnête, recherchée, qui s'occupe de la méditation de ce qu'il y a de plus subtil & de plus délié dans la religion (124).

Neither the meaning relating to the features of the 'spirit' (as compared with those of 'matter') nor the meaning referring to a devotional and meditative attitude of mind (as pertaining to religion) include the current, experiential definition of spirituality.

Dr Johnson offered four definitions of spirituality: '1) Incorporeity; immateriality; essence distinct from matter; 2) Intellectual nature; 3) *Spiritualité*, French), acts independent of the body; pure acts of the soul; mental refinement; and 4) That which belongs to any one as an ecclesiastic' (125). The first and second definitions refer to the qualities of the spirit, the third corresponds with the French usages, and the fourth relates to religion.

Roughly a century later, a popular English philosophy dictionary was defining spirituality as: 'of the nature of spirit, immateriality, as S of the soul' (126). It simply repeated the first definition of the French encyclopedia.

The new spirituality: its needs and its satisfactions

Based on the idea that spirituality should be considered as a primary human attribute/need, since early in the twentieth century, questions started to be asked as to how this attribute can be redefined and how the needs it engenders are satisfied.

Early in the century, Lucien Lévy-Bruhl suggested that these attributes/needs were the expression of a form of 'primitive' mentality, ever-present in the human:

---

[11] During the seventeenth century, angels and other divine creatures were often called 'célestes' in French. The Grand Robert (2005) defines Céleste: 'Qui appartient au ciel (IV.), considéré comme le séjour de la Divinité, des bienheureux. | *La gloire céleste.* | *La béatitude céleste.* | *La céleste patrie; la cité, la demeure, le royaume céleste. Les puissances célestes.* | *Les messagers célestes; l'armée, la milice céleste. Le Père; l'époux céleste:* Dieu; Jésus.' Thus, Furetiere's definition focuses on the religious aspects of the concept.

> In every human mind, whatever its intellectual development, there subsists an in-eradicable fund of primitive mentality. It is not likely that it will ever disappear, or become weakened beyond a certain point, and surely we ought not to wish that it might do so. For with it would disappear, perhaps, poetry, art, metaphysics, and scientific invention—almost everything, in short, that makes for the beauty and grandeur of human life (127).

In the cognitive sphere, philosophy has remained ready to offer, if not solutions to the deep questions, at least a repertoire of methods to tackle them.

In the moral sphere, systems of autonomous or contractual ethics began to be explored to replace forms of moral heteronomy or divine command ethics (128) that had been popular within the context of religion.

In the aesthetic sphere, artists with a conceptual bent (e.g. Kandinsky (129), Mondrian,[12] and Tisma (130)) have suggested that art and artistic expressions may be an important way to both represent and satisfy human spiritual yearnings (131).

Conclusions and pending issues

The concept of 'spirituality' can only be efficiently used if its origin and manifold meanings are identified. First and foremost, it needs to be established whether it is a primary/basic human attribute or whether it is just a term of art used to describe and/or enhance some aspects of human behaviour.

There are pending issues too: is spirituality fully definable as a deep and ir-resistible human yearning for information about the origins and meaning of everything? Is the observation that these general questions appear in each historical period enough to believe that they are innate to the human? Is there a cultural, environmental explanation for this observation? Is religion the answer or just one of the answers to the spirituality questions? Is it possible conceptually to deal with spirituality without bothering about religion? Should current forms of spirituality (secular, non-theistic, humanistic, non-religious, etc.) be taken seriously or are they just a hiding to nothing? This chapter's brief was to

---

[12] Mondrian wrote: 'Art and Reality. Art is higher than reality, and has no direct relation to reality. Between the physical sphere and the ethereal sphere there is a frontier where our senses stop functioning. Nevertheless, the ether penetrates the physical sphere and acts on it. Thus, the spiritual penetrates the real. But for our senses these are two different things—the spiritual and the material. To approach the spiritual in art, one will make as little use as possible of reality, because reality is opposed to the spiritual. Thus, the use of elementary forms is logically accounted for. These forms being abstract, we find ourselves in the presence of an abstract art' (quoted on p. 117 of Seuphor M. *Piet Mondrian, life and work*. New York: Harry Abrahams; 1956).

explore the historical epistemology of spirituality. These questions above will hopefully be dealt with in the rest of this book.

References

1. **Dupuy M, Solignac A.** Spiritualité. In: *Dictionnaire de Spiritualité*. Paris: Beauchesne; 1964.

2. **Jones C, Wainwright G, Yarnold SJ.** *The study of spirituality.* Oxford: Oxford University Press; 1986.

3. **Sheldrake P.** *A brief history of spirituality.* Oxford: Blackwell; 2007.

4. **Waaijman K.** *Spirituality: forms, foundations, methods.* Leuven: Peeters; 2002.

5. **Principe W.** Toward defining spirituality. *Studies in Religion/Sciences Religieuses.* 1983;**12**:127–41.

6. **Jacobs A.** Spirituality: history and contemporary developments—an evaluation. *Bulletin for Christian Scholarship.* 2013;**78**:1–12.

7. **Auvrey-Assayas C.** Religion. In: **B Cassin**, (ed.), *Dictionary of untranslatables.* Princeton: Princeton University Press; 2014, pp. 1399–402.

8. **Scheid J.** *An introduction to Roman religion.* Edinburgh: Edinburgh University Press; 2003.

9. **Durkheim E.** *The elementary forms of the religious life. A study in religious sociology.* London: George Allen and Unwin; 1915.

10. **Koenig HG** (ed.). *Handbook of religion and mental health.* London: Academic Press; 1998.

11. **Josephson AM, Peteet JR** (eds). *Handbook of spirituality and worldview in clinical practice.* Washington: American Psychiatric Publishing; 2004.

12. **Huguelet P, Koenig HG** (eds). *Religion and spirituality in psychiatry.* Cambridge: Cambridge University Press; 2009.

13. **Brown C.** *Dictionary of the New Testament theology* (vol. 2). Michigan: Regency Library; 1976, pp. 223–38.

14. **Benveniste E. Le Sacré.** In: *Le Vocabulaire des institutions indo-europées* (vol. 2). Paris: Éditions Minuit; 1969.

15. **Windelband W.** Das Heilige. In: *Präludien.* Tübingen: Mohr; 1907.

16. **Durkheim,** *Elementary forms.*

17. **Otto R.** *The idea of the holy.* London: Oxford University Press; 1923.

18. **Schlamm LCG.** Jung and numinous experience: between the known and the unknown. *European Journal of Psychotherapy and Counselling.* 2007;**9**:403–14.

19. **Huskinson L.** Holy, holy, holy: the misappropriation of the numinous in Jung. In: **A Casement & D Tacey**, (eds), *The idea of the numinous.* London: Routledge; 2006, pp. 200–212.

20. **Otto R.** *Das Heilige.* Gotta: Klotz; 1926.

21. **Chantraine P.** *Dictionnaire étymologique de la langue grecque.* Paris: Klincksieck; 1999, pp. 1294–5.

22. **Liddell HG, Scott R.** *A Greek-English lexicon.* Oxford: Clarendon Press; 1996, pp. 2026–2028.

23. **Urmson JO.** *Greek philosophical vocabulary.* London: Duckworth; 1990, pp. 145–6.

24. *Oxford Latin dictionary*. Oxford: Clarendon Press; 1968, pp. 1805–7.

25. **Kemmer E.** *Die polare Ausdrucksweise in der griechischen Literatur*. Würzburg: Stuber; 1900.

26. **Lloyd GER.** *Polarity and analogy. Two types of argumentation in Greek thought*. Cambridge, UK: Cambridge University Press; 1966.

27. **Bremmer JN.** *The early Greek concept of the soul*. Princeton: Princeton University Press; 1983.

28. **Goetz S, Taliafero C.** *A brief history of the soul*. London: Wiley-Blackwell; 2011.

29. **Frede D, Reis B.** *Body and soul in ancient philosophy*. Berlin: Walter de Gruyter; 2009.

30. **Heinämaa S, Reuter M** (eds). *Psychology and philosophy: inquiries into the soul from late scholasticism to contemporary thought*. Berlin: Springer; 2009.

31. **Onians RB.** *The origins of European thought. About the body, the mind, the soul, the world, time and fate*. Cambridge, UK: Cambridge University Press; 1951.

32. **Broadie S.** Soul and body in Plato and Aristotle. *Proceedings of the Aristotelian Society*. 2001;**101**:295–308.

33. **Berrios GE.** Historical epistemology of the body-mind interaction in psychiatry. *Dialogues in Clinical Neuroscience*. 2018;**20**:5–12.

34. **Augustine.** *On the Trinity*. Books 8–25. Cambridge, UK: Cambridge University Press; 2002.

35. **Rahner K.** *The Trinity*. London: Burns and Oates; 1970.

36. **Finger S, Piccolino M.** Animal spirits and physiology. In: S Finger & M Piccolino, (eds), *The shocking history of electric fishes: from ancient epochs to the birth of modern neurophysiology*. Oxford: Oxford University Press; 2011.

37. **Nelson JM.** *Psychology, religion, and spirituality*. Berlin: Springer; 2009.

38. **Cassaniti JL, Luhrmann TM.** The cultural kindling of spiritual experiences. *Current Anthropology*. 2014,**55**:33–43.

39. **Husserl E.** *Die Lebenswelt. Gesammelte Werke* (vol. 39). Dordrecht: Springer; 2008.

40. **Schutz A, Luckmann T.** *The structures of the life-world*. London: Heinemann; 1974.

41. **Langrebe L, Gaos J, Paci E, Wild J.** *Symposium sobre la noción husserliana de la Lebenswelt*, México: Universidad Nacional Autónoma de México; 1963.

42. **Blumenberg H.** *Teoría del Mundo de la Vida*. México: Fondo de Cultura Económica; 2013.

43. **San Martin J** (ed.). *Sobre el concepto del mundo de la vida*. Madrid: UNED; 1993.

44. **Zelić T.** On the phenomenology of the life world. *Synthesis Philosophica*. 2008,**46**:413–26.

45. **Horgan T, Woodward J.** Folk psychology is here to stay. *The Philosophical Review*. 1985;**44**:197–226.

46. **Bowker J.** *The Oxford dictionary of world religions*. Oxford: Oxford University Press; 1997, p. 334.

47. **Huss B.** Spirituality: the emergence of a new cultural category and its challenge to the religious and the secular. *Journal of Contemporary Religion*. 2014,**29**:47–60.

48. **Waaijman K.** Spirituality, a multifaceted phenomenon. *Studies in Spirituality*. 2007;**17**:1–113.

49. **McCarroll P, O'Connor T, Meakes E.** Assessing plurality in spirituality definitions. In: A Meier, T O'Connor, P VanKatwyk, (eds), *Spirituality and health*. Waterloo: Wilfried Laurier University Press; 2005.

50. **Scorgie GG.** *Guide to Christian spirituality.* Michigan: Zondervan; 2009.

51. **Sheldrake P.** *Spirituality and history.* New York: Crossroads; 1992.

52. **Sheldrake P.** *Spirituality, a very short introduction.* Oxford: Oxford University Press; 2012.

53. **Walach H.** *Secular spirituality.* Berlin: Springer; 2015.

54. **Harris S.** *Waking up: a guide to spirituality without religion.* New York: Simon & Schuster; 2014.

55. **Comte-Sponville A.** *The book of atheistic spirituality.* London: Bantam Press; 2007.

56. **Elkins DN.** Beyond religion: toward a humanistic spirituality. In: **KJ Schneider, JF Pierson, JFT Bugental,** (eds), *The handbook of humanistic psychology.* Second edition. California: Sage; 2014.

57. **Harré R, Moghaddam FM** (eds). *Questioning causality.* Santa Barbara: Praeger; 2016.

58. **Carsetti A** (ed.). *Causality, meaningful complexity and embodied cognition.* Berlin: Springer; 2010.

59. **Brunschvicg L.** *L'expérience humaine et la causalité physique.* Paris: Alcan; 1922.

60. **Collingwood RG.** On the so-called idea of causation. *Proceedings of the Aristotelian Society.* 1938;**38**:84–112.

61. **Ryle G.** Categories. *Proceedings of the Aristotelian Society.* 1938;**38**:189–206.

62. **Ryle G.** *The concept of mind.* London: Hutchinson; 1949.

63. **Dancy J.** Ryle and Strawson on category mistakes. In: **D Dolby,** (ed.), *Ryle on mind and language.* Basingstoke: Palgrave McMillan; 2014, pp. 9–25.

64. **Streib HY, Hood RW.** *Semantics and psychology of spirituality.* Berlin: Springer; 2016.

65. **Sponsel LE.** Ecology and spirituality. *Oxford Research Encyclopedia of Religion,* 2019.

66. **Crosson JB.** The politics of spirituality. *Oxford Research Encyclopedia of Religion,* 2019.

67. **Flanagan K, Jupp PC.** *Sociology of spirituality.* Aldershot: Ashgate; 2007.

68. **Houtman D, Aupers S.** The spiritual turn and the decline of tradition: the spread of post-Christian spirituality in 14 Western countries, 1981–2000. *Journal of the Scientific Study of Religion.* 2007;**46**:305–320.

69. **Possamai A.** Alternative spiritualities and the cultural logic of late capitalism. *Culture and Religion.* 2003;**4**:31–45.

70. **Saybold KS.** *Explorations in neuroscience, psychology and religion.* Aldershot: Ashgate; 2007.

71. **Feierman JR.** *The biology of religious behaviour.* Santa Barbara: Prager; 2009.

72. **Clayton P, Simpson Z** (eds). *Religion and science.* Oxford: Oxford University Press; 2006.

73. **Coles A, Collicut J** (eds). *Neurology and religion.* Cambridge, UK: Cambridge University Press; 2020.

74. **Danziger K.** *Naming the mind.* London: Sage; 1997.

75. **Symington N.** *Emotions and spirit. Questioning the claims of psychoanalysis and religion.* London: Karnac; 1998.

76. **Spezzano C, Gargiulo GJ** (eds). *Soul on the couch. Spirituality, religion, morality in contemporary psychoanalysis.* London: Analytic Press; 1997.

77. **Ostow M.** *Spirit, mind and brain. A psychoanalytic examination of spirituality and religion.* New York: Columbia University Press; 2007.

78. **Mancia M** (ed.). *Psychoanalysis and neuroscience.* Berlin: Springer; 2006.

79. **Hendrix JS.** *Unconscious thought in philosophy and psychoanalysis.* New York: Palgrave; 2015.

80. **Grünbaum A.** *The foundations of psychoanalysis. A philosophical critique.* Berkeley: University of California Press; 1984.

81. **Bowker,** *Oxford Dictionary,* p. 707.

82. p8, Otto, 1923, op. cit.

83. **McCalla A.** *The creationist debate.* London: Continuum; 2006.

84. **Numbers RL.** *The creationists. The evolution of scientific creationism.* Berkeley: University of California Press; 1993.

85. **Blancke S, Hjermitslev HH, Kjærgaard PC** (eds). *Creationism in Europe.* Baltimore: John Hopkins University Press; 2014.

86. **Austin JL.** *How to do things with words.* Oxford: Clarendon Press; 1962.

87. **Searle J.** *Speech acts.* Cambridge, UK: Cambridge University Press; 1969.

88. **Grewendorf G** (ed.). *Speech acts, mind and social reality.* Berlin: Springer; 2002.

89. **Kissine M.** *From utterances to speech acts.* Cambridge, UK: Cambridge University Press; 2013.

90. **Lash S.** *Experience.* Cambridge: Polity; 2018.

91. **Liddell** and **Scott,** *Greek-English Lexicon,* p. 544.

92. *Oxford Latin Dictionary,* p. 1343.

93. **Chantraine,** *Dictionnaire étymologique,* p. 870.

94. **Urmson,** *Greek Philosophical Vocabulary,* p. 52.

95. *Oxford English Dictionary,* 1992.

96. **Ritter J.** *Historisches Wörterbuch der Philosophie.* Basel: Schwabe Verlag; 1971–2007.

97. *Diccionario de la Real Academia Española,* Edición XXIII, 2014.

98. Ritter, *Historisches.*

99. *Diccionario.*

100. Otto, *Das Heilige,* p. 13.

101. **Zaehner RC.** *Mysticism sacred and profane.* New York: Galaxy Books; 1961.

102. **Alquié F** (ed.). *L'Expérience.* Paris: Albin Michel; 1963.

103. **Monk SH.** *The sublime: A study of critical theories in eighteenth-century England.* New York: Modern Language Association of America; 1935.

104. **Burke E.** *A philosophical enquiry into the origin of our ideas of the sublime and the beautiful.* London: Robertson; 1824.

105. **Van Eck C, Bussels S, Delbecke M, Pieters, J** (eds). Translations of the sublime. The early modern reception and dissemination of Longinus' *Peri Hupsous* in rhetoric, the visual arts, architecture and the theatre. Leiden: Brill; 2012.

106. **Rodgers D.** The sublime. In: *J Turner,* (ed.), *Dictionary of art* (vol. 29). Oxford: Oxford University Press; 1996, pp. 889–91.

107. **Wilton A.** Sublime or ridiculous? Turner and the problem of the historical figure. *New Literary History.* 1985;**16**(2):343–76.

108. **Wolf BJ.** A grammar of the sublime, or intertextuality triumphant in church, Turner, and Cole. *New Literary History.* 1985;**16**(2):321–41.

109. **Otto,** *Das Heilige,* p. 42.

110. **Boring EG.** A history of introspection. *Psychological Bulletin.* 1953;**50**:169–89.

111. **Danziger K.** The history of introspection reconsidered. *Journal of the History of the Behavioral Sciences.* 1980;**16**:241–62.

112. **Butler J.** *Rethinking introspection.* New York: Palgrave; 2013.

113. **Lyons WE.** *The disappearance of introspection.* Cambridge, Mass: MIT Press; 1986.

114. **Nisbett RE, Wilson TD.** Telling more than we can we: verbal reports on mental processes. *Psychological Review.* 1977; **84**:231–59.

115. **Scalon J.** Eidetic method. In: L Embree, EA Behnke, D Carr, (eds), *Encyclopedia of Phenomenology.* New York: Kluwer Academic Publishers; 1997, pp.168–71.

116. **Uehlein FA.** Eidos and eidetic variation in Husserl's phenomenology. In: **M Spitzer, FA Uehlein, MA Schwartz,** (eds), *Phenomenology language and schizophrenia.* Berlin: Springer; 1992, pp. 88–102.

117. **Levin DM.** Induction and Husserl's theory of eidetic variation. *Philosophy and Phenomenological Research.* 1968;**29**:1–15.

118. **Gutland C.** Husserlian phenomenology as a kind of introspection. *Frontiers in Psychology.* 2018;**9**:1–14.

119. **Ellenberger HF.** *The discovery of the unconscious: the history and evolution of dynamic psychiatry.* New York: Basic Books; 1970.

120. **Jung CG.** *The archetypes and the collective unconscious.* London: Routledge; 1991.

121. **Stevens A.** Archetypal theory. The evolutionary dimension. In: **R Withers,** (ed.), *Controversies in analytical psychology.* New York: Brunner-Routledge, 2003, pp. 252–64.

122. **Cassaniti, Luhrmann,** *Cultural Kindling.*

123. **Furetiere A.** *Dictionaire universel contenant generalment tous les mots François.* A la Haye: Chez Arnout & Reinier Leers; 1690.

124. **Diderot, D'Alambert** (eds). *Encyclopédie ou Dictionnaire Raisonné des Sciences, des Artes, et des Métiers, par une Société de Gens de Lettres.* (vol. 15). Paris: Briasson David, Le Breton, Durand; 1753–65.

125. **Johnson S.** *A dictionary of the English language* (2 vols). Sixth edition. London: JFC Rivington et al.; 1785.

126. **Krauth CP.** *A vocabulary of the philosophical sciences.* New York: Sheldon and Company; 1878, p. 879.

127. **Lévy-Bruhl L.** *Le mentalité primitive.* The Herbert Spencer Lecture delivered at Oxford 29 May 1931. Oxford: Clarendon Press; 1931.

128. **Harris,** *Waking up.*

129. **Kandinsky W.** *Concerning the spiritual in art.* New York: The Floating Press; 2008.

130. **Tisma A.** 'Art and Spirituality'. Available from: http://www.atisma.com/art_and_spir.htm

131. **Robertson J, McDaniel C.** Spirituality and art. In: **J Turner,** (ed.), *Grove dictionary of art online.* Available from: https://www.oxfordartonline.com/groveart/view/10.1093/gao/9781884446054.001.0001/oao-9781884446054-e-7002020414

Chapter 3

Conflicts and complexities: Medical science, exceptional experiences, and the perils of simplistic history

Andreas Sommer

Introduction

According to a popular narrative that continues to inform academic identities and public images of Western science and medicine, there is a perennial conflict between medical science and religion. In this view, science is taken to be an inherently objective, impartial, and thus self-correcting form of collective inquiry, which has given us a certain body of universally consistent and valid knowledge. In contrast, religion is considered a dogmatically closed magical belief system based on wilful ignorance of basic scientific facts (1–3).

Once we investigate science as it has historically been practised, however, claims of its inherent opposition to religion quickly run into severe problems. While scientific and medical research was sometimes indeed suppressed by theological censorship, we now know, for example, that many iconic representatives of the sciences ranging from Galileo and Isaac Newton to Michael Faraday and J. Clerk Maxwell, as well as physics Nobel Laureates like J.J. Thompson, Lord Rayleigh, and Werner Heisenberg, subscribed either to formal theological views or to more eclectic but equally committed holistic and spiritual philosophical outlooks.

Most professional historians of science and medicine now accept that scientific inquiry has often been motivated and guided by strong religious sentiments, which have included a wide range of beliefs from dogmatically theological positions to idiosyncratic theistic as well as non-theistic spiritualities. Modern notions of the eternal conflict of science with religion are in fact of fairly recent vintage and have their origins in nineteenth-century political struggles to secularize fledgling professionalized sciences. Despite its almost complete failure to inform ongoing science–religion polemics, the present state of the art of historical scholarship has demonstrated that the relationship of the sciences with various religions and spiritualities is more properly characterized by complexity than intrinsic opposition (4–6).

Perhaps most importantly, however, while it would be pointless to deny the self-professed dogmatism of orthodox theology, monolithic portrayals of religion as belief in 'magic' are as problematic as the popular assumption that religion and magic were simultaneously vanquished by secular science and medicine. Again, the historical record shows that from the Enlightenment to about the late twentieth century, claimed experiences that were incompatible with both religious orthodoxy and naturalistic maxims were rarely studied in an impartial manner, but were overwhelmingly ridiculed and pathologized (7–11). Moreover, present-day 'scientific naturalism' and its fundamental distrust of supposedly 'supernatural' experiences owes its pedigree to a long past of theological condemnations of certain reported spiritual experiences as heresies, and religiously motivated suppressions of empirical approaches to magic, faith healing, and a supposed spirit world as theologically and spiritually illicit and dangerous (7, 12, 13).

The problem of 'enthusiasm': spiritual experiences and 'naturalistic' medical science from Kant to James

There is a reference in the concluding lecture of William James's *The Varieties of Religious Experience* that modern readers may be excused for passing over because it seems unintelligible today. Summing up his emphasis on constructive social and clinical functions of transformative spiritual and mystical experiences, James briefly acknowledged that his audience might include 'enemies of what our ancestors used to brand as enthusiasm' (14). James himself referred to religious 'enthusiasm' throughout the *Varieties* overwhelmingly in a positive sense, stressing its constructive functions in terms of healthy-mindedness. Yet, his reference to unfavourable connotations of 'enthusiasm' in the past hints to a long history during which debates over spiritual experience constituted a fundamental political issue and were thus also integral to the making of Western secular science, medicine, and philosophy.

In fact, from the 'Scientific Revolution' to about the mid-nineteenth century, there was hardly a representative of science, medicine, or philosophy who did not express grave concerns over the dangers of 'enthusiasm'. Contrary to its modern positive connotations, the term was then used as a pejorative label for beliefs resting on claimed revelations and spiritual experiences that bypassed, if not contradicted, clerical and biblical authority. Generalizing from the very tangible dangers caused by destructive and morbid forms of religious fervour, early modern writers, themselves profoundly religious, used the term to denote mental instability and pathology (15, 16).

It is fair to say that there was never a time in the history of Western science and medicine when spiritual experiences constituted a strictly theoretical or empirical problem dispassionately discussed in the proverbial ivory tower. The social and political anxieties of the day have always shaped medical ideas and indeed the very conditions of scientific practice. From the Reformation and the French Revolution to smaller yet by no means bloodless religio–political revolts over the unholy alliance between church and state throughout the nineteenth century, debates over 'enthusiasm' (or *Schwärmerei* in German) were inseparably bound up with questions of religious and thus political authority. Modern notions of the supposedly inherent 'materialism' of science and medicine typically fail to consider that philosophical and political materialism has a long past predating the making of modern science. Indeed, present-day 'scientific materialism' cannot be understood without an acknowledgement of the political dimensions and specific historical contexts of its emergence (17, 18).

Actual responses to 'enthusiasm' indeed strikingly illustrate that 'scientific materialism' is a relatively recent invention and thus was not responsible for the marginalization of exceptional experiences in science and medicine since the Enlightenment—the supposed age of tolerance and humanism. This is illustrated, for example, in two responses to the writings of the now infamous 'arch enthusiast' of the Enlightenment, the natural philosopher and self-professed spirit-seer, Emanuel Swedenborg.

Swedenborg's contemporary role as a preeminent Swedish man of science (19, 20) is now largely forgotten, mainly thanks to a widely publicized polemical attack by the German philosopher Immanuel Kant in 1766. Like many other Enlightenment thinkers, Kant was a believer in the immortality of the soul and deeply hostile to materialism. He was no medical professional and never met Swedenborg in the flesh, yet he argued that Swedenborg and other 'enthusiasts' who claimed to see spirits were insane. Spectral visions, Kant believed, could indeed be caused by actual denizens of the spirit world, but the very predisposition of spirit-seership was a nervous disease that was bound to produce grotesque distortions of the original spiritual impetus. Kant's polemic was not beyond employing a joke involving flatulence to get his derision across: 'If a hypochondriac wind romps in the intestines it depends on the direction it takes; if it descends it becomes a f–––, if it ascends it becomes an apparition or sacred inspiration.' (21).

A second response came from another Enlightenment enemy of otherworldly visions, Joseph Priestley, a lay theologian who is now better known as a 'father' of modern chemistry. Priestley's critique of spirit-seership in 1791 did not advance scientific or empirical arguments either, but rested on biblical 'proof' that the only legitimate afterlife was the bodily resurrection of the dead (22). In fact, whereas nowadays 'materialism' is mostly synonymous with 'atheism', Priestley represented a genuinely Christian-theological materialist tradition often referred to as 'mortalism': based on scriptural exegesis, mortalist theologies in their strictest guises have taught that the soul or mind is indeed annihilated after bodily death, only to be miraculously recreated on Judgement Day by an act of God (23, 24).

About a century after Kant, Priestley and many other intellectuals dismissed and derided reports of spiritual experiences, William James participated in research on the first international census of hallucinations in non-morbid samples. The census was carried out in 1889–97 on behalf of the International Congress of Experimental Psychology, and drew on a sample of around 17,000 men and women (25). This survey showed that hallucinations—including visions of the departed—were remarkably widespread, thus severely undermining contemporary medical views of their inherent pathology. But the project was unorthodox in yet another respect: it scrutinized claims of 'veridical' impressions—that is, cases where people reported seeing or sensing the presence of a loved one suffering an accident or other crisis, which they had in fact undergone, but which the hallucinator couldn't have known about through 'normal' means (25–27).

While James is widely acknowledged by American psychologists as the founder of their profession, the results of his and subsequent heterodox psychologists' active investigations of telepathy and trance states (25, 28–31) are still openly derided by some of modern psychology's self-appointed metaphysical border guards (32). James, despite having early on rejected the eclectic Swedenborgianism of his father, and being well aware of the veritable thicket of deception, fraud, and genuine pathology associated with many spiritual and occult beliefs and practices, was certainly open to spiritual interpretations of certain alleged 'psychic' phenomena. What interested him far more than properly theological dimensions, however, were the constructive functions such experiences could serve—for example, as coping tools in the daily struggle with life (14, 33, 34).

While tackling the fundamental psychological question of the unity of the mind in the context of contemporary research on divided selves and multiple personalities, James was also pioneering the study of memory, volition, and creativity in altered states of consciousness, including hypnotic and mediumistic trance, psychedelic intoxication, and ordinary sleep (35–37). In opposition to James and his collaborators in psychical research, his German counterpart

Wilhelm Wundt—the 'founder' of modern experimental psychology at Leipzig—dismissed this particular brand of psychological investigation with 'enlightened' derision. In line with medical and anthropological standard views of the time, Wundt rejected trance and other altered states as improper venues of psychological experimentation, branding any belief in the very possibility of 'occult' phenomena—along with research on divisions of the self—as tell-tale signs of nervous as well as moral degeneration, and dangerous throwbacks to 'savage' stages of mental development (27, 38).

Resulting charges of 'materialism' by Catholic and other religious intellectuals notwithstanding, Wundt's psychological project did not adhere to materialistic maxims; on the contrary, it explicitly sought to establish the human psyche as an irreducible spiritual agent (39–41). Railing against materialism throughout his career, Wundt would in fact later claim that his psychology was motivated by a quasi-mystical experience he had had as a young man, and a subsequent perusal of writings by mystics and 'enthusiasts' such as Jakob Böhme (42). Yet, the year 1879 saw Wundt's simultaneous inauguration of experimental psychology at Leipzig University and his open attack on fellow scientists—including the founder of modern psychophysics, Gustav T. Fechner—who investigated the claimed marvels of spiritualism. While spiritualists usually argued that empirical evidence for 'occult' phenomena provided a weapon against materialistic doctrines, Wundt argued in his open letter that spiritualism was on the contrary a particularly dangerous and gross form of materialism, and that belief in spirit inference was proof of backward mental states characteristic of shamans and other members of the 'lower races' (43).

The transition of psychology from the science of the soul into a 'naturalistic' university profession in the late nineteenth century occurred against the backdrop of the diametrically opposed metaphysical sensitivities of its founders, none of whom was actually a materialist (44). Nor can the advent of an axiomatic 'naturalism' in Western science be understood without an appreciation of severe political crises caused by worries over the political exploitation of questions of the nature and destiny of the soul—such as the March Revolution of 1848, Bismarck's brutal war on Catholicism throughout the 1870s in Germany, and the anti-clerical upheavals during the Third Republic in France (18, 45–48).

While such dramatic instances of political unrest triggered by frustrations over the political power of the church were comparatively absent in British and American contexts, the German example in particular served as a template for efforts to free science from the strictures of theocratic politics and theological censorship through the creation of independently financed university professions in other countries. When considered within concrete political and cultural contexts of the time, it is therefore not surprising that most medical professionals and psychologists ignored or dismissed the Census of Hallucinations and related findings presented by James and fellow investigators of unorthodox questions without studying them. Lacking powerful ideological, metaphysical, and political lobbies and popularizers, impartial and discerning approaches to exceptional experiences remained scarce and under-represented, and the pathological interpretation of hallucinations, visions, and trance states continued to prevail until the late twentieth century.

Changing historiographies and constructive functions of transcendental experiences

It was only towards the end of the last century when academic sensibilities gradually began to change. This was reflected in fields including medicine and anthropology, but also in the historiography of the relationship between science and the occult. Whereas positivist frameworks and unquestioning science–religion dichotomies informed the work of previous generations of historians of science and medicine, it was not until about the 1970s that occult leanings of figureheads of the Scientific Revolution such as Copernicus, Galileo, Francis Bacon, Robert Boyle, and Isaac Newton, and major Victorian scientists such as evolutionary biologist Alfred Russel Wallace, became the object of more sustained and methodologically sophisticated discussion. Historians now began to reconstruct the past on its own terms rather than through the 'naturalistic' filters of the present, and to reveal the historically contingent nature of the very standards to which previous historical work had to conform (49–52).

Independent of these historiographical revisions, medical perspectives also slowly began to change at around the same time. For example, in 1971, the *British Medical Journal* published a study on 'the hallucinations of widowhood' by the Welsh physician W. Dewi Rees (53). Of the 293 bereaved women and men in Rees's sample, almost half reported encounters with their deceased spouses. Most importantly, 69% perceived these encounters as helpful, whereas only 6% found them unsettling. Many of these experiences, which ranged from a sense of presence to tactile, auditory, and visual impressions indistinguishable from interactions with living persons, continued over years. Rees's paper inspired a trickle of fresh studies (54–56) that confirmed his initial findings: these 'hallucinations' do not seem particularly rare, neither do they qualify as therapeutically undesirable let alone inherently pathological (57). On the contrary, whatever their ultimate causes, they often appear to provide the bereaved with much-needed strength to carry on.

Rees's study coincided with writings by a pioneer of the modern hospice movement, the Swiss–American psychiatrist Elisabeth Kübler-Ross. Her observations and emphasis of the prevalence of comforting other-worldly visions reported by dying patients were supported by later researchers. Indeed, a 2010 study in the *Archives of Gerontology and Geriatrics* addressed the need for special training for medical personnel regarding these experiences (58), and in recent years the medical literature on end-of-life care has recurrently examined and confirmed the constructive functions of death-bed visions in helping the dying come to terms with impending death (59–61).

Kübler-Ross was also among the first psychiatrists to write about 'near-death experiences' (NDEs) reported by survivors of cardiac arrests and other close brushes with death. Certain NDE elements have pervaded popular culture— impressions of leaving one's body, passing through a tunnel or barrier, encounters with deceased loved ones, a light representing unconditional acceptance, insights of the interconnectedness of all living beings, and so on. While the public discourse is typically dominated by exaggerated claims that scientists studying NDEs have either proven life after death or debunked the afterlife by reducing them to brain chemistry, the most comprehensive and balanced overview currently available (62) reveals a considerable amount of rigorous research published in medical journals, whose consensus is in line with neither of these popular polarizations but which seems to demonstrate the psychological import of the experiences.

While no two NDEs are identical, there is a strong consensus that they often cause lasting and significant personality changes. Regardless of survivors' preexisting spiritual inclinations, they usually 'come back' with the conviction that death is not the end. Understandably, this finding alone can make many people rather nervous, as one might fear threats to the secular character of modern science and medicine, or an abuse of NDE research in the service of fire-and-brimstone evangelism and its corresponding politics. But the specialist literature provides little justification for such worries. Other attested after-effects of NDEs include dramatic increases in empathy, altruism, and environmental responsibility, as well as strongly reduced competitiveness and consumerism (63, 64).

The professional literature also suggests that virtually all elements of NDEs can occur in psychedelic 'mystical' experiences induced by substances such as psilocybin and N, N-Dimethyltryptamine (DMT). Clinical trials at institutions such as Johns Hopkins University and Imperial College London have shown that these induced 'other-worldly' experiences can occasion similar personality changes as NDEs, most notably a loss of fear of death and a newfound purpose in life. Psychedelic therapies are now therefore becoming serious contenders in the treatment of severe conditions including substance addictions as well as treatment-resistant forms of post-traumatic stress disorder and depressions (65–67).

Outdated historiographies and clinical risks: historical evidence matters

This again brings us back to William James, who wrote concerning transformative spiritual experiences: 'If the *fruits for life* of the state of conversion are good, we ought to idealise and venerate it, even though it be a piece of natural psychology; if not, we ought to make short work with it, no matter what supernatural being may have infused it' (14). Yet, his pragmatic arguments for the constructive clinical and social functions and values of such transformative episodes have been mostly ignored by the scientific and medical mainstream.

If there really are tangible benefits of personality changes following 'mystical' and spiritual experiences, and if recent revisions in the historiography of medical science and the 'supernatural' are valid, together this might justify a question that is not usually raised: could it be harmful to blindly follow the standard narrative of Western modernity, according to which ontological naturalism is not only the default metaphysics of science but an obligatory philosophy of life demanded by centuries of supposedly linear progress based on allegedly impartial research?

Dangers of gullibility are evident enough in the tragedies caused by religious fanatics, medical quacks, and ruthless politicians. And while faith in the ultimate benevolence of the cosmos will strike many of us as hopelessly irrational, it should also be pointed out that spiritual world views are certainly not good, let alone healthy, for everybody. Yet, more than a century after James developed his pragmatist approach to transformative experiences, it might be time to restore a balanced perspective and to acknowledge the concrete damage that has been caused by stigma, misdiagnoses, and mis- or over-medication of individuals reporting exceptional experiences—which, after all, seem far more common than many appear to think and may therefore not be particularly 'exceptional,' at least in purely quantitative terms (26, 54, 68, 69). One can well be personally sceptical of the ultimate validity of spiritual beliefs and leave properly theological questions strictly aside, yet still investigate the salutary and prophylactic potential of these experiences.

By making this quasi-clinical proposal, I'm well aware that I could be overstepping my boundaries as a historian of Western science studying the actual means by which boldly empirical approaches to the transcendental have been rendered inherently 'unscientific' over time. However, questions of belief versus evidence are not the exclusive domain of scientific and historical research. In fact, it seems that orthodoxy is often crystallized collective bias starting on a subjective level, which, as James himself urged, is 'a weakness of our nature from which we must free ourselves, if we can' (33).

In the final analysis, it seems that regardless of whether we are committed to 'naturalistic' orthodoxy in medical science or to an open-minded perspective on otherworldly visions and related experiences, we must all cultivate scrutiny of the concrete sources that nourish our most fundamental convictions—including the religious and scientific authorities on which they rest perhaps a little too willingly. This will help us not only to put our empirical and conceptual houses in order, but also to stop projecting our modern ways of being in the world upon the past as well as on non-Western cultures. Coming to grips with ongoing claims of the supposedly eternal opposition between 'science' and 'religion' or 'spirituality' requires investigating how our 'naturalistic' cultural axioms emerged in their original contexts. And it seems that a basic precondition of such research is an ability to tolerate complexities of our findings, along with metaphysical uncertainty.

In this regard, it's often overlooked that clinicians and historians appear to share more in terms of professional ethos than meets the eye. After all, it's probably uncontroversial to demand that therapists as well as historians should strive to understand the biographical and cultural idiosyncrasies of the individuals they deal with: to work with our patients and historical actors, not as we insist they should be, but as we find them in the actual and the concrete (70).

Acknowledgements

Research for this chapter was supported by the Wellcome Trust, through a Junior Research Fellowship in History and Philosophy of Science at Churchill College, Cambridge. I am also grateful to Troy Tice for helpful editorial feedback.

This chapter is an elaboration of my article in Aeon magazine, 'Reasons not to scoff at ghosts, visions and near-death experiences' (6 January, 2020), https://aeon. co/ideas/ghosts-visions-and-near-death-experiences-can-be-therapeutic.

References

1. **Sagan C.** *The demon-haunted world: science as a candle in the dark.* New York: Random House; 1995.

2. **Shermer M.** *The believing brain: from ghosts and gods to politics and conspiracies.* New York: Times Books/Henry Holt & Co.; 2011.

3. **Pinker S.** *Enlightenment now. The case for reason, science, humanism and progress.* London: Allen Lane; 2018.

4. **Dixon T, Cantor G, Pumfrey S** (eds). *Science and religion.* New Historical Perspectives. Cambridge: Cambridge University Press; 2010.

5. **Brooke JH, Numbers RL** (eds). *Science and religion around the world.* Oxford: Oxford University Press; 2011.

6. **Harrison P, Roberts JH** (eds). *Science without God? Rethinking the history of scientific naturalism.* Oxford: Oxford University Press; 2019.

7. **Porter R.** Witchcraft and magic in Enlightenment, romantic and liberal thought. In: **Ankarloo B, Clark S** (eds), *Witchcraft and magic in Europe. Volume 5: The eighteenth and nineteenth centuries.* Philadelphia, PA: University of Pennsylvania Press; 1999, pp. 191–282.

8. **Fara P.** Marginalized practices. In: **Porter R** (ed.), *The Cambridge History of Science. Volume 4: The eighteenth century.* Cambridge: Cambridge University Press; 2003, pp. 485–507.

9. **Daston L, Park K.** *Wonders and the order of nature, 1150–1750.* New York: Zone Books; 1998.

10. **Hunter M.** Robert Boyle (1627–91): *Scrupulosity and science.* Woodbridge: Boydell; 2000.

11. **Sommer A.** Geisterglaube, Aufklärung und Wissenschaft—historiographische Skizzen zu einem westlichen Fundamentaltabu. In: **Schwenke H** (ed.), *Jenseits des Vertrauten Facetten transzendenter Erfahrungen.* Freiburg i. Br.: Verlag Karl Alber; 2018, pp. 183–216.

12. **Walker DP.** *Spiritual and demonic magic from Ficino to Campanella.* London: Warburg Institute; 1958.

13. **Copenhaver BP.** Magic. In: **Park K, Daston L** (eds), *The Cambridge History of Science. Volume 3: early modern science.* Cambridge: Cambridge University Press; 2006, pp. 519–40.

14. **James W.** *The varieties of religious experience. A study in human nature. Being the Gifford Lectures on natural religion delivered in Edinburgh in 1901–1902.* London: Longmans, Green, and Co.; 1902.

15. **Heyd M.** *'Be sober and reasonable'. The critique of enthusiasm in the seventeenth and early eighteenth centuries (Brill's studies in intellectual history, 63).* Leiden: Brill; 1995.

16. **Klein LE, La Vopa AJ** (eds). Enthusiasm and enlightenment in Europe, 1650–1850. *Huntington Library Quarterly.* 1997;60:1–203.

17. **Lange FA.** *Geschichte des Materialismus und Kritik seiner Bedeutung in der Gegenwart* (2 vols). Third edition. Iserlohn: Baedeker (first published in 1866); 1876–7.

18. **Gregory F.** *Scientific materialism in nineteenth century Germany (Studies in the history of modern science 1).* Dordrecht: Springer; 1977.

19. **Benz E.** *Emanuel Swedenborg. Naturforscher und seher.* Munich: Hermann Rinn; 1948.

20. **Schaffer S.** Swedenborg's lunars. *Annals of Science.* 2014;71:2–26.

21. **Kant I.** *Träume eines Geistersehers, erläutert durch Träume der Metaphysik.* Berlin: Schneider (first published in 1766); 1925.

22. **Priestley J.** *Letters to the members of the New Jerusalem Church, formed by Baron Swedenborg.* Birmingham: J. Thompson; 1791.

23. **Burns NT.** *Christian mortalism from Tyndale to Milton.* Cambridge, MA: Harvard University Press; 1972.

24. **Pfeffer M.** Christian materialism and the prospect of immortality. In: **Harrison P, Roberts JH** (eds), *Science without God? Rethinking the history of scientific naturalism.* Oxford: Oxford University Press; 2019, pp. 148–61.

25. James W. *Essays in psychical research.* Cambridge, MA: Harvard University Press; 1986.

26. Sidgwick H, Johnson A, Myers FWH, Podmore F, Sidgwick EM. Report on the census of hallucinations. *Proceedings of the Society for Psychical Research.* 1894;**10**:25–422.

27. Le Maléfan P, Sommer A. Léon Marillier and the veridical hallucination in late-nineteenth and early-twentieth century French psychology and psychopathology. *History of Psychiatry.* 2015;**26**:418–32.

28. Flournoy T. *From India to the planet Mars. A study of a case of somnambulism with glossolalia.* New York: Harper & Brothers; 1900.

29. Janet P. Note sur quelques phénomènes de somnambulisme. *Bulletin de la Société de Psychologie Physiologique.* 1885;**1**:24–32.

30. Janet P. Deuxième note sur le sommeil provoqué à distance et la suggestion mentale pendant l'état somnambulique. *Revue Philosophique.* 1886;**22**:212–23.

31. Cardeña E. The experimental evidence for parapsychological phenomena: a review. *American Psychologist.* 2018;**73**:663–77.

32. Reber AS, Alcock JE. Searching for the impossible: parapsychology's elusive quest. *American Psychologist.* 2019; Jun 13. Available from: https://psycnet.apa.org/doi/10.1037/amp0000486 [Epub ahead of print].

33. James W. *The will to believe and other essays in popular philosophy.* London: Longmans Green and Co.; 1897.

34. James W. Faith and the right to believe. In: **James H** (ed.), *Some problems in 'Philosophy: a beginning of an introduction to philosophy', by William James.* New York and London: Longmans, Green and Co.; 1911, pp. 221–31.

35. Taylor E. *William James on exceptional mental states. The 1896 Lowell lectures.* New York: Charles Scribner's Sons; 1983.

36. Sommer A. James and psychical research in context. In: **Klein A** (ed.), *The Oxford handbook of William James.* Oxford: Oxford University Press; 2020. doi:10.1093/oxfordhb/9780199395699.013.37 (Epub ahead of print).

37. Sommer A. *Crossing the boundaries of mind and body. Psychical research and the origins of modern psychology* (PhD thesis). London: University College London; 2013.

38. Wundt W. *Hypnotismus und suggestion.* Leipzig: Wilhelm Engelmann; 1892.

39. Mischel T. Wundt and the conceptual foundations of psychology. *Philosophy and Phenomenological Research.* 1970;**31**:1–26.

40. Danziger K. The positivist repudiation of Wundt. *Journal of the History of the Behavioral Sciences.* 1979;**15**:205–30.

41. Araujo SdF. *Wundt and the philosophical foundations of psychology. A reappraisal.* Heidelberg: Springer; 2016.

42. Wundt W. *Erlebtes und Erkanntes.* Second edition. Stuttgart: Alfred Kröner; 1921.

43. Wundt W. *Der Spiritismus. Eine sogenannte wissenschaftliche Frage. Offener Brief an Herrn Prof. Dr. Hermann Ulrici in Halle.* Leipzig: Wilhelm Engelmann; 1879.

44. Hatfield G. Remaking the science of mind: psychology as natural science. In: **Fox C, Porter R, Wokler R** (eds), *Inventing human science: eighteenth-century domains.* Berkeley, CA: University of California Press; 1995, pp. 184–231.

45. Junker T. Darwinismus, Materialismus und die Revolution von 1848 in Deutschland. Zur Interaktion von Politik und Wissenschaft. *History and Philosophy of the Life Sciences.* 1995;**17**:271–302.

46. **Goldstein J.** The hysteria diagnosis and the politics of anticlericalism in late nineteenth-century France. *Journal of Modern History.* 1982;**54**:209–39.

47. **Finkelstein G.** *Emil du Bois-Reymond. Neuroscience, self, and society in nineteenth-century Germany.* Cambridge, MA: MIT Press; 2013.

48. **Hopwood N.** *Haeckel's embryos. Images, evolution, and fraud.* Chicago, IL: University of Chicago Press; 2015.

49. **Yates FA.** *Giordano Bruno and the hermetic tradition.* London: Routledge and Kegan Paul; 1964.

50. **Webster C.** *From Paracelsus to Newton. Magic and the making of modern Science.* Cambridge: Cambridge University Press; 1982.

51. **Shapin S, Schaffer S.** *Leviathan and the Air-Pump. Hobbes, Boyle and the experimental life.* Princeton, NJ: Princeton University Press; 1985.

52. **Turner FM.** *Between science and religion. The reaction to scientific naturalism in late Victorian England.* New Haven, CT: Yale University Press; 1974.

53. **Rees WD.** The hallucinations of widowhood. *British Medical Journal.* 1971;**4**:37–41.

54. **Greeley AM.** *The sociology of the paranormal: a reconnaissance* (Sage Research Papers in the Social Sciences, vol. 3). Los Angeles: Sage; 1975.

55. **Olson PR, Suddeth JA, Peterson PJ, Egelhoff C.** Hallucinations of widowhood. *Journal of the American Geriatrics Society.* 1985;**33**:543–7.

56. **Streit-Horn J.** *A systematic review of research on after-death communication (ADC)* (PhD thesis). Denton, TX: University of North Texas; 2011.

57. **Stevenson I.** Do we need a new word to supplement 'hallucination'? *American Journal of Psychiatry.* 1983;**140**:1609–11.

58. **Fenwick P, Lovelace H, Brayne S.** Comfort for the dying: five year retrospective and one year prospective studies of end of life experiences. *Archives of Gerontology and Geriatrics.* 2010;**51**:173–9.

59. **Kerr CW, Donnelly JP, Wright ST, Kuszczak SM, Banas A, Grant PC, et al.** End-of-life dreams and visions: a longitudinal study of hospice patients' experiences. *Journal of Palliative Medicine.* 2014;**17**:296–303.

60. **Devery K, Rawlings D, Tieman J, Damarell R.** Deathbed phenomena reported by patients in palliative care: licnical opportunities and responses. *International Journal of Palliative Nursing.* 2015;**21**:117–25.

61. **Renz D, Reichmuth O, Bueche D, Traichel B, Schuett Mao M, Cerny T, et al.** Fear, pain, denial, and spiritual experiences in dying processes. *American Journal of Hospice & Palliative Medicine.* 2018;**35**:478–91.

62. **Greyson B.** Near-death experiences. In: **Cardeña E, Lynn SJ, Krippner S** (eds), *Varieties of anomalous experience: examining the scientific evidence.* Second edition. Washington, DC: American Psychological Association; 2014. pp. 333–67.

63. **Greyson B.** Near-death experiences and personal values. *American Journal of Psychiatry.* 1983;**140**:618–20.

64. **Klemenc-Ketis Z.** Life changes in patients after out-of-hospital cardiac arrest. *International Journal of Behavioral Medicine.* 2013;**20**:7–12.

65. **Mithoefer MC, Wagner MT, Mithoefer AT, Jerome L, Doblin R.** The safety and efficacy of 3,4-methylenedioxymethamphetamine-assisted psychotherapy in subjects with chronic, treatment-resistant posttraumatic stress disorder: the first randomized controlled pilot study. *Journal of Psychopharmacology.* 2010;**25**:439–52.

66. **Griffiths RR, Johnson MW, Carducci MA, Umbricht A, Richards WA, Richards BD,** et al. Psilocybin produces substantial and sustained decreases in depression and anxiety in patients with life-threatening cancer: a randomized double-blind trial. *Journal of Psychopharmacology.* 2016;**30**:1181–97.

67. **Carhart-Harris RL, Bolstridge M, Day CMJ, Rucker J, Watts R, Erritzoe DE,** et al. Psilocybin with psychological support for treatment-resistant depression: six-month follow-up. *Psychopharmacology.* 2018;**235**:399–408.

68. **Haraldsson E.** Survey of claimed encounters with the dead. *Omega: Journal of Death and Dying.* 1989;**19**:103–13.

69. **Cardeña E, Lynn SJ, Krippner S** (eds). *Varieties of anomalous experience: examining the scientific evidence.* Second edition. Washington, DC: American Psychological Association; 2014.

70. **Sommer A.** Are you afraid of the dark? Notes on the psychology of belief in histories of science and the occult. *European Journal of Psychotherapy & Counselling.* 2016;**18**:105–22.

Chapter 4

Can spirituality be a scientific topic and how?: A rigorous but open-minded scientific approach of studies on religion, spirituality, and mental health

Harald Walach

Why spirituality seems to be unscientific to most

Spirituality seems to be an unscientific topic to most scientifically minded people and a scientific fringe topic at best (1). Although quantitative surveys of whether scientists and scholars in the US are religious and spiritual regularly show that more than 50% of them would call themselves religious or spiritual (2, 3), spirituality seems to be a topic largely banned from scientific discourse. Mainstream and flagship journals do not publish opinion pieces. Empirical research on such topics is normally confined to third- or second-tier journals at best and, if published in first-tier journals, appears flanked with editorial caveats and highly critical voices (4). Those voices, more often than not, imply: spirituality and religion are topics not fit for scientific discourse, because the scientific world view does not cater for non-material entities and presupposes a world in which all events that happen can be accounted for through the effects of known material causes (5, 6), of which we currently know four—the electromagnetic force, the gravitational force, and the weak and the strong atomic interactions. There is no reason, so the mainstream narrative goes, to assume other forces at work, because this would entail a revision of our current physicalist model of the world, which is both extremely unlikely and cumbersome for it would turn our natural sciences upside down. Although some such efforts exist (7), they are not really prized highly. In addition, any non-physical intervention in our world would violate the laws of thermodynamics. And, after all, the grand narrative of evolution has done away with the necessity to assume an extra-material, divine entity as the creator and originator of our universe (8).

The progress of neuroscience has made it plausible that our consciousness can be explained, eventually, as an emergent property of a highly interconnected network or neuronal electric activity, and thus will also find, eventually, a physicalist interpretation in materialist terms. Thus, so the narrative goes, science really is a new world view, and not only a method to understand natural phenomena. It is a world view that is variably termed 'naturalistic', 'scientific', 'materialist', or in any conjunction of those three terms that are also normally used interchangeably (9).

The philosopher Baas van Fraassen has called people who hold such a world view 'naturalistic natives', because they subscribe to such a world view in an unreflected manner, without scrutinizing the presuppositions they are making (10). We will be doing exactly that in what follows. Because 'naturalistic natives' don't do that, they do not understand what they are actually doing. In that, they are similar to aboriginal natives who hold views about themselves and the world that seem completely natural to them. In order to disentangle these points, it might be useful to shortly review the history. Why has this stance become the default and mainstream one? And what is wrong with it, if anything at all?

A very short history of the scientific adage that spirituality and religion are unscientific

The common origin of our academic and scientific enterprise was the birth of universities in the Middle Ages in Europe, starting with the University of Paris, the Law School in Bologna, and the Medical Schools in Salerno and Montpellier (11–12). While informal processes of scholars assembling and giving themselves statutes started earlier, formalizations through papal bulls and royal diplomas started during the eleventh century. In rapid sequence, universities were founded in France, England, Italy, Germany, and Spain, such that in the fourteenth and fifteenth centuries there was a dense patchwork of universities all across Europe. All these universities started from the unquestioned presupposition that the basis of all scholarly and research activity should be theology, the knowledge and learned interpretation of the Holy Scriptures. Initially, there were hardly any natural sciences. These started in England with Robert Grosseteste (1175–1253) who began with optical experiments, reading and translating tracts on optics (13). It was followed by chemical experimenters, such as by Peter of Mahincourt (flourished 1269) in France and others. This effort was popularized and made prominent by Roger Bacon (1219–92) (14). Roger Bacon was a deft critic of his contemporaries and, apart from a few, he thought most academic writers shallow and badly educated. He wanted all scholarly and scientific activity to be founded on experience, flanked by good mathematical and linguistic knowledge, at least of Latin and Greek, but also Hebrew.

He set out to reform academic learning and put together what he thought was necessary for this on papal request in his 'Opus Majus', the larger work, which was a rough outline, written in haste and surreptitiously, because all Franciscan writers were under a ban to publish anything without prior permission from the General of their order (15). These sketches remained private, therefore, only available to the pope and probably a few fellow friars. Because the pope died quickly after having commissioned this work, it remained unread, except for those passages that were transcribed by later librarians and scribes, and until Pico della Mirandola discovered it in the papal library in the fifteenth century, some 200 years after it was written (16, 17). From there, the thoughts found their way to England where they were taken up by the chancellor of the English Queen Elizabeth, Francis Bacon, no relative of the older Bacon, and made their way into Francis Bacon's 'Novum Organon', 'New Instrument' (18). By then, the empirical enterprise of figuring out how nature operates was well underway. Economic and anthropological changes allowed the old ideas of Aristarchos of Samos that the sun was in the center of our planetary system to become viable again (19). With the cosmological view changing, the physical ideas also had to change from their old Aristotelean frame into what Galileo Galilei had worked out. From there it was a straight line, through Descartes' mathematical discoveries and philosophical stipulations to Newton's laws of gravity (20). While Descartes had codified the separation of mind and matter, making organismic entities like animals, but also the human body, an elaborate mechanical contraption, and mind an independent superior entity, Newton laid the foundation for a mechanical understanding of the whole universe. While Newton initially only tried to understand planetary motion, it became clear very quickly that this model, combined with Descartes' abstraction that organisms can be conceived as being mechanical in nature, could serve as a blueprint for the understanding of all-natural phenomena. Suddenly, a view opened itself that understood all of nature as natural machinery, governed by external laws. Naturalism was born: a stance that displaced the old-age creator, God, and allotted him a place and role outside this natural cosmos: as the one who once built the whole machinery, like a watchmaker, wound it and set it into motion, and since then watched it move (21). This naturalism was initially united with a kind of deism: God was still believed in as the aboriginal cause of the universe, but no longer involved in it, because the running of the whole machinery could be understood through natural laws (22). At least this was the promise.

When Darwin's discovery made evolution a universal option for understanding how development of species from one into another might have happened, he opened a new chapter (23, 24). Now, it might be possible to understand the whole universe's development as a story of self-evolution, where not even an aboriginal maker and creator was necessary, who made this whole machinery in the first place. The machinery was conceived in modern times as one that was bootstrapping itself into existence, perhaps once in the aboriginal Big Bang, perhaps more frequently in various such events. At any rate, science, it seems now, has brought about a new Grand Narrative of natural self-creation and evolution that has got rid of any divine entity. Although there are still a few unknowns and irregularities in these narratives, the promise goes that these will be sorted eventually, as other unknowns have been figured out in the past as well.

This Grand Narrative of self-creation and evolution of the material world has replaced the creation myth of religion in most of the enlightened Western world, except in those pockets of fundamentalist religious resistance in the US Bible belt, where people are trying to hold fast to the religious beliefs and have created an alternative narrative called 'Intelligent Design'. They point to holes in the Grand Narrative and demand that these holes can only be filled if some intelligent agent is postulated—of course, the naturalist version of their creator god—who can make the narrative work. Because, in the US, these fights are not only scientific discourses but social–political, intensely tied to religious and cultural stances, scientists are often very weary when spirituality is made a scientific topic. They suppose that intelligent design, and thereby creationism, are entering the scientific discourse through the back door. My stance here is that this is a very American problem, and that making spirituality a scientific topic has nothing to do, in principle and in general terms, with championing creationism. Certainly, I am not doing that, neither implicitly nor explicitly.

While natural scientists developed the blueprint for a purely mechanical universe in the seventeenth and eighteenth centuries, philosophers in France and later in Germany were probably most radical in combining this with a purely materialist world view, probably for the first time in human history, if we neglect some early starters in the Middle Ages, when such positions were also occasionally held (25). The idea was that the analysis of matter alone was sufficient to understand the world. The mechanistic abstraction that Descartes had produced in his posthumous book, *Traité de l'homme*, published in 1664, was radicalized by La Mettrie in his book *L'homme machine*: man, and all that can be seen from the outside as human can be understood as a reflex of mechanical workings. The philosophers of the eighteenth-century enlightenment movement, such as Diderot, d'Holbach, d'Alembert, all championed such a mechanistic, materialist view of the world. This was not a scientifically necessary consequence of new developments, but a choice of a world view that was in stark contrast to the old, politically oppressive clericism that was liaised with a politically obsolete monarchy denying dignity and freedom to the majority of the population. This modern naturalism was politically progressive and in liaison with revolutionary enlightenment movements. Naturalism offered a new religion, fitting to the general political and cultural stance of an intelligentsia that was at the same time scientifically minded and politically progressive. This can be nicely seen in a letter that Voltaire wrote in 1732 to the physicist and biologist Maupertuis, who had given him some lessons in Newtonian physics:

> Pardon Monsieur. Mes tentations sont allées au diable d'ou elles venaient. Votre première lettre m'a baptisé dans la religion Newtonienne; votre seconde m'a donné la confirmation. En vous remerciant de vos sacraments. Brûlez, je vous prie, mes ridicules objections, elles sont d'un infidèle. Je garderai à jamais vos lettres, elles sont d'un grand apôtre de Newton, lumen ad revelationem gentium ...—Excuse me, sir. My temptations have gone to the devil, where they belong. Your first letter has baptized me in the Newtonian religion. The second has given me the confirmation. I am grateful for your sacraments. Please burn my ridiculous objections of an infidel. I will guard your letters, since they come from a great apostle of Newton, light to enlighten the gentiles ...' (26, p. 320)

Despite his general tendency towards irony, I think it is worthwhile to take the religious language here seriously. Voltaire points to Newton in the words of Simeon in the gospel according to Luke, announcing the new messiah. The new messiah is Newton and with him the world view of a rationally structured, understandable mechanical universe.

This world view, married with the politically progressive idea of freeing man from dogmatic bondage, allowing him his own world view and choices, empowering him to use his rationality, as Kant has demanded (27), set the stage for modern naturalistic atheism. God was no longer necessary to understand how the world came about and operated. Extra-material entities, such as spirit, soul, or mind, let alone ghosts, demons, and angels, were no longer necessary as explanatory entities, neither for the world at large nor for personal individual lives. All, it seems, can be explained naturalistically. This opens the scene for the triumph of rationalism over obscurantism, humanism over theistic concepts, and makes humans the new Gods: *homo deus* (28).

The philosopher Charles Taylor has pointed out that the standard narrative of replacement of religion by science is too short-sighted, and so is my shorthand history here (29). There are many other factors operative, since the Grand Narrative is very deficient: too many things are unclear to make it really convincing. But it is very suggestive, and it ties in with an economic drive to profit making, a political one to improving living conditions here and now and not to wait for a transcendent perfect world to come, and it links up with a profound distrust in religious narratives after all the disasters the world has seen since 1900. One can point to many failures of the churches over the ages, to the link between economic flourishing and a certain type of Protestantism, and the failure of Catholic dogma to offer new interpretations for scientific findings. The net result will not change: the Grand Narrative of a loving God that made the world and is taking care of His creatures has been displaced by the Grand Narrative of a cold and indifferent spontaneous and largely accidental evolution process as a result of which we have now evolved as we are, purely by accident, improbable as this might be, and are now the creators of our own fate and future, which will happen here, on earth (or maybe one day in outer space), but not in a transcendent heaven.

The consequence of this history

Now, it is pretty clear that in such a world view there is no place for religion and spirituality except as a relict of an archeology of mental history, or even as a persistence of delusory thinking. Spiritual experiences, powerful as they may be, can only be seen as a mental merry-go-round of a mind gone astray or entertaining itself while nothing more useful is happening. If mind is nothing but the result of electric activity in the brain, and, hence, a product of matter, mental events that do not have an outside referent can only be hallucinations. Hence, the only plausible scientific way of studying religion or spirituality is by their psychological function—How does it help people cope with their lives and its problems? How may it foster social coherence but nothing else? Why is it still persisting despite all our enlightened knowledge? But even that is more of a study of defect than a study of strength. At any rate, spirituality and religion cannot have a positive and constructive role in such a world view, and they are certainly not central to the scientific enterprise. It might be interesting to study relicts and remnants of a culture long gone, and those are certainly worthwhile topics of archeology, but they are not central to filling in the gaps of the Grand Narrative.

Why spirituality and, as a consequence, religion should be a more prominent topic

This new Grand Narrative about Nature bootstrapping itself into existence with all its laws, principles, and consequences in place has a lot of gaps. Many details of the evolution process, starting from cosmology and ending with the details of the biological processes, are unclear (23). That does not mean that intelligent design is a better or more viable alternative. It simply means that the new Grand Narrative is less clear than most would have it. Iain McGilchrist has pointed out that our whole intellectual endeavour of the past centuries has a strong cognitive mental bias in that it neglects holistic aspects and focuses on details, separated entities, and graspable things (30). Put very succinctly: it deals with dead things that can be clearly delineated and studied, and neglects the live and fluid processes of relationship and creation. This is because one cognitive function of our brain, the more logical, linear, and conceptual has taken over from the more intuitive, holistic, and artistic one, thereby making itself the dominant mode. The old image of the servant making itself master is a fitting image for this. Put differently: it is unclear to what extent our scientific findings are really truthful representations of the full and whole reality.

I have made a lengthier argument that I can only hint at here (31). There is a general consensus in the research community of science studies that every intellectual activity has to rest on presuppositions that come from outside the system itself. These are assumed to be rational or true without any possibility to prove this within and through the system itself. The philosopher Collingwood has called these 'absolute presuppositions' and has pointed to the fact that they come from the cultural background of a society (32). Thus, the materialist assumptions made by the Grand Narrative are such absolute presuppositions. They are necessary for this narrative to function, but they cannot be proven true by it, because this would involve circularity. The fact that they work well to produce this narrative is nothing but a proof of consistency, but not a proof of truth. While consistency is necessary for truth, it is not sufficient. In that sense, the Grand Narrative and the seemingly necessary, implicit materialism of science is such an absolute presupposition and results in the stance of scientific naturalism. It is important to realize: it is a stance, not a truth, and, in the same sense, a new kind of religion. Everyone is entitled to their religion, as the Declaration of Human Rights states. But no religion should dominate another one, and in the same sense some modesty would be in place regarding the viability of the new Grand Narrative. It is a possible stance, and in some respects our scientific world view, or rather our modern science, has provided some important and true insights into the working of the material world. But it has by no means elucidated the workings of the world as such in totality. On the contrary, by focusing on the material aspects only, it has, by the same token, obscured others.

Another way of saying the same thing might be to state: perhaps there are other modes of gaining knowledge about the world that are not dependent on the major epistemic mode of our current science—namely, sense experience and its analysis. Another, complementary mode could be the inner experience that we normally call a spiritual experience of enlightenment (33, 34). It might offer a different set of insights into the deep structure of the world from within. To make this clearer, let me go back to Roger Bacon and his Opus Majus, written in 1267. There, as I said, he stated that experience should be the basis of science, scholarship, and learning. Experience, he said, comes in two modes:

an outer mode, through sense experience, by which we learn about the material world. But there is also an inner mode, inner experience, he calls it—experientia interior—which he aligns with spiritual experience or divine enlightenment. Putting aside the adjective 'divine' for a moment and trying to understand what he means in purely secular terms, we could put it in the following way: spiritual experience might be a mode of getting into touch with reality—our own personal individual reality, but also reality as such, from within. This is something that has been described as enlightenment experience in various traditions or as spiritual experience in more theistic traditions (34–39). Neglecting those differences for a moment, one might be able to say that such experiences reveal something about the underlying unity of reality. In order to make this more understandable, we could use the inner experience of meaningfulness and purpose.

Victor Emil Frankl pointed out that the experience of meaning might occur even in the most untoward circumstances, in his case while being imprisoned in a Nazi concentration camp (40). Such experiences happen from within. When we discover the meaning of some life situation, this is normally, phenomenologically speaking, felt as something that reveals itself from within. It is accompanied by a sense of clarity and insight, and normally also by some positive emotion, like joy. Such experiences normally occur spontaneously and rarely through a rational reflection process. On the contrary, it seems that such rational, linear reflections are rather detrimental (41). It seems necessary that we halt such processes and become one with whatever we do—be it some sports, or some social encounter, or some leisure activity—without reflecting (42). In the terminology introduced by McGilchrist, we need to let go of our sequential, language-based cognitive processes and immerse ourselves in the experiential, image-based processes. Then the experience of meaning comes to us and reveals something about the totality of a situation—for instance, about being in love with someone and wanting to spend more time with him or her.

In the same sense, we can conceive of a spiritual experience. The referent here is not our individual life, as in the experience of meaning and purpose. The referent is reality as such, in one or another aspect, experienced from within, as it were, or, put differently, in its deep structure. What could that be? It could be, for instance, some abstract structure, as is sometimes found by great theoreticians who offer an abstract mathematical theory—for instance, as in Einstein's 'finding' relativity theory. Einstein used to say, 'Ideas come from God' (43, p. 61). Because Einstein was an agnostic, he did not mean a personal creator God, but he was referring to such a process of insight into the deep structure of reality. It could be an experiential understanding of the connectivity between beings and the consequences for our societal and personal ways of relating with others and our environment. While our scientific analysis—for instance, through modelling climate data and ecological interdependencies— shows us clearly how strong this connectivity is, this clear, rational knowledge does not seem to be enough to inspire change and actions, not because we lack knowledge but because we lack experience. This experience of mutual dependence and interconnectivity is a standard example of the deep structure of reality and of the content of a spiritual experience of unity. While in spiritual traditions such an experience is then formulated and interpreted within a religious framework, by its very nature it is the experiential counterpart of an otherwise rationally founded insight. The point is: the rational insight is normally not enough, but needs to be bolstered by experience in order to create enough momentum to inform our actions. This experience, however, is not an experience of the outside, material world through our senses. It is an experience of the deep structure of our world through our conscious mind, which needs to be prepared in a certain mode to be able to access this reality from within. Spiritual traditions normally have some ideas of such a preparation of our consciousness, and offer practice and exercises to foster such a stance. Meditation or contemplation are examples of such practices. It seems to be necessary that we lay our discursive conceptual mind to rest for a while to let the experience of holistic interrelationship emerge. Because our conceptual, discursive mind is so dominant, this is not a trivial task and requires some effort and practice. Sometimes this happens naturally, inadvertently, and spontaneously. William James has studied such cases within religious contexts (44). But they happen also spontaneously to atheists and agnostics, such as astrophysicist Lightman, himself an agnostic, describes (45, p. 6). We conducted a survey of a representative sample of nearly 900 German psychotherapists and found that only one-third of them reported never to have had such a spiritual experience (46). The rest said they had had such an experience at least once in their lives, some even multiple times. Sometimes, such experiences have very strong impacts on the lives of those who have them, such as in the historic Gautama Buddha, or in saintly figures of ecclesiastical history such as Saint Francis or Saint Ignatius. Sometimes, they are the backdrop to simple content lives. But do they have a place in science other than as curiosities of human experience? I think they could, if we wanted them to.

How spirituality and religion could inform science and to what extent they might be useful for mental health practitioners

I have hinted at the epistemic role of such inner experiences: They might be sources of inspiration for scientists. Historical examples are many, once we open our eyes. The initial experiences of important figures in the history of science can be interpreted in this way. Descartes reports such experiences (19, p. 69f). One can see the story of the apple falling on Newton's head as a chiffre for such a holistic insight into the nature of things. Many scientists were inspired by such insights that I would call spiritual by their phenomenology, except that the context was science, not spirituality. Barbara McClintock, studying her maize plants and discovering jumping genes, immersed herself into the inner life of those plants (47, 48). Kekulé dreamt of the structure of the benzole ring he discovered (49). Examples could be multiplied to say: Such inner experiences of reality could help science to reach a deeper understanding of the structure of reality itself, in the theories it develops and the consequences thereof. Nick Maxwell has pointed out for decades that science needs to develop into a science of wisdom, really, and not only into a science of knowledge, in order to foster human flourishing (50–52). This is exactly the point: How do we decide what kind of science is useful, and what is not? What helps us flourish? Here we touch an important area, the field of ethics and value.

The current stance is to leave this to philosophy, which uses rational argument. As the history of moral philosophy and the current state of it show: there is no consensus and every possible position, even if completely contrary to others, can be rationally defended, depending on what presuppositions someone makes about humans and their nature. Perhaps inner experience is a way of accessing the deep structure of the world, which also opens insight about moral structures? We do not know, but the teachings of spiritual traditions might suggest this, because they all involve ethical imperatives that are derived on deeper inspection from the spiritual experience of their founders. Thus, a consciousness trained in accessing the deeper aspects of reality might actually be able to experience some of these structures whose consequences are values and morals, or at least moral tendencies that might inform our decision-making processes.

To be sure: inner experience is, similar to the experience of the outer world through our senses, not free from deception, error, and doubt. It is not as simple as some might have it: just sit down on your cushion, quiet your mind, and you will see what it is like and can pluck the fruits of contemplative wisdom from the tree of knowledge. This would be spiritual positivism of the worse kind (53). We have taken more than 500 years to develop a solid methodology of purging the outer experience of our senses with which we experience the material world from error to reach some scientific knowledge. It is surely even more difficult to arrive at a methodology of purging individual inner experience from aspects of deception and error to arrive at unequivocal knowledge of such deep structures of reality. The processes some religions have employed through the ages might help, but are likely not enough in a secular, multicultural, multiethnic, and, by the same token, multireligious and multispiritual world. Perhaps it is the task of a future science of consciousness to move this process forward in the secular spirit of science, without bias, without prejudice, and in radical openness regarding the outcome.

Traditionally, spiritual experiences can be said to be at the basis of each and every religion. Those experiences, when communicated and immersed into a cultural and political environment would have given rise to certain interpretations, made easier or possible through language, but also confined and limited through such structures. Religions are the outcome of this process. Thus, in this view, spiritual experiences were the basis for religions, and religions are communal cultural practices to communicate, purge, and stabilize the impact of spiritual experiences and make them available for a certain culture within a certain political and historical situation. In that sense, science and religion are not enemies, but complementary aspects of our human endeavour to understand the world and live in it. While science has honed the capacity of our senses to understand the world from outside, mostly pertaining to its material aspects, religion has used spiritual experiences—that is, experiences of the world from within and thus pertaining to its deep structure to convey meaning about the world. They are complementary aspects of our human meaning-making of the world, because they are both necessary but radically incompatible with each other. Therefore, both need to be reinforced in their own right. Neither should science have to bow to any religion, nor should religion be ridiculed by science. Both have the same parent: experience. Science as experience of the outside world, religion as spiritual experience of the world from within. It is interesting to observe that this insight stood already at the cradle of modern science in Roger Bacon's writings in 1267. While we have used one strand of this insight, we forgot about the other one. Perhaps it is time now to take it up again?

Spirituality and spiritual experience within mental health

While the above ideas are comparatively abstract and complex, they do have very practical reverberations. Humans, we saw, have spiritual experiences, sometimes spontaneously, sometimes through specific practices, sometimes willingly, sometimes unwillingly. While, for some people, such experiences come with benefits, others might feel disturbed. This may be due to the fact that they are impinging on their current world view and thus upsetting it. This may be because their personality is a bit more fragile and cannot hold and live up to the implications. In such a situation we speak of a spiritual crisis: An experience unsettles a previously solid life. The psychiatrist Roberto Assagioli was the first to point to this fact (54). In order to harness the potential benefits, such experiences need to be integrated into the lives of the experiencers through diligent psychological work. Sometimes, practitioners are not up to that task because they remain beholden to the stance that all such experiences are hallucinatory and detrimental to normal functioning. They then treat them as psychotic episodes. While some practitioners fall in the other extreme, treating all psychotic experiences as spiritual ones, the truth is likely in the middle, here too. The discerning element, it seems, is whether people can manage their everyday lives. Some experiential reports of people who have had such experiences spontaneously show that, if they were truly spiritual experiences, the experiencers were able to manage their lives as parents, or partners, or in their jobs, despite the unsettling nature of their experiences (55). If personalities are not really strong enough, it might happen that the experience is also accompanied by some psychotic mentations. Practitioners who know about this might help strengthen and support the person without battling the experience. This is not the place to give recipes but it might be useful to consult the specialized literature knowing that this might happen (56–59).

In the end, it might be helpful to also engage the supportive power of spiritual practice. The recent movement of integrating mindfulness practices, such as breathing meditation, body scans, and mindfully observing the content of one's consciousness, might be good examples and have shown effects such as in mindfulness-based prevention of depression relapse (60, 61). On a more individual and personal basis, if patients are stable enough, practitioners might invite or suggest spiritual or contemplative practice as a complement to psychotherapeutic work.

Similar to the pathologization of spiritual experience, there is also the danger of spiritualization of psychological shortcomings and pathologies. Especially, spiritual practice and the environment of spiritual communities are in danger of fostering narcissistic ways of dealing with reality that can be counterproductive (62). Where psychological pathology is concerned, spirituality is no replacement for solid therapy, nor is psychology or psychotherapy a replacement for spiritual longing.

It is useful to know and acknowledge that having spiritual experiences is a human constant: it is as human as sexuality. Only the convoluted history of spirituality within our Western scientific mode has made it a deviance in the eyes of some. Knowing this will help practitioners to deal a little bit more realistically with such experiences, neither extolling them nor ridiculing them.

And finally another aspect: in an interesting study, psychotherapists in training were randomized to practise meditation each morning with a Soto Zen master, without their patients knowing (63). The results of their patients were nearly four times as good at discharge as those of the patients of therapists who did not meditate. The knowledge of patients could not have been the decisive element here, because they were blind to this intervention. So what was it that made these therapists more effective? Perhaps they were more creative? Perhaps they were better able to empathize and communicate this empathy? Perhaps they were more relaxed and less stressed-out themselves? We don't know, but it appears as if spiritual practice, in the sense of some regular spiritual activity like meditation, can be a resource for mental health practitioners. A while ago, we studied a large sample of people with a special questionnaire we had developed to measure exceptional human experiences, spiritual ones and also psychiatric ones, called the Exceptional Human Experiences Questionnaire (64–67). This instrument assesses experiences in four dimensions: positive spiritual experiences, negative spiritual experiences of deconstruction and problems, and visionary and psychiatric experiences. We assessed these experiences twice together with a measure of psychiatric symptomatology, the SCL90. We found that those participants who had a regular spiritual practice suffered much less distress as a consequence of unsettling spiritual experiences, while positive spiritual experiences served as a buffer against psychological stress. We condensed these findings in the adage: not having a spiritual practice is a risk factor for mental health.

Spirituality within an enlightened and open science

Spirituality is a mode of experiencing the world and our lives from within. As such, it might bear some promise that is largely undiscovered, because religion has been disparaged during the course of enlightenment by science as one of the prime movers of this enlightenment process. I have argued that this need not be the final word and have tried to show that there is a role for spirituality. One possibility is to study the effect of spiritual and religious stances and experiences on people's lives, and this is what has traditionally been done in spirituality and religion research. Another option is to develop interventions that are derived from spiritual practices and offer them as therapeutic modules, as has been done by the implementation of mindfulness into various treatment programmes. Yet another completely unexplored arena is what I have argued for: to see spirituality as having a part even in the scientific process of discovery. The implicit presupposition that I have made without elaborating on it is that consciousness is likely dependent on, but not produced by, the brain and hence can likely have its own access route to reality. I have elaborated on this elsewhere (31, 68). Accepting this as a rational position allows a special role for spirituality.

It offers experiential access to the deep structure of reality from within. This can be general structures, such as abstract mathematical structures or ethical values. They can be individual ones, such as meaning and purpose. This makes spirituality also an asset for patients and practitioners. It might be one of the routes to touching forgotten sounds of wholeness within. When these experiences happen spontaneously, they could and should be supported without forgetting the standard knowledge of clinical psychology and psychiatry. Such a stance also invites spiritual practice, perhaps as a therapeutic intervention, but probably much more as a preventive measure against the fragmentation and flooding of our minds with irrelevant information, motives, and impulses. In that sense, spirituality is a challenge in terms of understanding and implementation for the future, rather than a relict of the past.

References

1. **Stirrat M, Cornwell RE.** Eminent scientists reject the supernatural: a survey of the Fellows of the Royal Society. *Evolution: Education and Outreach.* 2013;6(1):33.

2. **Howard Ecklund E.** Religion and spirituality among scientists. *Contexts.* 2008;7:12–5.

3. **Smith DP, Orlinsky DE.** Religious and spiritual experience among psychotherapists. *Psychotherapy: Theory, Research, Practice, Training* 2004;41:144–51.

4. **Seeman TE, Dubin LF, Seeman M.** Religiosity/spirituality and health: a critical review of the evidence for biological pathways. *American Psychologist.* 2003;58:53–63.

5. **Reber AS, Alcock JE.** Searching for the impossible: parapsychology's elusive quest. *American Psychologist.* 2020;75:391–9.

6. **Dawkins R.** *The blind watchmaker.* London: Longmans; 1986.

7. **Carr BJ.** Hyperspatial models of matter and mind. In: **Kelly EF, Crabtree A, Marshall P**, editors. *Beyond physicalism: Toward reconciliation of science and spirituality.* Lanham, MD: Rowman & Littlefield; 2015, pp. 227–73.

8. **Rees M.** *On the future. Prospects for humanity.* Princeton: Princeton University Press; 2018.

9. **Pinker S.** *Enlightenment now: the case for reason, science, humanism, and progress.* London: Penguin; 2018.

10. **van Fraassen B.** Naturalism in epistemology. In: **Williams RN, Robinson DN,** (eds), *Scientism: the new orthodoxy.* London: Bloomsbury; 2016, pp. 64–95.

11. **Leff G.** *Paris and Oxford universities in the thirteenth and fourteenth centuries. An institutional and intellectual history.* New York and London: Wiley; 1968.

12. **Randall H.** The Universities of Europe in the Middle Ages. **Volume 1**: Salerno, Bologna, Paris. Cambridge: Cambridge University Press; 1895.

13. **Southern RW.** *Robert Grosseteste. The growth of an English mind in medieval Europe.* Oxford: Clarendon Press; 1986.

14. **Power A.** *Roger Bacon and the defence of Christendom.* Cambridge: Cambridge University Press; 2012.

15. **Bacon R.** *The 'Opus Majus' of Roger Bacon* (2 vols). **Bridges JH,** (ed.),Clarendon: Oxford; 1897, orig. 1267.

16. **Mandonnet P.** Roger Bacon et le Speculum Astonomiae (1277). *Revue Néoscolastique de Philosophie.* 1910;**17**(67):313–35.

17. **Newbold WR.** The Voynich Roger Bacon manuscript. *Transaction of the College of Physicians of Philadelphia.* 1921;**43**(3rd series):431–74.

18. **Bacon F.** *Neues Organon. Lateinisch-deutsch. Hrsg. und mit einer Einleitung von. W. Krohn.* **Krohn W** (ed.). Hamburg: Meiner; 1990.

19. **Burtt EA.** *The metaphysical foundations of modern physical science: a historical and critical essay.* London: Routledge and Kegan Paul; 1932.

20. **Maxwell N.** *In praise of natural philosophy. A revolution for thought and life.* Montreal: McGill-Queen's University Press; 2017.

21. **Plantinga A.** *Where the conflict really lies: science, religion, and naturalism.* New York: Oxford University Press; 2011.

22. **Dupré L.** *The Enlightenment and the intellectual foundations of modern culture.* New Haven: Yale University Press; 2004.

23. **Hands J.** *Cosmosapiens. Human evolution from the origin of the universe.* London: Duckworth; 2015.

24. **Nagel T.** *Mind and cosmos: why the materialist neo-Darwinian conception of nature is almost certainly false.* Oxford: Oxford University Press; 2012.

25. **Buckley MJ.** *At the origins of modern atheism.* New Haven: Yale University Press; 1987.

26. **Voltaire FMA de.** *Correspondance Tome 1.* **Beuchot M** (ed.). Paris: Lefèvre; 1830, orig. 1732.

27. **Kant I.** *Kants Werke. Studienausgabe.* Damtstadt: Wissenchaftliche Buchgesellschaft; 1983 ff.

28. **Benedikter R.** *Homo deus?* Das Zusammenwachsen von Mensch und Maschine. *Analysen und Argumente—Konrad Adenauer Stiftung.* 2017(270):1–13.

29. **Taylor C.** *A secular age.* Cambridge, MA: Harvard University Press; 2007.

30. **McGilchrist I.** *The master and his emissary: the divided brain and the making of the Western world.* New Haven: Yale University Press; 2009.

31. **Walach H.** *Beyond a materialist worldview: Towards an expanded science.* London: Scientific and Medical Network; 2019.

32. **Collingwood RG.** *An essay on metaphysics.* Revised edition. Oxford: Clarendon Press; 1998, orig. 1940.

33. **Walach H.** Secular spirituality—what it is. Why we need it. How to proceed. *Journal for the Study of Spirituality.* 2017;**7**(1):7–20.

34. **Walach H.** Secular spirituality: the next step towards enlightenment. In: **Walach H, Schmidt S** (eds), *Neuroscience, consciousness, spirituality.* Cham, Heidelberg, New York, Dordrecht: Springer; 2015.

35. **Kapleau P.** *The three pillars of Zen: teaching, practice, enlightenment.* New York: Harper; 1969.

36. **MacPhail J.** Vertical hierarchy and the invariance principle in four models of consciousness/spirituality. *Journal for the Study of Spirituality.* 2017;**7**:99–113.

37. **MacPhail J.** *Learning in depth: a case study in twin 5x5 matrices of consciousness.* Frankfurt (Oder): Europa-Universität Viadrina; 2013.

38. **Lancaster BL.** The hard problem revisited: From cognitive neuroscience to Kabbalah and back again. In: **Walach H, Schmidt S, Jonas WB** (eds), *Neuroscience, consciousness and spirituality.* Dordrecht, Heidelberg: Springer; 2011, pp. 229–51.

39. **Lancaster BL.** *Approaches to consciousness: the marriage of science and mysticism.* Basingstoke: Palgrave Macmillan; 2004.

40. **Frankl VE.** *Man's search for meaning: an introduction to logotherapy.* London: Hodder & Stoughton; 1964.

41. **Kuhl J.** *Volition and personality: action versus state orientation.* Seattle: Hogrefe & Huber; 1994.

42. **Csikszentmihalyi M.** *Flow: the psychology of optimal experience.* New York: Harper-Collins; 1990.

43. **Brian D.** *Einstein—a life.* New York: Wiley; 1996.

44. **James W.** *The works of William James. The varieties of religious experience.* Cambridge, MA: Harvard University Press; 1985.

45. **Lightman A.** *Searching for stars on an island in Maine.* London: Corsair; 2018.

46. **Hofmann L, Walach H.** Spirituality and religiosity in psychotherapy—a representative survey among German psychotherapists. *Psychotherapy Research.* 2011;**21**:179–92.

47. **Keller EF.** *A feeling for the organism. The life and work of Barbara McClintock.* New York: Freeman; 2003, orig. 1983.

48. **Comfort NC.** *The tangled field. Barabara McClintock's search for the patterns of genetic control.* Cambridge MA: Harvard University Press; 2001.

49. **Bowers KS.** On being unconsciously influenced and informed. In: **Bowers KS, Meichenbaum D,** (eds), *The unconscious reconsidered.* New York: Wiley; 1984, pp. 227–72.

50. **Walach H.** Nicholas Maxwell: in praise of natural philosophy—a revolution for thought and life (book review). *Journal for General Philosophy of Science.* 2019;**50**(4):603–9.

51. **Maxwell N.** How can life of value best flourish in the real world? In: **McHenry L,** (ed.), *Science and the pursuit of wisdom: studies in the philosophy of Nicholas Maxwell.* Frankfurt: Ontos Verlag; 2009, pp. 1–56.

52. **Maxwell N.** *From knowledge to wisdom: a revolution in the aims and methods of science.* Oxford: Blackwell; 1984.

53. **Ferrer JN.** *Revisioning transpersonal theory: a participatory vision of human spirituality.* Albany: SUNY Press; 2002.

54. **Assagioli R.** Spiritual development and its attendant maladies. *Hibbert Journal.* 1937;**36**:69–88.

55. **Roberts B.** *The experience of no-self. A contemplative journey.* Boulder & London: Shambala; 1984.

56. **Kelly SM.** Space, time and spirit: the analogical imagination and the evolution of transpersonal theory. Part one: contexts—theoretical and historical. *Journal of Transpersonal Psychology.* 2002;**34**:73–86.

57. **Kelly SM.** Space, time and spirit: the analogical imagination and the evolution of transpersonal theory. Part two: contemporary models. *Journal of Transpersonal Psychology.* 2002;**34**:87–99.

58. **Grof S.** *Psychology of the future. Lessons from modern consciousness research.* Albany, NY: State University of New York Press; 2000.

59. **Grof S.** *The adventure of self-discovery.* Albany, NY: State University of New York Press; 1988.

60. Kuyken W, Warren FC, Taylor RS, Whalley B, Crane C, Bondolfi G, et al. Efficacy of mindfulness-based cognitive therapy in prevention of depressive relapse: an individual patient data meta-analysis from randomized trials. *JAMA Psychiatry*. 2016;**73**:565–74.

61. Williams M, Teasdale J, Segal Z, Kabat-Zinn J. *The mindful way through depression: freeing yourself from chronic unhappiness*. New York: Guilford Press; 2007.

62. Walach H. Narcicissm: the shadow of transpersonal psychology. *Transpersonal Psychology Review*. 2008;**12**(2):47–59.

63. Grepmair L, Mitterlehner F, Loew T, Bachler E, Rother W, Nickel M. Promoting mindfulness in psychotherapists in training influences the treatment results of their patients: a randomized, double-blind, controlled study. *Psychotherapy and Psychosomatics*. 2007;**76**:332–8.

64. Kohls N, Walach H, Lewith G. The impact of positive and negative spiritual experiences on distress and the moderating role of mindfulness. *Archive for the Psychology of Religion*. 2009;**31**:357–74.

65. Kohls N, Walach H, Wirtz M. The relationship between spiritual experiences, transpersonal trust, social support, and sense of coherence—a comparison between spiritually practising and non-practising samples. *Mental Health, Religion & Culture*. 2009;**12**:1–23.

66. Kohls N, Hack A, Walach H. Measuring the unmeasurable by ticking boxes and opening Pandora's Box? Mixed methods research as a useful tool for investigating exceptional and spiritual experiences. *Archive for the Psychology of Religion*. 2008;**30**:155–87.

67. Kohls N, Walach H. Exceptional experiences and spiritual practice: a new measurement approach. *Spirituality and Health International*. 2006;**7**:125–50.

68. Walach H. Naturalising religion—spiritualising science: the role of consciousness research. *Journal of Consciousness Studies*. 2020;**27**(7–8):165–94.

Chapter 5

Differentiating spiritual experiences from mental disorders

Leonardo Machado and
Alexander Moreira-Almeida

Introduction

It is not uncommon for patients with mental disorders to have symptoms with religious or spiritual (R/S) contents (e.g. delusions, hallucinations, obsessions, and pathological guilt) and, on the other hand, spiritual experiences often involve dissociative and psychotic-like phenomena (e.g. hearing voices, visions, trances, and thought insertion). This frequently creates difficulties in differentiating between a non-pathological R/S experience and a mental disorder (MD) (1, 2).

Because most people with R/S experiences are culturally adapted in their contexts, it is not so difficult, in most cases, to perceive those who actually suffer from MD from those who report sound R/S experiences. However, there are some shady areas that deserve clinical and scientific research, especially given that in the past there was a tendency to pathologize R/S experiences, regardless of the context in which they were presented (3, 4). Even today, there is a risk of encountering this clinical tendency because of lack of knowledge by clinicians, lack of training, or historical institutional rivalry between religion and science (5, 6).

Anyway, clinical differentiation between a non-pathological R/S experience and an MD with R/S content brings risks in both extremes: to pathologize normal R/S experience (promoting iatrogenic suffering) or neglecting pathological symptoms (delaying proper treatment, such as in a first psychotic episode). In an attempt to mitigate these risks, this chapter will gather the best current scientific evidence in order to help the clinical distinction between R/S experiences and mental disorders with R/S content.

Psychotic experiences in the general population

A consistent and growing body of epidemiological evidence has shown that psychotic experiences (PEs) are very common in the community and are not usually linked to psychotic disorders, with a recent meta-analysis yielding a prevalence of 7.2% (2, 7). In fact, this reality was noticed and investigated more than a century ago at the pioneering 'Census on Hallucination' conducted by the Society for Psychical Research (8, 9). More recently, a World Health Organization study (8) involving more than 250,000 subjects in 52 countries found that 12.5% of world population reported at least one 'psychotic symptom' over the past 12 months, not including those happening under substance use or during sleep–wake transition. Fewer than 1/10 of these 12.5% had a lifetime diagnosis of schizophrenia. A large cross-sectional study evaluated samples from 18 countries throughout the world, from 2001 through 2009. Respondents included 31.261 adults (18 years and older) who were asked about lifetime and 12-month prevalence and frequency of six types of PEs (two hallucinatory experiences and four delusional experiences). In this study, the mean lifetime prevalence of ever having a PE was 5.8%, with hallucinatory experiences (5.2%) much more common than delusional experiences (1.3%) (10).

Besides this, approximately 20% of people with PEs report persistent, rather than transient, experiences. Although a minority of this subgroup may eventually develop a psychotic disorder, in most cases, these experiences are not associated with distress and do not lead to a malign outcome (11). However, regardless of the exact prevalence of PEs in the general population, this subpopulation of healthy voice-hearers may have much to teach us about the neurobiology, cognitive psychology, and ultimately the treatment of voices that are distressing (12).

Nomenclatures

The fact that most people reporting 'psychotic symptoms' in the general population are neither psychotic nor have a symptom of a MD raises the challenge of how to name these experiences. One important question is how to name these experiences in the population that does not need treatment. Naming them the same way psychopathology does in psychotic disorders (e.g. hallucination, psychotic symptoms) would not bring an a priori pathological attribution in a population that will never meet diagnostic criteria? On the other hand, creating a new nomenclature would not risk neglecting the early detection of a possible disease in this population?

One possibility would be referring to these phenomena not related to MD as PEs and the phenomena happening in clinical populations, including ultra-high-risk (UHR) and attenuated psychotic syndromes, as 'psychotic symptoms' (13). The word 'symptom' would indicate the pathological nature of the phenomena. One possible problem, however, is that the very word 'psychotic' in PEs already brings in itself an idea of pathology.

Another possibility would be to call 'anomalous experience' those experiences that are uncommon (14) or deviate from the usually accepted explanations of reality. One could even call spiritual experiences 'anomalous experiences with spiritual/transcendent content'. One difficulty is that anomalous and spiritual experiences can also occur in clinical populations.

One of the leaders in this field, the psychiatrist Ian Stevenson, drew attention in an article published in 1983 in the *American Journal of Psychiatry* to the fact that 'unshared sensory experiences' are common among those who are and those are not mentally ill (15). In addition, he raised the challenging idea that some of these unshared sensory experiences actually may provide evidence of veridical (paranormal) communication (e.g. correspond veridically to some physically distant event). So, the author suggested the neutral term 'idiophany' (meaning private apparitions, from the Greek words *idios* [private] and *phainomai* [appear]) to designate all unshared sensory experiences. Hallucination would be the subgroup of unshared sensory experiences (ideophany) related to perceptual error in mental disorders. The ideophanies that convey veridical information would be called 'veridical paranormal idiophanies'. In the past decades, there has been an increasing interest in alleged veridical perceptions during a specific type of spiritual experience: near-death experience. An example of this claim of 'veridical idiophany' during cardiac arrest was reported by van Lommel et al. (16) Holden published a review of reported veridical perceptions in near-death experience (17). For a recent review of experimental evidence for parapsychological phenomena in general, see Cardena, 2018 (18).

At any rate, it seems, so far, that there is no nomenclature that can encompass all the angles of this complex relationship between symptoms found in clinical populations and experiences reported by populations who do not need clinical care. It is important, in this sense, to be aware of the limitations of the current nomenclature and to keep an open mind to advances in the understanding of this field as new research emerges.

Dimensional and categorical models of psychotic experiences

In order to make sense of the large prevalence of PE in the general population, several models have been proposed. The continuum view of psychosis proposes that psychotic symptoms are the severe expression of 'schizotypal' traits that are normally distributed in the general population. For some authors, in the past decades, the concept of psychosis was consolidate as a dimensional manifestation instead of an all-or-nothing event (7, 19).

However, some authors have argued that subclinical or psychosis-like experiences in the general population are distinct from true symptoms of psychosis, because they are often too mild and transient to be clinically meaningful (11). This could be called a 'categorical model of PE'.

The continuum model of psychosis predicts that the higher the number, intensity, or frequency of PEs, the sicker the person, and the closer to the fully psychotic pole of the continuum (19). In this sense, they should have more markers of mental disorders such as functional impairment and worse quality of life. Indeed, large populational studies have found these correlations on a global level. However, a major challenge arises when we take a closer look at specific groups with high levels of PEs, especially people from groups that foster 'PEs in spiritual environments (2, 11). As an example, we have investigated 115 spiritist mediums with high levels of PEs. They had normal level of social adjustment and low levels of common mental disorder symptoms. And, contrary to the continuum model predictions, the higher the frequency of auditory hallucinations, the better the social adjustment (20). Other evidence suggesting that psychotic experience may not be a marker of mental disorder is provided by a prospective study with 115 subjects who seek help in spiritual groups because of distressing anomalous experiences. The intensity of 'unusual experiences' was not a predictor of quality of life one year later. However, cognitive disorganization was (21).

We propose that we can have both continuum and categorical distribution of PEs in the general population. We hypothesize that people with these experiences form a heterogeneous group. Unshared sensory experiences, for example, would be a final common phenomenological experience that may have many diverse causes, some pathological and others not—something similar to tachycardia whose causes may vary from severe heart failure to sudden joy. So, a proportion of people with PEs in general population would fit on the psychotic continuum, but another group would have anomalous experiences of a different nature, not related to psychosis or mental disorders (2).

The definitive answers still seem to be coming. Until then, it is important to keep an open mind to the emerging evidence.

Brief overview of studies

The interplay between religiousness and psychosis has long been studied (22). In early psychiatry, Phillipe Pinel stated that religious fanaticism might be a causative factor of madness. Emil Kraepelin described a high frequency of mystical and religious content in his psychotic patients, and Kurt Schneider reported a heightened religiousness in schizophrenia patients (7). Nowadays, this field has been growing at a great speed allowing some data to have clinical utility (23). We summarize some recent studies tackling different aspects of the interplay of PEs, psychotic disorders, R/S, and sociobiological factors.

Another paper reported a functional imaging study with eight mentally healthy spiritual mediums and eight matched healthy controls. The mediums' brains were scanned during a mediumistic-trance state (when they reported seeing and hearing spirits as well as out-of-body and telepathic experiences) and in a control condition, when they were instructed to re-enact the same mediumistic experiences that they had had during the mediumistic-trance condition but in a non-trance (imaginative-trance) state. In addition, both mediums and controls took part in a resting state scanning session. Results indicated stronger activation in the lateral occipital cortex (LOC), posterior cingulate cortex (PCC), temporal pole (TP), middle temporal gyrus (MTG) and orbitofrontal cortex (OFC) during the mediumistic-trance state. We also observed increased functional connectivity within auditory and sensorimotor resting state networks (RSNs) during mediumistic-trance compared with resting and imaginative-trance conditions. Comparing spiritual mediums and controls, no differences in RSN were found. These data show preserved engagement of prefrontal cortex (PFC) and connectivity of the default-mode network (DMN) that indicate maintained introspective control over non-pathological psychotic-like experiences (24).

In an experiment published in the journal *Science*, Powers et al. recruited four groups of subjects: people with a diagnosed psychotic illness who heard voices (n = 15); those with a similar illness who did not hear voices (n = 14); an active control group who heard daily voices, but had no diagnosed illness (n = 15)—they attributed their experiences metaphysically; and, last, controls without diagnosis or voices (n = 15). Using a Pavlovian learning task, the authors induced conditioned hallucinations in these four groups of people. All groups demonstrated conditioned hallucinations. However, those with daily hallucinations endorsed more conditioned hallucinations than those without, regardless of diagnosis. Hallucinators were more confident in their conditioned hallucinations than non-hallucinators. Both conditioned hallucinations and confidence correlated with hallucination severity outside the laboratory. Whole-brain analysis revealed that conditioned hallucinations also engaged the anterior insula cortex (AIC), inferior frontal gyrus, head of caudate, anterior cingulate cortex (ACC), auditory cortex, and posterior superior temporal sulcus (STS). There were no significant between-group differences in brain responses during conditioned hallucinations. However, hallucinators deactivated ACC more during correct rejections compared with non-hallucinators (25).

The same group of researchers conducted a study with clairaudient psychics who received daily auditory messages. They conducted phenomenological interviews with these subjects, as well as with patients diagnosed with a psychotic disorder who heard voices, people with a diagnosis of a psychotic disorder who did not hear voices, and matched control subjects (without voices or a diagnosis). They found the hallucinatory experiences of psychic voice-hearers to be very similar to those of patients who were diagnosed. The authors employed techniques from forensic psychiatry to conclude that the psychics were not malingering. Critically, they found that this sample of non-help-seeking voice-hearers were able to control the onset and offset of their voices, that they were less distressed by their voice-hearing experiences and that, the first time they admitted to voice-hearing, the reception by others was much more likely to be positive (12).

Another group of researchers studied religiosity in individuals at risk for psychosis in a Brazilian sample. They assessed the interplay between religion and prodromal symptoms in 79 UHR and 110 control individuals. Organizational religious activity, a measure of how often someone attends churches/temples, was positively related to perceptual abnormalities/hallucinations. Intrinsic religious activity was negatively correlated with suspiciousness, and non-organizational religious activity was correlated with higher ideational richness. The authors hypothesized that subjects with subclinical psychosis may possibly use churches and other religious organizations to cope with hallucinations (7).

An experimental study investigated how people with PE make sense of unusual experiences. The study involving 84 people with diagnosed psychotic disorders (clinical group), 92 participants from the general population with persistent psychotic experiences but without a need for care (non-clinical group), and 83 controls from the general population without persistent psychotic experiences. When asked to explain how each task worked, participants in the non-clinical group were likely to offer appraisals that were spiritual, normalizing, and non-personal in nature. By contrast, those in the clinical group appraised the experiences as negative, dangerous, and personal. As the authors noted, these data support the underlying logic and clinical relevance of this kind of research, showing that 'the way in which psychotic experiences are interpreted, rather than merely their presence, is important to clinical status'

(26). Another paper, a qualitative one, showed the same conclusions: it is not the PE itself that determines the development of a clinical condition, but rather the wider personal and interpersonal contexts that influence how this experience is subsequently integrated (27).

Differentiating spiritual experiences from psychotic disorders

Generally speaking, the main difficulty in differential diagnosis is between spiritual experiences and psychotic and dissociative disorders. A study compared non-clinical voice-hearers with controls and showed that higher schizotypy scores, lower education, and higher family loading for psychiatric disorders, but not presence of voices, were associated with lower global functioning. Besides that, auditory verbal hallucinations in non-clinical and clinical samples are broadly phenomenologically similar (10, 28, 29), but differ in content, emotional valence, and appraisals about their omnipotence. In general, intense spiritual experiences reported by some individuals could not be distinguished phenomenologically from psychotic symptoms; the differences lay in the interpretation and meaning given to these experiences, and in their emotional and behavioural correlates. Similarly, other authors found that the positive symptoms present in psychotic patients and individuals at ultra-high-risk for psychosis were similar to the PEs reported by a non-clinical group, with only 'cognitive' anomalies (inability to concentrate, loss of automaticity of thinking skills) being more common in both help-seeking groups. Specifically, several studies suggest that PEs occur in the absence of paranoid appraisals in people with no need for care (11, 29).

A more recent study seems to have also been one of the largest on this topic. The authors evaluated 259 participants recruited in one urban and one rural area in the United Kingdom. The non-clinical group had a younger age of onset of their PEs than the clinical group, and had lived with their experiences for longer. Both groups reported hallucinations in all modalities, although commenting and conversing voices were rare in the non-clinical individuals, while somatic/tactile and (at trend level) olfactory hallucinations were more frequent in the non-clinical sample. Schneiderian first-rank symptoms, especially thought insertion, mind reading, and feelings of being controlled, were also commonly reported in the non-clinical group, although they had a higher lifetime (but not current) frequency in the clinical group. The non-clinical individuals showed few signs of being paranoid or deluded, apart from ideas of reference, which were commonly reported, but still less frequently than in the clinical group. Compared with the clinical group, the non-clinical sample reported fewer negative symptoms and cognitive difficulties, both currently and over their lifetime; and they were lower on bizarre behaviour and thought disorder (although these were not common in the clinical group either) (11).

On the other hand, childhood and interpersonal trauma have been consistently associated with the presence of voices and other PEs, irrespective of need for care. However, the clinical individuals reported significantly having suffered more lifetime discrimination than non-clinical individuals (11). In another study, the sample of non-help-seeking voice-hearers were able to control the onset and offset of their voices, were less distressed by their voice-hearing experiences, and reported that, the first time they admitted to voice-hearing, the reception by others was much more likely to be positive. Patients had much more negative voice-hearing experiences and were more likely to receive a negative reaction when sharing their voices with others for the first time, and this was subsequently more disruptive to their social relationships (12).

In addition, people with untreated PEs, when compared with the clinical population, appeared to have the highest IQ, a higher educational level, and more likely to be employed or in training, with higher professional grades; they were more likely to be in/have had a long-term relationship and to have children; they were less likely to use drugs. On the other hand, those in the clinical group were more anxious, depressed and stressed, reported lower self-esteem, and scored higher in negative schemas about the self and others (11).

Another study investigated 115 participants who reported a high frequency of PEs. The instruments used were the Temperament and Character Inventory the Structured Clinical Interview for DSM-IV, and the Oxford–Liverpool Inventory of Feelings and Experiences. In this study, personality features seemed to be an important criterion to distinguish between pathology and mental health in individuals presenting high levels of PEs. While self-directedness is a protective factor, both harm avoidance and novelty seeking were predictors of negative mental health outcomes. The authors suggested that the impact of PEs on mental health is moderated by personality factors (30).

Other important clinical data are that non-help-seeking voice-hearers have relatively intact verbal and executive functioning, though the neural circuitry engaged during voice-hearing experiences appears to be broadly similar (12).

In summary, the presence of positive psychotic symptoms, even those of the first-rank proposed by Kurt Schneider, does not seem to be a good criterion for differentiating spiritual experiences from psychotic disorders. Negative symptoms and cognitive symptoms seem to be better parameters for making such a differentiation. The following Table 5.1 summarizes the studies.

Table 5.1 Summarizing the studies

Name of article	Countries	Characteristics of individuals and samples
Psychotic experiences in the general population: a cross-national analysis Based on 31,261 respondents from 18 countries	Colombia, Mexico, Peru, Brazil, United States, Nigeria, Iraq and Lebanon, China, New Zealand, Belgium, France, Germany, Italy, the Netherlands, Portugal, Romania, and Spain.	31,261 adults (18 years and older)
Clinical, socio-demographic and psychological characteristics in individuals with persistent psychotic experiences with and without a 'need for care'	United Kingdom	259 adults (18 years and older)
Varieties of voice-hearing: psychics and the psychosis continuum	United States	67 adults
How to tell a happy from an unhappy schizotype: Personality factors and mental health outcomes in individuals with psychotic experiences	Brazil	115 adults
Dissociative and psychotic experiences in Brazilian spiritist mediums	Brazil	24 adults
Hearing spirits? Religiosity in individuals at risk for psychosis—results from the Subclinical Symptoms and Prodromal Psychosis (SSAPP) cohort	Brazil	189 participants

Criteria for differential diagnosis

Based on the available scientific and clinical evidence, we have proposed the criteria below for the distinction between healthy R/S experience and mental disorder (1, 2):

◆ Absence of psychological suffering: the individual does not feel disturbed by the experience them having.

◆ Absence of social and occupational impediments: the experience does not compromise the individual's relationships and activities.

◆ The experience has a short duration and happens occasionally, and it does not have an unwilled, invasive character in consciousness or in the individual's daily activities. There are some experiences that may have a long duration but can be seen as a stage within the previous spiritual development of the person.

◆ There is a discerning attitude about the experience. The capacity to perceive the unusual/anomalous character of the experience is preserved along with the insight that it may not be everyone's experience.

◆ Compatibility with some religious tradition. The individual's experience might be understood within the concepts and practices of some established cultural or religious practice, even if it is not the local tradition.

◆ Absence of psychiatric co-morbidities. There are no other mental disorders or other symptoms suggestive of mental disorders besides those related to spiritual experiences. Regarding psychotic experiences, although there may be reports of hallucinations or unusual beliefs, there is a lack of negative or disorganization symptoms.

◆ Control over the experience. The individual is capable of limiting his/her experience to the right time and place for its occurrence—for instance, within a ritual rather than in an inappropriate setting.

◆ The experience promotes personal growth over time; it enriches the personal, social, and professional life of an individual. It is directed towards self-integration and helping others.[1]

The presence of these criteria suggests a non-pathological spiritual experience, but, on the other hand, there is a lack of well-controlled studies testing these criteria (1). Whereas pathological counterexamples can be found for all of them (e.g. catatonic episodes without psychological suffering), the variables described in these criteria generally speak against the presence of mental disorder. The more elements present, generally speaking, the less likely is the experience to be related to a MD (2).

----

[1] Reproduced with permission from Moreira-Almeida A, Cardeña E. Differential diagnosis between non-pathological psychotic and spiritual experiences and mental disorders: a contribution from Latin American studies to the ICD-11. *Braz J Psychiatry.* 2011;33 Suppl 1:S21-36.

Case reports

Case report 1

M., 51 years old, female, completed high school, was taken to the psychiatrist by her husband because, two months after the initial consultation, she had ideas that she wanted to kill herself and her family members (31). As she left the house, she had a clear perception that cars, motorcycles, and even guards were watching her. So, on some occasions, she ran down the streets as if she were being chased. At the same time, she began to isolate herself from her family members and to present with initial insomnia, anorexia, and weight loss. The patient only agreed to go to an appointment with a psychiatrist after her husband prevented her from killing herself with a knife. The episode left her very shaken because she could not quite understand the reason for this attitude. At the time of the first consultation, M. was adequately groomed, clean, and oriented. She was very suspicious, even insinuating that the doctor knew everything and had made some arrangement with her husband. She did not present alterations in perception, psychomotricity, nor flow of thinking. She was euthymic and denied her husband's complaints, she had no insight into her condition and answered many questions tangentially. Asked directly about the suicide attempt with a knife, M. denied wanting to kill herself, stating that the episode was motivated by an impulse of uncertain origin for her. Prior to the onset of symptoms, M. was planning a trip to Europe with her husband. However, near the trip, her mother revealed that M. would be killed if she travelled and that she (the mother) had obtained this information through a spiritual revelation. The trip was cancelled and, from then on, the patient began to present the described psychotic picture. M.'s mother was an 81-year-old woman who claimed to be a medium, although she did not regularly attend any religious institution. Likewise, she did not undergo any psychiatric or neurological treatment. However, on that occasion, she had some forgetfulness perceived by family members. Mother and daughter lived close together, were sympathetic to spiritism (a religion based on mediumship), and the mother had a great influence on M.'s attitudes. Unfortunately, the patient's mother refused to go to any appointment. In fact, she said that her daughter was also a medium and that neither needed psychiatric assistance. M. was not on any medication, did not use psychoactive substances, and had adequate recent premorbid functioning. Nevertheless, after the birth of her last child 26 years ago, she had puerperal psychosis. At that time, her mother had alleged spiritual revelations of ill omen for the baby. Then M.'s husband came up with delusional ideas about his son, thinking that he was some bad spirit and even trying to kill him. She improved from the puerperal psychosis with pharmacological treatment and remained asymptomatic until this present consultation. Although there was no opportunity to consult with the mother of M., the diagnostic hypothesis of induced delusional disorder was raised. The patient was prescribed risperidone 2 mg and advised to stay away from being with her mother during the treatment. After 14 days, the patient had no psychotic symptoms, and in two months she presented insight about her condition. After six months, the risperidone was gradually withdrawn and the patient remained well at the two-year follow-up evaluation.

Despite the patient's mother claiming spiritual revelations to other family members, only the patient developed a psychotic condition. This fact, associated with the previous puerperal psychosis that she presented, shows the biological susceptibility she had, which is described in secondary psychotic individuals. Persecutory delusion is the type of delusion most commonly found in this syndrome, although religious content may be present and make it difficult to differentiate where faith ends and where psychosis begins. However, the phenomenon described in the case generated suffering, was not shared by others, happened out of a religious context, was shown to be out of control by those involved and did not provide personal growth. Thus, it can be classified as pathological.[2]

Case report 2

S. is a 55-year-old woman whose first unusual experiences, at the age of 7, were characterized by intrusive thoughts: 'I started having these experiences very young, odd experiences like something came into my mind, an idea about something happening to someone. I'd tell this to my family, and 3 or 4 days later the event happened. This usually concerned a health problem or even the death of people who were close to my family, friends and neighbors' (32). In addition, she eventually had involuntary possession trances that she felt to be frightening but pleasant. She had grown up in a Catholic family that was not supportive of her experiences and forbade her to talk about them. From the age of 13 to 25, Dona Sara gradually developed a way of dealing with the premonitions and possession. She would keep to herself, not disclosing what she experienced to her family, and praying for the experiences to stop. She felt lonely and distressed. The intrusive thoughts, or 'messages', started being preceded by marked physical symptoms, including body tremors and heart palpitations. When her body started 'acting' like this, she knew a message was coming. When S. turned 26, her unusual experiences intensified and she decided to seek help

[2] Source: Data from Machado, L., Cantilino, A., Petribú K, Pinto, T. (2015). Folie à deux (transtorno delirante induzido). *J Bras Psiquiatr.* 64(4):311–4.

from the leader of an Umbanda group (an African–Brazilian religion). She was then told that she had a spiritual gift and ought to develop it. 'Meeting this Umbanda leader', S. said, 'was like being in the presence of a medical doctor who knows exactly what you're going through.' S. reported that during the first three years of regular Umbanda attendance, her possession trance was 'gradual, like a smokescreen'; she could see people around her and listen to them, though it all felt distant. Although she had no control over some parts of her body, usually the legs, she did not lose her sense of self involuntarily any more. She was still afraid of the spirits that possessed her and of having her body 'taken over', but generally after the ritual she felt relaxed and at peace, 'like coming back from a deep sleep'. She was also pleasantly surprised by the positive comments of the people who had been healed by her. S. reported that, since turning 30, she started being fully unconscious during a possession trance 'like being under general anesthesia'. S. now leads Umbanda rituals. After a short lecture, usually on a moral topic (e.g. happiness, faith, love), she leads the group in prayers and directs the music and dance to start. As soon as the dance begins, some individuals show physical tremors or laugh loudly and she then turns to the whole group to greet them: 'I'm here!' 'Good evening!' or 'I've come to heal and work with you.' S., after overseeing the possession of these individuals, then goes into a trance that may last for up to four hours. For many years, S. has led Umbanda groups providing regular counselling and healing to more than 150 people. At the time she was interviewed (for research purposes, at 55 years old), she had never been to a psychiatrist or clinical psychologist. She also reported not taking drugs or alcohol, though when in a possessed state she often drinks wine or *cachaça* (a distilled alcoholic Brazilian drink).

The authors analyzed the case based on the DSM-5 diagnostic criteria and reached the following conclusions: 'Her experiences of possession can be broken into two distinct stages. In the first stage (childhood and early adulthood), she displayed intrusive thoughts and a lack of control over possession states, which were associated with a heightened state of anxiety, loneliness, amnesia, and family conflict (meeting all five criteria for dissociative identity disorder [DID]). In the second stage (late 20s up to the present), she regularly experienced possession states but felt in control of their onset and found them religiously meaningful. In this second stage, she only fulfilled three criteria for DID' (32).

In addition, analysing the case history, the authors made the following summary (32): 'If she had been seen by a clinician during the first stage of her experiences, it is very likely she would have been diagnosed with DID. But would this be an accurate diagnosis? There are two ways in which we can interpret the evolution of S.'s possession experiences. We may argue that for the first part of her life she suffered from DID, but this disorder eventually subsided when she entered a religious group, which provided her with social support, a spiritual framework to interpret her experiences, and the necessary training to control and develop them. If we consider the positive attachment to the group as mirroring that of an individual therapist, this would help explain the remission of her DID symptoms. However, S.'s consistent characterization of possession states as positive—pleasant, good, peaceful—despite the suffering derived from their social unacceptability and the ensuing loneliness, as well as her later development as a leader in a possession-based religion, all suggest that a diagnosis of DID in her earlier life would be clinically inappropriate'(p.331).[3]

Conclusions

There are increasing literature reports showing a high prevalence of psychotic, dissociative, or other anomalous experiences in the general population, but most people who experience such events do not have mental disorders (2). Therefore, it seems that positive psychotic experiences such as hallucinations and thought interference are not good parameters for the differential diagnosis between psychiatric disorders and non-pathological spiritual phenomena. The presence of cognitive dysfunction and negative psychotic symptoms are better criteria. In addition, personality factors (such as high self-directedness), good social adjustment, control over the experience, lack of suffering or impairment related to experience, and having a cognitive framework and social support that help to make sense and deal with the PE are indicators of non-pathological experience.

It is important that clinicians be aware of these data and the clinical differentiation between people who will not need care and those who have psychiatric diagnoses, especially psychotic and dissociative disorders. It is also important to foster scientific studies in people who have spiritual experiences, especially investigations of the phenomenology, neurobiology, precipitants, and outcomes in order to enlarge the empirical base needed to advance the criteria for this differential diagnosis. Because these phenomena happen so often in these individuals, studying them seems to be a window of opportunity to better understand the clinical and biological differentiation between psychiatric disorders and spiritual phenomena (12).

....

[3] Source: Reproduced from Delmonte, R., Lucchetti, G., Moreira-Almeida, A., Farias, M. (2016). Can the DSM-5 differentiate between nonpathological possession and dissociative identity disorder? A case study from an Afro-Brazilian religion. *J Trauma Dissociation.* 17(3):322–37.

References

1. De Menezes Jr A, Moreira-Almeida A. Differential diagnosis between spiritual experiences and mental disorders of religious content [O diagnóstico diferencial entre experiências espirituais e transtornos mentais de conteúdo religioso]. *Revista de Psiquiatria Clínica* [Internet]. 2009;**36**(2):75–82. Available from: https://www.scopus.com/inward/record.uri?eid=2-s2.0-67649616553&doi=10.1590%2FS0101-60832009000200006&partnerID=40&md5=705a983ecde832d28ace5b4950893716

2. Moreira-Almeida A, Cardeña E. Differential diagnosis between non-pathological psychotic and spiritual experiences and mental disorders. *Revista Brasileira de Psiquiatria*. 2011;**33**(1):29–36.

3. Lukoff D, Lu F, Turner R. Toward a more culturally sensitive DSM-IV: psychoreligious and psychospiritual problems. *Journal of Nervous and Mental Disease*. 1992;**180**:673–82.

4. Alexander Moreira-Almeida, Angélica A Silva de Almeida, Francisco Lotufo Neto. History of 'Spiritist madness' in Brazil. *History of Psychiatry*. 2005;**16**(61 Pt 1):5–25.

5. Curlin FA, Lawrencer RE, Odell S, Chin MH, Lantos JD, Koenig HG, et al. Religion, spirituality, and medicine: psychiatrists' and other physicians' differing observations, interpretations, and clinical approaches. *American Journal of Psychiatry*. 2007;**164**(12):1825–31.

6. Pargament KI, Lomax JW. Understanding and addressing religion among people with mental illness. *World Psychiatry*. 2013;**12**(1):26–32.

7. Loch AA, Freitas EL, Hortêncio L, Chianca C, Alves TM, Serpa MH, et al. Hearing spirits? Religiosity in individuals at risk for psychosis—results from the Brazilian SSAPP cohort. *Schizophrenia Research*. 2019;**20**:353–9. Available from: https://doi.org/10.1016/j.schres.2018.09.020

8. Nuevo R, Chatterji S, Verdes E, Naidoo N, Arango C, Ayuso-Mateos JL. The continuum of psychotic symptoms in the general population: a cross-national study. *Schizophrenia Bulletin*. 2012;**38**(3):475–85.

9. Sidgwick H, Johnson A, Myers FWH, Podmore F, Sidgwick EM. Report on the census of hallucinations. *The Unconscious in Psycho-analysis*. 1894;**10**:25–422.

10. McGrath JJ, Saha S, Al-Hamzawi A, Alonso J, Bromet EJ, Bruffaerts R, et al. Psychotic experiences in the general population: a cross-national analysis based on 31 261 respondents from 18 countries. *JAMA Psychiatry*. 2015;**72**(7):697–705.

11. Peters E, Ward T, Jackson M, Morgan C, Charalambides M, McGuire P, et al. Clinical, socio-demographic and psychological characteristics in individuals with persistent psychotic experiences with and without a 'need for care'. *World Psychiatry*. 2016;**15**(1):41–52.

12. Powers AR, Kelley MS, Corlett PR. Varieties of voice-hearing: psychics and the psychosis continuum. *Schizophrenia Bulletin*. 2017;**43**(1):84–98.

13. Menezes A Jr, Moreira-Almeida A. Religion, spirituality, and psychosis. 2010;(April):174–9.

14. Etzel Cardeña, Steven Jay Lynn, Stanley Krippner. *Varieties of anomalous experience: examining the scientific evidence*. Washington, DC: American Psychological Association; 2000.

15. Stevenson I. Do we need a new word to supplement 'hallucination'? *American Journal of Psychiatry*. 1983;**240**:1609–11.

16. **van Lommel P, van Wees R, Meyers V, Elfferich I.** Near-death experience in survivors of cardiac arrest: a prospective study in the Netherlands. *Lancet.* 2001;**358**(9298):2039–45.

17. **Holden JM.** Veridical perception in near-death experiences. In: **Holden JM, Greyson B, James D** (eds), *The handbook of near-death experiences: Thirty years of investigation.* Praeger: ABC-CLIO; 2009. p. 185–211.

18. **Cardeña E.** The experimental evidence for parapsychological phenomena: a review. *American Psychologist.* 2018;**73**(5):663–77.

19. **Guloksuz S, Van Os J.** The slow death of the concept of schizophrenia and the painful birth of the psychosis spectrum. *Psychological Medicine.* 2018;**48**(2):229–44.

20. **Moreira-Almeida A, Lotufo Neto F, Greyson B.** Dissociative and psychotic experiences in Brazilian spiritist mediums [1]. *Psychotherapy and Psychosomatics.* 2006;**76**(1):57–8.

21. **Alminhana LO, Farias M, Claridge G, Cloninger CR, Moreira-Almeida A.** Self-directedness predicts quality of life in individuals with psychotic experiences: a 1-year follow-up study. *Psychopathology.* 2017;**50**(4):239–45.

22. **Koenig HG.** Religion, spirituality and psychotic disorders. *Revista de Psiquiatria Clínica.* 2007;**34**(Suppl. 1):95–104.

23. **Huguelet P.** Psychiatry and religion: a perspective on meaning. *Mental Health, Religion & Culture.* 2017;**20**(6):567–72. Available from: https://doi.org/10.1080/13674676.2017.1377956

24. **Mainieri AG, Peres JFP, Moreira-Almeida A, Mathiak K, Habel U, Kohn N.** Neural correlates of psychotic-like experiences during spiritual-trance state. *Psychiatry Research: Neuroimaging.* 2017;**266**(August 2016):101–7. Available from: http://dx.doi.org/10.1016/j.pscychresns.2017.06.006

25. **Powers AR, Mathys C, Corlett PR.** Pavlovian conditioning–induced hallucinations result from overweighting of perceptual priors. *Science.* 2017;**357**(6351):596–600.

26. **Woods A, Wilkinson S.** Appraising appraisals: role of belief in psychotic experiences. *Lancet Psychiatry.* 2017;**4**(12):891–2. Available from: http://dx.doi.org/10.1016/S2215-0366(17)30434-0

27. **Heriot-Maitland C, Knight M, Peters E.** A qualitative comparison of psychotic-like phenomena in clinical and non-clinical populations. *British Journal of Clinical Psychology.* 2012;**51**(1):37–53.

28. **Albert R. Powers III.** Psychotic experiences in the general population symptom specificity and the role of distress and dysfunction. *JAMA Psychiatry.* 2019 Dec 1;**76**(12):1228–9. doi:10.1001/jamapsychiatry.2019.2391

29. **Johns LC, Kompus K, Connell M, Humpston C, Lincoln TM, Longden E, et al.** Auditory verbal hallucinations in persons with and without a need for care. *Schizophrenia Bulletin.* 2014;**40**(Suppl. 4).

30. **Alminhana LO, Farias M, Claridge G, Cloninger CR, Moreira-Almeida A.** How to tell a happy from an unhappy schizotype: personality factors and mental health outcomes in individuals with psychotic experiences. *Revista Brasileira de Psiquiatria.* 2017;**39**(2):126–32.

31. **Machado L, Cantilino A, Petribú K, Pinto T.** Folie à deux (transtorno delirante induzido). *Jornal Brasileiro de Psiquiatria.* 2015;**64**(4):311–4.

32. **Delmonte R, Lucchetti G, Moreira-Almeida A, Farias M.** Can the DSM-5 differentiate between nonpathological possession and dissociative identity disorder? A case study from an Afro-Brazilian religion. *Journal of Trauma & Dissociation.* 2016;**17**(3):322–37.

Chapter 6

The light and the bulb: The psychology and neurophysiology of mystical experience

Etzel Cardeña and Lena Lindström

M'illumino d'Immenso (I'm alight by Immensity).

Mattina (Morning), Giuseppe Ungaretti, 1917

The self

In a way, defining the *self* is as easy as posing the question, 'Who am I?', but complications ensue when seeking a deeper understanding. 'Self' and the related term 'ego' encompass many aspects, varying in focus according to the discipline (1). A good starting point is William James's (2) basic taxonomy of self and its relation to consciousness. In it, the *self* was divided into two major components. First, the 'self as knower', or 'I-self', in which the stream of thought (or consciousness) is experienced as owned by an experiencing entity. James posited that consciousness is personal and mental events occur to a particular, not directly shareable, experiencing centre: 'The universal conscious fact is not 'feelings and thoughts exist' but 'I think' and 'I feel' (2, p. 226). This form of self might not even require specific mental content, as described in episodes of pure consciousness/emptiness (3), such as 'I experienced a silent inner state of no thoughts; just pure awareness and nothing else' (4, p. 27). Whether there can be self-less awareness is a contested issue (5).

James's I-self is close to the core or 'minimal' self of Gallagher: 'a consciousness of oneself as an immediate subject of experience, unextended in time' (6, p. 15). Typically, however, there is a certain implicit spatiality and temporality, a perspectival viewpoint, to this self, which also partly corresponds to the 'ecological self' of Neisser (7), based on proprioception and sensorimotor processes. In the usual spatial perspective of consciousness, the self is egocentrically experienced as being within the cranium of a sensed body located within a specific sur-rounding. There is also typically a temporal context to the minimal self, in which every conscious moment includes some awareness of the past moment and an anticipation of the future one (8), inconsistent with the contention that the minimal self is 'devoid of temporal extension' (6, p. 14). Lack of tem-poral continuity in the self is momentarily experienced when coming out of deep sleep, anaesthesia, or coma, only to be re-established almost immediately in the case of waking up. This temporal continuity can fail, as in the case of Clive Wearing, who suffers from severe hippocampal and perhaps frontal lobe damage. Every few minutes, he experiences emerging from unconsciousness with no autobiographic memory at all, despite maintaining normal procedural and semantic memories (9).

The self is not only the *subject* of awareness, however, but can also be the *object* of experience, knowledge, attitudes, and so on. This is the 'Me-self' of William James (2). The constituents of this objectified self include the body and material possessions, the self in interaction with others, the self extended across time through memory, and the conceptual or narrative self, including self-attributions, social roles, and so on (2, 6, 7). The 'Me-self' encompasses iden-tity and concepts, attitudes, and other implicit or explicit attributions about the self, which undergo transformations throughout one's life. Developmentally, from an emergent self, the infant gradually organizes the array of bodily and external stimuli into a core and a subjective self, which includes distinguishing self from others, and eventually includes a verbal narrative of the self (7, 10). One final point about the constituents of the self is that they can be more or less implicit, and that the person may engage in meta-cognition of these various constituents—for instance, by not only being vaguely aware of a spatial position but becoming reflectively aware of it.

Alterations of the self

There are many types of alterations of the self, including those related to neuro-pathological (11) and psychological (12) processes. To give but two examples, in simple out-of-body experiences, the spatial situatedness and ecological self change, whereas the sense of identity (the narrative self) remains unaltered, while in mediumship/spirit possession it is the latter that is transformed (12). There are as well minor quotidian changes, such as in 'losing oneself' in a movie, in the sense that reflective awareness of, for instance, the spatial and temporal contexts are peripheral. The 'I-self' continues to have personal experiences, but other components may fade into the background, such as awareness of the situatedness of the body in the cinema. Such experiences of 'losing oneself' may be pleasant and sought-after in religious and spiritual (13, 14), athletic and artistic (15), and hypnotic (16, 17) activities.

Because of their various potential interpretations, terms such as *ego dissolution*, *ego death*, *ego loss*, *selflessness*, and so on, say very little unless they are clearly defined with regard to the different aspects of self. Each of those terms could refer to such different events as being fully absorbed in an experience, a non-dual experience of not making a distinction between subject and object, experiencing the self as part of everything else, a temporary retrograde amnesia, decrease in self-importance, and so on (18).

Self-transcendence is a broad term referring to decreased self-salience or importance and/or a sense of connectedness or unity with something beyond and larger than the self. Connectedness is a complex construct that may include different experiences such as interconnective (aspects of reality linked by a common nature) or communal unity (a sense of kinship with others in a community) (19).

Another broad construct is *hypo-egoicism*, which involves low identification with the self-as-object, including low self-preoccupation, in contrast with egocentrism and egoism (20). Examples of hypo-egoicism not involving qualitative alterations of consciousness include being absorbed in an event or activity, and having an allo-inclusive identity, in which self-identity is extended to larger constituents such as all living beings. Hypo-egoicism is not necessarily positive and may include deindividuation, in which a person does not experience personal responsibility and engages in destructive acts along with others. An example of the opposite construct, *hyper-egoicism* can be exemplified by narcissism and an exaggerated sense of self-importance. A sense of unity and hypo-egoicism can co-occur (21), but they are not necessarily synonymous (see Fig. 6.1).

Mystical experiences

In what remains in this chapter, we will focus on the intense instances of self-transcendence and hypo-egoicism known as 'mystical experiences (ME)', which typically occur during an altered state of consciousness (see Fig. 6.1). Stace (22) characterized ME as including an overwhelming sense of unity, abeyance of the usual sense of space and time, positive affect, a sense of sacredness, experienced insight into ultimate reality, paradoxical mental content, and ineffability. To these, Hood (23) added perceptual enhancement and a sense of life in everything (see also (19, p. 21)). ME have been divided into an 'introvertive' type, characterized by a sense of pure consciousness, not located in time or space and lacking mental content, and an 'extrovertive' type, in which there is an experience of interconnectedness or merging with the outside world or

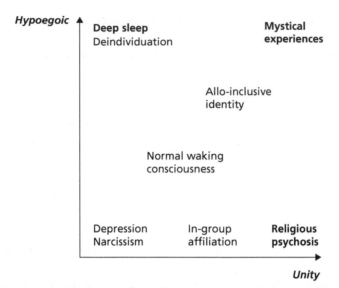

Fig. 6.1 Some examples of states of consciousness and traits along axes of hypo- versus hyper-egoicism and a sense of unity versus isolation. **Bold** font indicates an altered state.

a transcendent being (24). Marshall (19) has sought to clarify these distinctions by positing that the experiences can be 'this-wordly,' (e.g. a sense of direct union with all of nature), 'other-wordly' (e.g. union with a transcendent being or reality), and 'no-wordly' (e.g. pure consciousness without an object), with an occasional mixture of them.

It is important to distinguish between the mystical *experiences* themselves and the sometimes years-long contemplation and elaboration of them with potentially ensuing changes in self-image and world view (bringing about an altered *trait*). Nonetheless, simultaneous reports of the experience are consistent with those described in retrospective recollections. For instance, a contemporaneous report of the spontaneous experience of a highly hypnotizable person during 'deep hypnosis' included many of the same elements that are reported retrospectively: 'This is the best place to be ... I am out in the brightness ... I'm not matter anymore ... I'm part of [the light] ... Things do not happen here ... here there is no time and no space' (25, pp. 136–7).

Marshall (19, p. 25) lists 13 potential triggers of ME, including exposure to art or nature, ingestion of psychedelics, and contemplative practices such as meditation. To these should be added hypnosis, which can induce ME either spontaneously (26–28) or in response to suggestions (29). Psychological turmoil is also a common trigger, as described by Arthur Koestler (30, p. 350) in his autobiography: ' ... I noticed some slight mental discomfort nagging at the back of my mind—some trivial circumstance that marred the perfection of the moment ... I was, of course, in prison and might be shot. But this was immediately answered by a feeling whose verbal translation would be 'So what? ... ' Then I was floating on my back on a river of peace ... Then there was no river and no I. The I has ceased to exist.'

To what extent ME induced by different means are to be regarded as similar is debated, but accumulating evidence supports similarities above differences (21, 24, 31, 32). In an online survey of encounters with an 'experience of the divine', for non-drug and drug (psilocybin, lysergic acid diethylamide (LSD), ayahuasca, or N,N-Dimethyltryptamine (DMT)) respondents, a sense of unity or transcendence of time and space were similarly represented in both groups, with drug experiences being slightly more intense in this regard (33).

Individual differences and demographic variables

Three methods are commonly used to measure ME: open-ended responses to specific questions, questions in survey research, and scales to measure mysticism (34). More rarely, open-ended, phenomenological interviews have been used, whereby individuals are asked about their experience within a context that may give rise to self-transcendent experiences (see, e.g. (27, 35); for a discussion of the importance of an integration of various methodological strategies, see (36)).

Questionnaires include the Mysticism Scale (an operationalization of Stace's mysticism criteria) and the Religious Experience Episode Measures (which include brief narratives of the experiences assessed), both by Hood (34), and the Mystical Experience Questionnaire (37). The integration of multiple methods, including interviews and qualitative approaches in addition to neuroscientific ones, will likely provide a more complete perspective on ME (36).

Surveys have shown that ME happen very rarely and have to be distinguished from more general religious/spiritual experiences. A review found that around 20%–50% of the general public in the US have had a strong religious/spiritual experience, with aspects of self-transcendence, during their lifetime (38), but the incidence of full ME are very likely much lower. For instance, Hood et al. (34, p. 341) write that fewer than 6% of the reports sent to the Hardy Centre concerning a query about being 'close to a powerful spiritual force' could be classified as involving 'feelings of unity', and in two studies with a random sample in England the percentages were even smaller (2% and 1%). Even in a self-selected sample of people responding to a query about 'awakening' experiences, out of 90 reports no more than 11 seemed to qualify as an ME (39).

Environmental setting and cognitive processes such as expectations can have an important effect on facilitating ME, but personality traits relating to the propensity to have alterations of consciousness such as absorption, thin boundaries, self-transcendence, and hypnotizability likely have a stronger impact (40–43).

As for demographics, studies have revealed the following correlates of ME: being a woman, educated and affluent, of middle age or older, and psychologically healthy (24, 34). Religiosity also correlates with ME (38), which nonetheless occur most often in non-religious contexts. Contemplative practices/meditation are more strongly linked to ME than religious practice generally, unsurprisingly given meditation's goal to enhance a non-discursive experience of the present moment. In a non-random survey of 1,130 meditators of different traditions, over 70% reported having had an experience of 'fusion of their personal self into a larger whole' more than once during meditation, and over half reported having had this experience 'many times' or 'almost always' (44). Similar results were obtained for experiences such as 'freedom from the limitations of your personal self' and 'experience of an insight that "all is one"'. Indeed, ME are at the very core of many meditation traditions, however divergent at the surface, as both an associated feature or an ultimate goal.

Mystical experience and mental health

At times, ME have been considered pathological by definition, a product of malfunctioning psychological and/or brain processes. This is not an unreasonable speculation because some psychotic episodes with religious content resemble the pronouncements of mystics not known to have had psychosis. Compare for instance this recollection: 'Suddenly my whole being was filled with light and loveliness ... I was in a state of the most vivid awareness and illumination ... I was in touch with a reality beyond my own' (Coate, 1965 in (45, p. 516)) with 'As I reached the source of light I could see in. I cannot begin to describe in human terms the feeling I had at what I saw. It was a giant infinite world of calm, and love, and energy, and beauty' (Ring, 1958, in (19, p. 58)). The first is the description of the onset of a psychotic episode; the second is an account by a 14 year old as he was about to drown and had a transcendent experience.

William James in his foundational book on religious experience (46, p. 36) remarked that a 'psychopathic temperament' (by which he meant something like a hypomanic disposition that included 'ardor and excitability') could intensify an inner religious life, a similar conclusion to that of Pierre Janet (47). Leuba (48) went considerably farther and opined that ME were essentially delirious

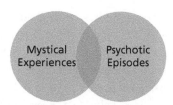

Fig. 6.2 The overlaps consists of mystical experiences with psychotic features and of psychotic disorders with mystical features.
Source: Based on 50.

and fully explainable through pathophysiology, similar to a later pronouncement by Rose (49, p. 334) that schizophrenics and mystics suffer from faulty brains whose experiences have no validity or importance.

Nonetheless, psychotic disorders do not necessarily include religious ideation and, even when they do, it often takes a very different expression than in ME and includes egocentric delusions and dysphoria (see Fig. 6.1 and Fig. 6.2).

Studies have distinguished ME from psychotic experiences with religious content by, among other things, the former entailing a sense of connectedness rather than grandiosity, and being briefer; more pleasant or at least serene; associated with visual rather than auditory hallucinations; part of a tradition; and not being associated with cognitive impairment (51, 52). The grandiosity and delusion typical of religious psychosis is evident in the example of the jurist Daniel Paul Schreber, on whom Freud based his theory of paranoia. The former declared that God had impregnated him and was sending him 'miracles' that caused him great pain: '*every ... thing that happens is in reference to me ...* I became in a way for God the only human being, or simply the human being around whom everything turns' (in (53, p. 56)).

Arbman (51) devoted a whole volume to 'religious trance' (alterations of consciousness with a spiritual/religious content) and psychopathology, and, in a chapter comparing ME and schizophrenia, concluded that 'only in rare, exceptional cases can religious ecstasy have been connected with the forms of mental abnormality designated as schizophrenia' (51, p. 385).

After Arbman arrived to this conclusion, a few studies have compared transcendent experiences of people with and without psychoses. In an impressionistic paper, Buckley (54) concluded that, despite some similarities, mystical accounts do not evidence the thought disorganization found in acute psychosis and, if they include hallucinations, they tend to be visual rather than auditory. In more elaborate research, a scale of various mystical aspects did not differentiate people with psychoses who had profound religious experiences from undiagnosed religious contemplatives, but the former evidenced more 'ego-grasping' (e.g. having strong desires, being rigid, wanting to exert control) and narcissistic tendencies (55). A study did a computerized content analysis of autobiographical reports by individuals describing schizophrenic, hallucinogenic, mystical, or important personal experiences (56). The mystics differed from all other groups in using language related to religiosity such as 'God' and 'holy', and to the category of 'Ideal value' (e.g. 'peace' and 'experience'), whereas the schizophrenic narratives had greater verbalizations related to 'deviation' and 'medical content' than the other groups. A phenomenological comparison of mystical and schizophrenic experiences concluded that, although they may share some 'affinities' such as the revelation of a hidden order, 'we are dealing with very distinct conditions' (57, p. 85).

In sum, ME are not intrinsically associated with pathology (34) but there is a small overlap between the two (Fig. 6.2; see also (58)). As pointed out by Schoenberg and Barendregt (59), the 'disintegration of the self' that can take place under pathological conditions, such as psychosis and depersonalization, are fundamentally different from that taking place in ME because of the lack of *insight* and *reintegration* in the former.

Mystical experience and positive psychology

In spiritual traditions, long-term positive after-effects are an expectable outcome of a contemplative life (24) and the few related experiments have supported this contention. This is not to deny, however, that some individuals who have had ME induced through drugs or meditation may have transient or even chronic negative effects (e.g. (60, 61)). More needs to be known about the interaction of diverse sociocultural and psychological variables as predictors of positive versus negative outcomes (62).

In a recent online survey of self-selected participants, experiences classified as mystical/unitive (rather than just exceptional) were associated with positive personal transformations (63). ME have often been rated as among the most important events in a person's life and may provide long-term benefits that include perceptual enhancement, enhanced positive emotions and well-being; greater openness to experience; a sense of connectedness, love, and compassion with other sentient beings and the environment; increased interpersonal closeness; and decreased fear of death (19, 34, 60, 64, 65). These after-effects are similar to those reported in near-death experiences that fulfil many or most criteria of ME (66).

In perhaps the first systematic study of this issue, individuals who had been administered psilocybin within a religious context reported after the session and six months later significantly more long-term changes in attitudes and behaviour than a control group administered an inert drug (67), This effect was also found in a follow-up after about 25 years (68). Hood, Hill, and Spilka (34, p. 357) compared the percentage of the experimental and control groups in the studies (67, 68) for different features such as a sense of unity after the session, six months later, and 25 years later. To give but one example, an internal sense of unity was reported at these three time points by 70%, 60%, and 77% of experimental participants, as compared to 8%, 5%, and 5% of control ones .

A series of more recent and better designed studies by Griffiths and associates using psilocybin have shown that most participants exposed to it, as compared with a psychoactive but not psychedelic substance, declared that it had been one of the most important experiences in their lives, producing a sense of unity and other characteristics of ME, and later positive effects in attitudes, mood, behaviour and social interactions; the positive self-reports were ratified independently by those close to the participants (60). Participants at times felt negative emotions such as fear or anxiety, but within the experiment's supportive environment these dissipated.

Follow-up studies by that research group (69, 70) have replicated their basic finding, with the addition that higher doses of the drug were tied to more complete ME. In still another study, MacLean, Johnson, and Griffiths (71) found an enduring increase in the personality trait of openness to experience, mediated by having had more complete ME and seeking to maintain it through a discipline such as meditation (72). In agreement with this finding, in a mixed-methods study, having a spiritual practice made it more likely that an ME would be interpreted as positive (73) (see also (74)).

Whether ME provide beneficial effects likely depends on factors such as sociocultural support; personal factors including cognitive organization and lack of negative affect; factors preceding the experience, such as ongoing mood, expectation, and desire (i.e. 'set'); and immediate contextual factors, such as the setting and the characteristic of the inducing agent (e.g. amounts of a psychedelic drug) (75). The characteristics of the experience are also germane, with pleasant or at least serene content, some control, short-term duration, and sociocultural support related to a positive outcome (76). Personality traits including being self-directed and social make it more likely that a predisposition to experience self-transcendence will be associated with a positive outcome (77).

Finally, some experiences that may be dysfunctional at a certain stage in life may become adaptive at another stage. For instance, manifestations interpreted emically as spirit possession had negative personal and social consequences when a devotee was a child, but became prized by the community as he became adept to have some control and use them for the communal good (78).

Neural correlates

The past few years have seen a surge in research on the neural correlates of psychedelic intoxication, which often have included measures of phenomena associated with ME. Several of these studies have focused on the activity and interaction of brain networks, particularly the internally oriented 'default mode' (DMN) and the externally oriented, or 'task positive', networks (TPN). They usually show opposite activity to one another: while TPN are engaged in attention-demanding tasks, the DMN is more active when there is no task at hand (79). Activity in DMN has been associated with self-related processing (e.g. self-awareness, self-reflection) (80, 81) and it encompasses areas implicated in different aspects of self-reference such as the medial prefrontal cortex (mPFC), posterior cingulate cortex (PCC), and inferior parietal lobe (IPL) (82). fMRI studies have found that decreased internal connectivity of the DMN (83), increased functional connectivity between networks (84), and complex changes in the connectivity of DMN and TPN (85) correlate with subjectively evaluated 'dissolving of self or ego' under LSD intoxication. Similarly, magnetoelectroencephalography (MEG) studies of psilocybin (86) and LSD (83) intoxication have shown a correlation between decreased alpha power (synchronized neural oscillation in the 8–12 Hz range, associated with sensory inhibition) in the DMN hub PCC and ratings of 'ego-disintegration'. Here, the conceptual ambiguity mentioned in the earlier section, 'Alterations of the self', has to be acknowledged: it is far from clear just what these terms refer to in the minds of the participants and/ or the researchers (see (18)).

It should be mentioned that psychoactive drugs present a serious confound in studies of neural correlates of ME because they alter brain dynamics in various ways besides the potential induction of ME. For this reason, it is important to look for parallels to the neural correlates of ME induced by other means. Decreased network anticorrelation has been seen in studies of several different kinds of meditation (without targeting ME specifically) (87), including nondual awareness meditation with self-transcendent qualities (88). Less intense experiences of hypo-egoicism, such as flow and forgiveness, have been linked to decreased activity in DMN areas and to changes in DMN–TPN interaction (89, 90). An EEG study found decreased activity of the DMN and central areas of the TPN in four self-transcendent meditative states compared with baseline (91). Similarly, in a MEG study, Dor-Ziderman et al. (35, 92) found decreased beta power (ca. 12–25 Hz oscillatory activity associated with ordinary active processing) in DMN areas PCC and IPL as meditators entered a mode of self-less experience (35) and boundarylessness (92). Dor-Ziderman et al. (35) found that narrative self-thoughts correlated with gamma activity (activity of ca. 30

Hz and above) in medial and lateral frontal areas, including both the DMN hub mPFC and several TPN areas—activity that slowed down to beta in experiences of minimal self and with a marked decrease in beta power as meditators entered a selfless state. However, an EEG study of a single meditator restricted to the gamma band found greater activation of the lateral frontal cortex, part of the TPN, to coincide with experiences of 'self-dissolution' (93), and a few studies have found *increases* in DMN-areas during ME: in positron emission tomography (PET) studies using ketamine and psilocybin, Vollenweider et al. (94, 95) found increased glucose metabolism in the right mPFC as a correlate of ME, and increased activity of the two DMN areas, mPFC and IPL, was reported from an fMRI study of re-experienced ME (96). However, neither of these studies addressed network function as a whole but only activity in specific areas.

Most studies of self-transcendence induced by meditation have used methods that measure activity patterns for the entire brain rather than for specific areas or networks, with results for overall brain synchronization showing equivocal results. In two early EEG studies on transcendental meditation (97, 98), episodes of 'pure consciousness' were found to correlate with increased global synchronization across frequency bands (delta, theta, alpha, and beta), and Berkovich-Ohana (99) found that spontaneous episodes of contentless ME related to increases in long-range gamma synchronization.

In an LSD study using multiple brain-imaging techniques, Carhart-Harris et al. (83) reported that global decrease in the power of low-frequency delta and alpha brainwaves, and decreased connectivity between the parahippocampus and retrospenial cortex related to experiences of 'ego dissolution'. In contrast, episodes of contentless 'non-duality' of meditators correlated with global activity increases for the lower frequencies (delta, theta, and alpha) whereas gamma power decreased (100), suggestive of decreased global synchronization. The only study we know of evaluating the neural correlates of hypnosis-related ME also found decreased global synchronization related to spontaneous transcendent and imaginal experiences (27). In terms of within- and between-network synchronicity, however, measures of average global synchronicity are not very illuminating.

The partly disparate neural findings suggest that there are several neural paths to the same type of experience, a case of 'multiple realizations' (101), or the discrepancy might be due to the experiences in fact not being very similar, consistent with the considerable complexity both of ordinary self-experience and ME (31). Much of the discrepancy is also likely due to individual differences among participants, the large variety of measurements, induction methods, comparison conditions, and neuroimaging techniques, not to mention the limited reliability of these techniques (e.g. (102, 103)).

A central question concerns whether self-transcendence corresponds to eliminative or generative neural processes. Is it the case that self-related neural activity is reduced during ME, or that new patterns corresponding to a feeling of unity and connection emerge? Perhaps it is either, or both. In light of the 'default' character of the default mode network and its role in self-related processing, reductions in its internal integrity and activity reasonably correspond to decreases in self-experience. At the same time, findings of increased connectivity between networks that are usually anticorrelated, and of increased global synchronization, may correspond to new patterns of functioning that—both on a neuronal and experiential level—could be interpreted as more integrative.

The ontology of mystical experience

In a lucid categorization, Hood and colleagues (34) listed three interpretations of mysticism. In the first one, ME are erroneous attributions or interpretations, be it of pathological processes (e.g. (48)) or of psychological regressions to an idealized infantile state of unity (104). We have already shown that there is no empirical support for considering ME to be pathological per se, and they do not seem to be similar to what we know of infantile cognition, although this hypothesis warrants some attention. The second view proposes that ME represent forms of a progressive evolution of consciousness, in which nature is gradually achieving self-consciousness of its underlying connection, with Teilhard de Chardin (105) being the best-known proponent of this view. The positive after-effects of ME would seem to support the notion that a sense of union entails personal benefits, but in a limited, personal way. Given the cosmological breadth of this view, it is difficult to see how it could be ascertained or falsified.

The third view, and the one we devote greater attention to here, considers mysticism a form of heightened (at least partly) accurate awareness. The thesis here is that ME reveal aspects of reality that are commonly hidden, including its underlying unity and the illusion of an isolated self. This is the interpretation favoured by some religious thinkers (see (106)) and, in a secular context, was championed at the inception of psychology as a science by F.W.H. Myers (107) and William James (46). In the past few decades, some proposals and findings within both physics and parapsychology research have been consistent with this view. Theoretical physicists Bernard d'Espagnat (108) and David Bohm (109) wrote of a unity of all as 'veiled reality' or 'implicit order', respectively, and D'Espagnat mentioned that the insight of mystics and artists may reveal something about this aspect of reality (108, p. 433). Bohm also discussed parapsychological or psi phenomena, which seem to provide valid information that is temporally and/or spatially distant and unmediated by the senses or reason, within his physical model of reality. Relatedly, there is supportive evidence that alterations of consciousness (although not necessarily ME) facilitate awareness of information that is temporally or spatially distant (64) and that this information is more likely to be apprehended in connection with meditation and/or by long-term meditators (110). Thus, the notion that ME (or some aspects of them) may provide a valid view of aspects of reality is an empirically defensible hypothesis. A possible explanation of how this may happen is that ordinary states of consciousness impose biases and limitations, explainable by evolutionary demands (e.g. (111, 112)) whereas some alterations of consciousness provide alternate forms of cognition that might bypass these limitations and/or provide greater availability of usually unconscious information (46, 107).

Conclusion

ME can have profound positive personal and social consequences, yet have received scant attention by the scientific community until recently. There are some areas in which there is fairly consistent knowledge about them, such as their triggers, individual differences in who is likely to have them, and their rarity. No such consistency is found in research on studies of their neural correlates. A possible explanation is that ME might be realized by different neural activation patterns. But, before contemplating that hypothesis, researchers need to have precise descriptions of the phenomena they study through questionnaires and other measures, and make sure that they are comparing the same kind of experience. Theory-driven neurophenomenological investigations need to be developed with individuals and under circumstances that are likely to produce ME. Finally, the ontological implications of these experiences for our understanding of consciousness and its relation to reality deserve serious discussion.

References

1. **Snodgrass JGE, Thompson RL.** *The self across psychology: self-recognition, self-awareness, and the self concept.* New York: Annals of the New York Academy of Sciences; 1997.
2. **James W.** *The principles of psychology.* New York: Henry Holt; 1890.
3. **Shear J.** Eastern approaches to altered states of consciousness. In: **Cardeña E, Winkelman M** (eds), *Altering consciousness: Multidisciplinary perspectives.* Santa Barbara, CA: Praeger; 2011, pp. 139–58.
4. **Forman RKC.** Introduction: Mysticism, constructivism, and forgetting. In: **Forman RKC** (ed.), *The problem of pure consciousness: Mysticism and philosophy.* Oxford: Oxford University Press; 1990, pp. 3–49.
5. **Gallagher S.** Introduction: A diversity of selves. In: *The Oxford handbook of the self.* Oxford; Oxford University Press; 2011, pp. 1–30.

6. **Gallagher S.** Philosophical conceptions of the self: implications for cognitive science. *Trends in Cognitive Sciences.* 2000;**4**(1):14–21.

7. **Neisser U.** Five kinds of self-knowledge. *Philosophical Psychology.* 1988;**1**(1):35–59.

8. **Husserl E.** *The phenomenology of internal time-consciousness.* **Heidegger M,** (ed), Bloomington, IN; Indiana University Press; 1964. Orig. 1928.

9. **Sacks, O.** The abyss. The New Yorker [Internet]. 2007 Sep 24 [cited 2019 Sep 16]. Available from https://www.newyorker.com/magazine/2007/09/24/the-abyss

10. **Stern D.** *The interpersonal world of the infant.* New York: Basic Books; 1985.

11. **Noirhomme Q, Laureys S.** Altering consciousness and neuropathology. In: **Cardeña E, Winkelman M,** (es). *Altering consciousness: Multidisciplinary perspectives. Volume 2: Biological and psychological perspectives.* Santa Barbara, CA; Praeger; 2011, pp. 263–78.

12. **Cardeña E, Alvarado CS.** Anomalous self and identity experiences. In: **Cardeña E, Lynn SJ, Krippner S** (eds), *Varieties of anomalous experience: Examining the scientific evidence.* (Seconddition). Washington: American Psychological Association; 2014, pp. 273–301.

13. **Lifshitz M, van Elk M, Luhrmann TM.** Absorption and spiritual experience: a review of evidence and potential mechanisms. *Conscious and Cognition.* 2019;**73**:102760.

14. **Yamashiro J.** Brain basis of samadhi: the neuroscience of meditative absorption. *New School Psychology Bulletin.* 2015;**13**(1):1–10.

15. **Csikszentmihalyi M.** *Beyond boredom and anxiety.* San Fransisco—Washington—London: Jossey-Bass Publishers; 1975.

16. **Cardeña E, Spiegel D.** Suggestibility, absorption, and dissociation: An integrative model of hypnosis. In: **Schumaker J** (ed.), *Human suggestibility: advances in theory, research, and application.* New York; Routledge; 1991, pp. 95–107.

17. **Shor RE.** Hypnosis and the concept of the generalized reality-orientation. *American Journal of Psychothery.* 1959;**13**(3):582–602.

18. **Millière R.** Looking for the self: phenomenology, neurophysiology and philosophical significance of drug-induced ego dissolution. *Frontiers in Human Neuroscience.* 2017;**11**(May):1–2.

19. **Marshall P.** *The shape of the soul: what mystical experience tells us about ourselves and reality.* Lanham, MD; Rowman & Littlefield; 2019.

20. **Brown KW, Leary MR,** (eds), *The Oxford handbook of hypo-egoic phenomena.* First edition. New York: Oxford University Press; 2016.

21. **Yaden DB, Haidt J, Hood RW, Vago DR, Newberg AB.** The varieties of self-transcendent experience. *Review of General Psychology.* 2017;**21**(2):143–60.

22. **Stace WT.** *The teachings of the mystics.* New York: The New American Library; 1960.

23. **Hood RW.** The construction and preliminary validation of a measure of reported mystical experience. *Journal for the Scientific Study of Religion.* 1975;**14**(1):29.

24. **Wulff MD.** Mystical experiences. In: **Cardeña E, Lynn SJ, Krippner S** (eds), *Varieties of anomalous experience: Examining the scientific evidence.* Second edition. Washington, DC: American Psychological Association; 2014, pp. 369–40.

25. **Cardeña E.** *The phenomenology of quiescent and physically active deep hypnosis* (Doctoral dissertation, unpublished). Davis: University of California; 1988.

26. **Cardeña E.** The phenomenology of deep hypnosis: quiescent and physically active. *International Journal of Clinical and Experimental Hypnosis.* 2005;**53**(1):37–59.

27. Cardeña E, Jönsson P, Terhune DB, Marcusson-Clavertz D. The neurophenomenology of neutral hypnosis. *Cortex*. 2013;**49**(2):375–85.

28. Sherman SE. *Very deep hypnosis: sn experiential and electroencephalographic investigation* (Doctoral dissertation; unpublished). Stanford, CA: Stanford University; 1971.

29. Lynn SJ, Evans J. Hypnotic suggestion produces mystical-type experiences in the laboratory: a demonstration proof. *Psychology of Consciousness: Theory, Research, and Practice*. 2017;**4**(1):23.

30. Koestler A. *The invisible writing*. New York, Macmillan; 1954.

31. Millière R, Carhart-Harris RL, Roseman L, Trautwein FM, Berkovich-Ohana A. Psychedelics, meditation, and self-consciousness. *Frontiers in Psychology*. 2018;**9**(Sept.):1475.

32. Wahbeh H, Sagher A, Back W, Pundhir P, Travis F. A systematic review of transcendent states across meditation and contemplative traditions. *Explore*. 2018;**14**(1):19–35.

33. Griffiths RR, Hurwitz ES, Davis AK, Johnson MW, Jesse R. Survey of subjective 'God encounter experiences': comparisons among naturally occurring experiences and those occasioned by the classic psychedelics psilocybin, LSD, ayahuasca, or DMT. *PLoS One*. 2019;**14**(4):e0214377.

34. Hood RW, Hill PC, Spilka B. *The psychology of religion: an empirical approach*. Fourth edition. New York: Guilford Publications; 2009.

35. Dor-Ziderman Y, Berkovich-Ohana A, Glicksohn J, Goldstein A. Mindfulness-induced selflessness: a MEG neurophenomenological study. *Frontiers in Human Neuroscience*. 2013;**7**(Sept.):1–17.

36. Cardeña E, Pekala RJ. Methodological issues in the study of altered states of consciousness and anomalous experiences. In: **Cardeña E, Lynn SJ, Krippner S**, (eds), *Varieties of anomalous experience: examining the scientific evidence*. Second edition. Washington, DC: American Psychological Association; 2014, pp. 21–56.

37. MacLean KA, Leoutsakos JS, Johnson MW, Griffiths RR. Factor analysis of the mystical experience questionnaire: a study of experiences occasioned by the hallucinogen psilocybin. *Journal for the Scientific Study of Religion*. 2012;**51**(4):721–37.

38. Yamane D, Polzer M. Ways of seeing ecstasy in modern society: experiential-expressive and cultural-linguistic views. *Sociology of Religion*. 2007;**55**(1):1.

39. Taylor S, Egeto-Szabo K. Exploring awakening experiences: A study of awakening experiences in terms of their triggers, characteristics, duration and aftereffects. *Journal of Transpersonal Psychology*. 2017;**49**(1):45.

40. Cardeña E, Terhune DB. Hypnotizability, personality traits, and the propensity to experience alterations of consciousness. *Psychology of Consciousness, Theory, Research, and Practice*. 2014;**1**(3):292–307.

41. Cloninger CR, Svrakic DM, Przybeck TR. A psychobiological model of temperament and character. *Archives of General Psychiatry*. 1993;**50**:975–90.

42. Hartmann E, Harrison R, Zborowski M. Boundaries in the mind: past research and future directions. *North American Journal of Psychology*. 2001;**3**(3):347–68.

43. Lifshitz M, van Elk M, Luhrmann TM. Absorption and spiritual experience: a review of evidence and potential mechanisms. *Consciousness and Cognition*. 2019;**73**:102760.

44. Vieten C, Wahbeh H, Cahn BR, et al. Future directions in meditation research: recommendations for expanding the field of contemplative science. *PLoS One.* 2018;**13**(11):1–30.

45. Buckley P. Mystical experience and schizophrenia. *Schizophrenia Bulletin.* 1981;7(3):516–21.

46. James W. *The varieties of religious experience: a study in human nature.* New York: New American Library; 1958. Orig. 1902.

47. Janet P. *De la angustia al éxtasis* (2 vols). México City, México: Fondo de Cultura Económica; 1991. Orig. 1926.

48. Leuba JH. *The psychology of religious mysticism.* New York: Harcourt, Brace; 1925.

49. Rose S. *The conscious brain.* Revised edition. Middlesex, UK: Penguin Books; 1976.

50. Lukoff D, Lu F, Turner R. Toward a more culturally sensitive DSM-IV: Psychoreligious and psychospiritual problems. *Journal of Nervous and Mental Disease.* 1992;**180**(11):673–82.

51. Arbman E. *Ecstasy, or religious trance: In the experience of ecstatics and from the psychological point of view. Volume 3: Ecstasy and psychological states.* Uppsala; Svenska bokförlaget; 1970.

52. Austin JH. *Zen and the brain: toward an understanding of meditation and consciousness.* Cambridge, MA: MIT Press; 1999.

53. Landis C. *Varieties of psychopathological experience.* Fred A. Mettler (ed.). New York: Holt, Rinehart and Winston; 1964.

54. Buckley P. Mystical experience and schizophrenia. *Schizophrenia Bulletin.* 1981;7(3):516–21.

55. Stifler K, Greer J, Sneck W, Dovenmuehle R. An empirical investigation of the discriminability of reported mystical experiences among religious contemplatives, psychotic inpatients, and normal adults. *Journal for the Scientific Study of Religion.* 1993;**32**(4):366–72.

56. Oxman TE, Rosenberg SD, Schnurr PP, Tucker GJ, Gala G. The language of altered states. *Journal of Nervous and Mental Disease.* 1988;**176**:401–8.

57. Parnas J, Henriksen MG. Mysticism and schizophrenia: a phenomenological exploration of the structure of consciousness in the schizophrenia spectrum disorders. *Consciousness and Cognition.* 2016;**43**:75–88.

58. Kerns JG, Karcher N, Raghavan C, Berenbaum H. Anomalous experiences, peculiarity, and psychopathology. In: *Varieties of anomalous experience: examining the scientific evidence.* Second edition. Washington, DC: American Psychological Association; 2014, pp. 57–76.

59. Schoenberg PLA, Barendregt HP. Mindful disintegration and the decomposition of self in healthy populations: conception and preliminary study. *Psychological Studies (Mysore).* 2016;**61**(4):307–20.

60. Griffiths RR, Richards WA, McCann U, Jesse R. Psilocybin can occasion mystical-type experiences having substantial and sustained personal meaning and spiritual significance. *Psychopharmacology.* 2006;**187**(3):268–83.

61. Lindahl JR, Fisher NE, Cooper DJ, Rosen RK, Britton WB. The varieties of contemplative experience: a mixed-methods study of meditation-related challenges in Western Buddhists. *PLoS One.* 2017;**12**(5):e0176239.

62. **Cardeña E, Lynn SJ, Krippner S.** *Varieties of anomalous experience: examining the scientific evidence.* Washington: American Psychological Association; 2014.

63. **Tassell-Matamua NA, Frewin KE.** Psycho-spiritual transformation after an exceptional human experience. *Journal of Spirituality in Mental Health.* 2018;**21**(4):1–22.

64. **Cardeña E.** The experimental evidence for parapsychological phenomena: a review. *American Psychologist.* 2018;**73**:663–677.

65. **Ross S.** Therapeutic use of classic psychedelics to treat cancer-related psychiatric distress. *International Review of Psychiatry.* 2018;**30**(4):317–30.

66. **Greyson B.** Near-death experiences. In: **Cardeña E, Lynn SJ, Krippner S,** (eds), *Varieties of anomalous experience: examining the scientific evidence.* Second edition. Washington, DC: American Psychological Association; 2014, pp. 333–67.

67. **Pahnke WN.** Drugs and mysticism. *International Journal of Parapsychology.* 1966;**8**(2):295–313.

68. **Doblin R.** Pahnke's 'Good Friday experiment': a long-term follow-up and methodological critique. *Journal of Transpersonal Psychology.* 1991;**23**(1):1–28.

69. **Griffiths RR, Johnson MW, Richards WA, Richards BD, McCann U, Jesse R.** Psilocybin occasioned mystical-type experiences: immediate and persisting dose-related effects. *Psychopharmacology.* 2011;**218**(4):649–65.

70. **Griffiths RR, Richards WA, Johnson MW, Mccann UD, Jesse R.** Mystical-type experiences occasioned by psilocybin mediate the attribution of personal meaning and spiritual significance 14 months later. *Journal of Psychopharmacology.* 2008;**22**(6):621–32.

71. **MacLean KA, Johnson MW, Griffiths RR.** Mystical experiences occasioned by the hallucinogen psilocybin lead to increases in the personality domain of openness. *Journal of Psychopharmacology.* 2011;**25**(11):1453–61.

72. **Griffiths RR, Johnson MW, Richards WA,** et al. Psilocybin-occasioned mystical-type experience in combination with meditation and other spiritual practices produces enduring positive changes in psychological functioning and in trait measures of prosocial attitudes and behaviors. *Journal of Psychopharmacology.* 2018;**32**(1):49–69.

73. **Kohls N, Hack A, Walach H.** Measuring the unmeasurable by ticking boxes and opening Pandora's Box: mixed methods research as a useful tool for investigating exceptional and spiritual experiences. *Archive for the Psychology of Religion.* 2008;**30**(1):155–87.

74. **Walsh RN, Grob CS.** *Higher wisdom: eminent elders explore the continuing impact of psychedelics.* New York: State University of New York Press; 2005.

75. **Tart CT.** *States of consciousness.* New York: EP Dutton; 1975.

76. **Moreira-Almeida A, Cardeña E.** Differential diagnosis between non-pathological psychotic and spiritual experiences and mental disorders: a contribution from Latin American studies to the ICD-1. *Revista Brasileira de Psiquiatria.* 2011;**33**(Suppl. 1):S29–S36.

77. **Cloninger CR.** Completing the psychobiological architecture of human personality development: Temperament, character, and coherence. In: **Staudinger UM, Lindenberger U** (eds), *Understanding human development.* Boston, MA; Kluwer; 2003, pp. 159–81.

78. **Cardeña E, Schaffler Y.** 'He who has the spirits must work a lot': a psycho-anthropological account of spirit possession in the Dominican Republic. *Ethos.* 2018;**46**(4):457–76.

79. **Fox MD, Snyder AZ, Vincent JL, Corbetta M, Essen DC Van, Raichle ME.** The human brain is intrinsically organized into dynamic, anticorrelated functional networks. *Proceedings of the National Academy of Sciences.* 2005;**102**(27):9673–8.

80. **Andrews-Hanna JR.** The brain's befault network and its adaptive role in internal mentation. *Neuroscientist.* 2012;**1**(3):233–45.

81. **Bressler SL, Menon V.** Large-scale brain networks in cognition: emerging methods and principles. *Trends in Cognitive Sciences.* 2010;**14**(6):277–90.

82. **Qin P, Northoff G.** How is our self related to midline regions and the default-mode network? *Neuroimage.* 2011;**57**(3):1221–33.

83. **Carhart-Harris RL, Muthukumaraswamy S, Roseman L,** et al. Neural correlates of the LSD experience revealed by multimodal neuroimaging. *Proceedings of the National Academy of Sciences.* 2016;**113**(17):4853–8.

84. **Tagliazucchi E, Roseman L, Kaelen M,** et al. Increased global functional connectivity correlates with LSD-induced ego dissolution. *Current Biology.* 2016;**26**(8):1043–50.

85. **Atasoy S, Roseman L, Kaelen M, Kringelbach ML, Deco G, Carhart-Harris RL.** Connectome-harmonic decomposition of human brain activity reveals dynamical repertoire re-organization under LSD. *Scientific Reports.* 2017;**7**(1):1–18.

86. **Muthukumaraswamy SD, Carhart-Harris RL, Moran RJ,** et al. Broadband cortical desynchronization underlies the human psychedelic state. *Journal of Neuroscience.* 2013;**33**(38):15171–83.

87. **Brewer JA, Worhunsky PD, Gray JR, Tang Y-Y, Weber J, Kober H.** Meditation experience is associated with differences in default mode network activity and connectivity. *Proceedings of the National Academy of Sciences.*2011;**108**(50):20254–9.

88. **Josipovic Z, Dinstein I, Weber J, Heeger DJ, Schultheiss OC.** Influence of meditation on anti-correlated networks in the brain. *Frontiers in Human Neuroscience.* 2012;**5**(Jan.):1–11.

89. **Farb N, Desormeau PA, Dinh-Williams L-A.** The neuroscience of hypo-egoic processes. In: **Brown KW, Leary MR,** (eds), *The Oxford handbook of hypo-egoic phenomena.* New York: Oxford University Press; 2016, pp. 109–31.

90. **Ulrich M, Keller J, Hoenig K, Waller C, Grön G.** Neural correlates of experimentally induced flow experiences. *Neuroimage.* 2014;**86**:194–202.

91. **Schoenberg PLA, Ruf A, Churchill J, Brown DP, Brewer JA.** Mapping complex mind states: EEG neural substrates of meditative unified compassionate awareness. *Consciousness and Cognition.* 1 January 2018;**57**:41–53.

92. **Dor-Ziderman Y, Ataria Y, Fulder S, Goldstein A, Berkovich-Ohana A.** Self-specific processing in the meditating brain: a MEG neurophenomenology study. *Neuroscience of Consciousness.* 2016;(1):1–13.

93. **Lehmann D, Faber PL, Achermann P, Jeanmonod D, Gianotti LRR, Pizzagalli D.** Brain sources of EEG gamma frequency during volitionally meditation-induced, altered states of consciousness, and experience of the self. *Psychiatry Research: Neuroimaging.* 2001;**108**(2):111–21.

94. Vollenweider FX, Leenders KL, Scharfetter C, et al. Metabolic hyperfrontality and psychopathology in the ketamine model of psychosis using positron emission tomography (PET) and [18F]fluorodeoxyglucose (FDG). *European Neuropsychopharmacology.* 1997;**7**(1):9–24.

95. Vollenweider F, Leenders K, Scharfetter C, Maguire P, Stadelmann O, Angst J. Positron emission tomography and fluorodeoxyglucose studies of metabolic hyperfrontality and psychopathology in the psilocybin model of psychosis. *Neuropsychopharmacology.* 1997;**16**(5):357–72.

96. Beauregard M, Paquette V. Neural correlates of a mystical experience in Carmelite nuns. *Neuroscience Letters.* 2006;**405**(3):186–90.

97. Badawi K, Wallace RK, Orme-Johnson D, Rouzere AM. Electrophysiologic characteristics of respiratory suspension periods occurring during the practice of the transcendental meditation program. *Psychosomatic Medicine.* 1984;**46**(3):267–76.

98. Farrow JT, Hebert RJ. Breath suspension during the Transcendental Meditation technique. *Psychosomatic Medicine.* May 1982;**44**(2):133–53.

99. Berkovich-Ohana A. A case study of a meditation-induced altered state: increased overall gamma synchronization. *Phenomenology and the Cognitive Sciences.* 2017;**16**(1):91–106.

100. Berman AE, Stevens L. EEG manifestations of nondual experiences in meditators. *Consciousness and Cognition.* 2015;**31**:1–11.

101. Putnam H. Psychological predicates. In: Capitan WH, Merrill DD, (eds), *Art, mind, and religion.* Pittsburgh: University of Pittsburgh Press; 1967, pp. 37–48.

102. Hinterberger T. I am I from moment to moment: methods and results of grasping intersubjective and intertemporal neurophysiological differences during meditation states. In: Schmidt S, Walach H, (eds), *Meditation—neuroscientific approaches and philosophical implications.* New York: Springer; 2014, pp. 95–113.

103. Tallis R. *Aping mankind.* Durham, UK: Routledge; 2016.

104. Freud S. *Civilization and its discontents.* New York: WW Norton & Company; 1989. Orig. 1930.

105. de Chardin PT. *The phenomenon of man.* New York: Harper & Row; 1959.

106. Huxley A. *The perennial philosophy.* New York: Harper Colophon Books; 1945.

107. Kelly EF, Kelly EW, Crabtree A, Gauld A, Grosso M. *Irreducible mind: toward a psychology for the 21st century.* Lanham, MD: Rowman & Littlefield; 2007.

108. d'Espagnat B. *On physics and philosophy.* Princeton, NJ: Princeton University Press; 2006.

109. Bohm DJ. A new theory of the relationship of mind and matter. *Journal of the American Society for Psychical Research.* 1986;**80**:113–35.

110. Roney-Dougal SM. Ariadne's thread: meditation and psi. In: Cardeña E, Palmer J, Marcusson-Clavertz D, (eds), *Parapsychology: a handbook for the 21st century.* Jefferson, NC: McFarland; 2015, pp. 125–38.

111. Hoffman D. Conscious realism and the mind-body problem. *Mind Matter.* 2008;**6**(1):87–121.

112. Ornstein R. *The psychology of consciousness.* Revised edition. New York: Penguin; 1986.

Chapter 7

Evidence for the influence of religiosity and spirituality on mental health

Giancarlo Lucchetti,
Rodolfo Furlan Damiano,
Alessandra Lamas Granero Lucchetti, and
Mario Fernando Prieto Peres

Introduction

According to Sigmund Freud, in his Introductory Conferences about Psychoanalysis (1), the advent of psychoanalytical theory was so revolutionary that it shook human narcissism. In *The future of an illusion* (2), he presented what is referred to as intrinsic religiosity (connection of humans with a superior divinity) as a kind of a childhood neurosis. In other words, when one realizes that one's father, hitherto almighty, cannot explain many human dilemmas, such as death, one creates God as a way of recreating the idea of an omniscient, omnipotent, and omnipresent father. This notion, according to Freud, was more than an illusion, rather a social/collective delusion, because it was not based on reason but on helplessness and dogmatic and irreducible ideas, seeming like a delusional idea. Therefore, religion to Freud was doomed to failure and oblivion through the development of reason.

Along with Freud's ideas, there has been growing scepticism within the scientific community over spiritual or religious beliefs, where all knowledge, practices, or values derived from religious traditions have been shunned by researchers. Religion started being treated almost as a mental disease and kept separate from psychiatry practice (3–5). However, contrary to expectations, religion is growing and set to carry on growing, in absolute and relative terms, up to 2050 (6). This implies that even more patients will want their spirituality/religiosity (S/R) addressed, while fewer mental health workers are able or willing to deal with these emerging issues (7–12).

Thus, this chapter aims to discuss the scientific evidence, proposed mechanisms, and possible interventions supporting the relationship between R/S and mental health, in order to encourage health professionals to reflect on their practice and promote a more integral model of care.

Spirituality, religiosity and clinical practice

According to Celmo Celeno Porto (13), the perfect medical act consists of a combination of three basic components: technical competence, ethical principles, and humanistic virtues. Based on this principle, addressing spirituality and/or religiosity in clinical practice might have an impact on these three domains.

First, it is well known that almost 85% of the world population identifies with some religious tradition (6) and, when sick, most want their spirituality addressed (9–11, 14). Moreover, researchers have also shown that addressing S/R might reduce care costs at end of life (15) and is strongly associated with physical and mental health (16). Therefore, according to a number of medical organizations, knowing how to address S/R in clinical practice is a basic technical competence that physicians should develop and perform with confidence and without fear of imposing their own beliefs (12). These organizations include the Association of American Medical Colleges (17), the World Health Organization (18), the World Psychiatry Association (19), the NANDA (20), and Division 36 of the American Psychological Association (21).

Second and third, caregiving is a moral and humanistic experience (22) and, for most people, being spiritual also means being moral (23). Classical and theological virtues intertwine to form a large cluster of ethical principles, such as prudence, justice, courage, temperance, faith, hope, and charity (24). There principles are deeply embodied in clinical practice, as evident from the Hippocratic Oath (25). Thus, for most scholars, dealing with spirituality is reassuming the moral art of medicine, and considering each patient as the central focus of this practice (26).

Relationship between spirituality/religiosity and mental health

In order to conclude that S/R is an important technical competence that all mental healthcare professionals must address, we need to deepen our knowledge about the latest science about the impact of these factors on human mental health. The evidence is summarized in Table 7.1 compiling the results of two reviews (27, 28). A summary of the most important findings for each mental health issue is given below.

Table 7.1 Summary of scientific evidence on religion, spirituality, and mental health

Dimension	Number of original studies evaluated	Study outcomes
Depression	444	61%—inverse relationship/6%—direct relationship
Suicide	141	75%—inverse relationship/3%—direct relationship
Anxiety	299	49%—inverse relationship/11%—direct relationship
Psychotic disorders	43	33%—inverse relationship/23%—direct relationship
Substance use disorders	278	86%—inverse relationship/1%—direct relationship
Crime/delinquency	104	79%—inverse relationship/3%—direct relationship
Stress	75	61%—inverse relationship/12%—direct relationship
Marital instability	79	86%—inverse relationship/0%—direct relationship

Source: Data from Lucchese, F.A., Koenig, H.G. (2013). Religion, spirituality and cardiovascular disease: research, clinical implications, and opportunities in Brazil. *Brazilian Journal of Cardiovascular Surgery*. 28:103–28.

Depression, addiction, and suicide are among the most studied mental health issues, and there is good evidence for a positive association between higher levels of S/R and lower levels of these mental health disorder symptoms (supported by at least 66% of studies published) (27, 28). Furthermore, there is some evidence for the association of S/R with dementia and stress-related disorders, yet weak evidence for schizophrenia and bipolar disorders, and little evidence for other International Classification of Diseases-10 (ICD-10) mental health disorders and their association with mental health issues (29). The three most studied areas are outlined below.

Smith et al. (30) conducted a systematic review and meta-analysis of the studies involving religiousness and depressive symptoms. The authors found 147 independent studies, showing a weak but significant (correlation = −0.096, p<0.001) association between greater religiousness and depressive symptoms, regardless of age, gender, or ethnicity. When analysing each moderator variable separately, there was a negative and significant association between depressive symptoms and the intrinsic aspect of religiosity, and a positive and non-significant association between extrinsic religiosity and depression symptoms. This finding was later confirmed by McCullough and Larson (31). Recently, Braam and Koenig published a systematic review of prospective studies only, and found 152 studies with major heterogeneity. Of these studies, 49% reported at least one negative association between depressive symptoms and higher levels of R/S over time, with 41% showing no association and 10% presenting a positive association, supporting the role of R/S in depressive symptoms.

Substance use disorder is another important aspect highly studied in the area of R/S and mental health (32), even giving rise to a special edition of the *Substance Use and Misuse Journal* on this relationship (33). Evidence suggests there is a robust positive association between religiousness and lower levels of alcohol/drug use and abuse (Table 7.1) (34), and also of internet addiction (35). According to Borras et al. (34), there are four causal models to explain this association: (a) a personal belief experience may fill some essential need, decreasing the need to use substances; (b) continued exposure to church doctrines might influence behaviours; (c) religion might function as a social supportive group and; (d) religion might offer alternative coping strategies to deal with stress, reducing the need for substance use to manage painful emotions. Conversely, a neutral relationship was found in a qualitative study evaluating the impact of religiosity and meaning of death on suicidal ideation, substance abuse, and alcoholism in a sample of homeless people (36).

Suicide, as shown in Table 7.1, is also one of the most important aspects studied in the area of S/R and health (a 75% inverse relationship). Lawrence et al. (37) conducted a systematic review analysing several aspects of the religious dimension (affiliation, involvement, doctrine), and suicidal behaviour. They found 89 articles published in the past 10 years and concluded that, although data remains inconsistent, there is good evidence that religious attendance protects against suicide attempts, and possibly against suicide, even after adjusting for social support measures. Moreover, Wu et al. (38), in a meta-analysis, also found a protective pattern of religiosity against completed suicide (Odds Ratio (OR): 0.38; 95% Confidence Interval (CI): 0.21–0.71), confirmed by subanalyses with Western cultures, areas with religious homogeneity, and among older populations. Not surprisingly, in Eastern religious traditions and among young populations, religiosity did not appear to be a protective factor. There are several studies investigating the high rates of suicide in Eastern cultures (39, 40), and a different view of the significance of suicide in these areas (e.g. honour of dying by suicide) might play a role (41).

Despite all this evidence for the positive impact of S/R on mental health, there are some inverse associations between mental health issues and aspects of spirituality and/or religiosity (see Table 7.1). To give some examples, Leurent et al. (42) followed 8,318 general practice attendees across several countries, and evaluated S/R beliefs and mental health diagnoses of major depression. They found that people with more spiritual understanding had a higher risk of being depressed in the following year. Similarly, King et al. (43), in a cross-sectional study of 7,403 people from England, found that individuals who had a spiritual understanding of life without a religious root exhibited higher levels of mental health issues. This notion that being spiritual, but not religious, is a risk factor for psychiatry disorders was not confirmed by other studies (44, 45).

Religious and spiritual coping

With the release of the book, *The Psychology of Religion and Coping: Theory, Research, and Practice* (46), Pargament initiates a great discussion on how people use their religion/spiritual beliefs and practices to cope with life's stressful events and traumas. To date, many articles and scientific output have been published in this emerging area (47), with some scales developed to quantitatively investigate this subjective phenomena (48, 49). Kremer and Ironson (50), assessing 177 people living with HIV for 10 years, showed that the vast majority of patients (94%) used some kind of spiritual coping, with 85% using positive coping strategies (from some connection to a higher power to spiritual growth/transformation) and only 9% used negative coping strategies (from spiritual guilt to severe spiritual struggle). It is important to point out that most of these negative coping strategies could have been ameliorated if these patients had been given good spiritual support by care providers or religious leaders.

A number of articles have shown the association of positive R/S coping with lower levels of depression in HIV-infected gay men (51), lower cognitive symptoms of depression in elderly medical inpatients (52), better psychological adjustment at 3 and 12 months after kidney transplantation (53), and many others (54). Furthermore, negative spiritual coping has been associated with depressed mood in women at 3, 6, and 12 months after breast cancer diagnosis (55), and with higher severity of post-traumatic stress disorder in Iraq and Afghanistan war veterans (56). Similar associations between negative R/S coping and worse mental health outcomes were found in a sample of patients dealing with active Crohn's disease (57) and in a sample of family caregivers of paediatric cancer patients (58).

To better understand some R/S coping strategies used by most people, Pargament et al. (48) developed a scale to objectively evaluate these issues. Positive strategies used include religious purification/forgiveness, religious direction/conversion, religious helping, seeking support from clergy/members, collaborative religious coping, religious focus, active religious surrender, benevolent religious reappraisal, spiritual connection, and marking religious boundaries. Negative strategies were also used such as spiritual discontent, demonic reappraisal, passive religious deferral, interpersonal religious discontent, reappraisal of god's powers, punishing god reappraisal, and pleading for direct intercession and its frustration.

Religion and spirituality interventions on mental health

Religious and spiritual interventions are hard to conceptualize, and even harder to interpret, in clinical practice. First, there is no consensus on the definition of R/S (59, 60). Second, fitting both concepts within a group of practices referred to as 'R/S interventions' is challenging (61). And third, the issue of whether physicians should prescribe these practices or not is under debate (5).

Systematic reviews with meta-analysis addressing R/S interventions and their impact on patients' mental health have been conducted (61–66). McCullough (62) and Smith et al. (64) focused their review on psychological interventions, such as counselling and psychotherapy. The former found that religion-accommodative counselling, compared with standard approaches for depression, were not more efficacious and should be a matter of patient choice. The latter, not comparing with other standard interventions, found a beneficial effect of spirituality-oriented psychotherapy approaches in treating some kinds of psychiatry disorders, such as depression, anxiety, stress, and eating disorders.

Oh et al. (65) and, more recently, Xing et al. (66) evaluated the effects of spiritual interventions in patients with cancer. Both groups of authors concluded that, despite the high heterogeneity of data, there is weak evidence that spiritual interventions might reduce depression, anxiety, and hopelessness, and improve meaning and quality of life of cancer patients.

Gonçalves et al. (61), in an effort to reduce the heterogeneity of the data, conducted a meta-analysis of R/S interventions on mental health (healthy population, use/abuse of alcohol/drugs, post-trauma stress, schizophrenia, migraine, depression, and anxiety), grouping them into four groups of practices: pastoral services, spiritual/religious meditation, psychotherapy, and audiovisual sources. Meta-analysis was possible only for depression and anxiety.

Despite the lack of studies found by Gonçalves et al. (61), there was positive evidence of the impact of R/S interventions on the mental health of the healthy population (67, 68), patients with alcohol use disorder (69), post-trauma stress disorder (70, 71), schizophrenia (72), and migraine (73). For anxiety and depression, a meta-analysis was conducted. Authors found a statistically significant impact of R/S interventions for reducing anxiety symptoms, with important differences for two subgroups: spiritual medication and psychotherapy. However, there was only a tendency (not significant) for the impact of R/S interventions in reducing depressive symptoms.

Proposed mechanisms of religion and spirituality influence on mental health

Studies seek to elucidate the mechanisms by which R/S influences mental health. The most accepted and studied mechanism available for the influence of R/S on mental health was proposed by Koenig et al. (74). According to these authors, spiritual and religious beliefs are associated with human virtues, such as honesty, forgiveness, altruism, gratefulness, patience, dependability, and diligence. All these human virtues may be potentially related to social relationships/support, and ultimately responsible for positive or negative mental health. Finally, factors such as genetics, temperament, and character could also influence this relationship.

Besides this model, other factors might have an impact on this relationship, such as adherence to therapy, risky behaviours, and use and abuse of substances. In research identifying biological markers for the impact of R/S on health, researchers have found that individuals with higher spiritual and religious beliefs have lower levels of cortisol (75), C-reactive protein (76), fibrinogen (77), inflammatory interleukins (e.g. IL–6) (78), better immunity (79), and autonomic control (80). However, it remains unclear how these biological factors have an impact on mental disorders or mental health issues.

Recently, authors have attempted to identify more specific markers of the relationship between spiritual and religious beliefs and mental health. Individuals with higher R/S had higher levels of brain-derived neurotrophic factor (81), while individuals with higher levels of self-transcendence had higher serotonin transporter (SERT) availability in brainstem raphe nuclei. There are also possible genetic correlates for the genes for dopamine, serotonin, their vesicular transporter, and oxytocin, which could play a potential role in this relationship (82). All these studies are preliminary and results should be interpreted with caution.

Implications for clinical practice

Arguably, there are many implications for clinical practice, especially for mental health practitioners. As seen above in section 2, most patients want their S/R addressed. However, few mental health practitioners are able and/or trained to fulfil this need (7–11). In spite of this unmet need, there is a large body of evidence suggesting that addressing S/R might improve patient satisfaction following treatment (11, 83), and also reduce medical costs (15). Furthermore, the evidence associating S/R and mental health (positively and negatively) is solid and physicians should address this issue in clinical encounters to provide more integrative care.

Conclusion

There is a large body of evidence with regard to the impact of R/S on mental health, particularly for the impact on suicidal behaviour, substance use and abuse, and depression. Furthermore, a growing number of studies suggest that R/S might also be a positive coping behaviour after a stressful/painful event, with studies promoting spiritual or religious interventions in individuals with mental health issues. Finally, R/S can also have a negative impact on mental health for some patients. Mental health professionals should be trained to deal with all human dilemmas and issues (physical, mental, social, spiritual) in order to provide the best medical care applying knowledge on the best technical competences, while also observing ethical principles and humanistic virtues.

References

1. Freud S. *Introductory lectures on psychoanalysis*. New York: Norton; 1977.
2. Freud S. *The future of an illusion*. New York: Norton; 1927.
3. Dein S. Against the stream: religion and mental health—the case for the inclusion of religion and spirituality into psychiatric care. *BJPsych Bulletin*. 2018;**42**(3):127–9.
4. Sloan RP, Bagiella E, Powell T. Religion, spirituality, and medicine. *Lancet*. 1999;**353**(9153):664–7.
5. Sloan RP, Bagiella E, VandeCreek L, Hover M, Casalone C, Hirsch TJ, et al. Should physicians prescribe religious activities? *New England Journal of Medicine*. 2000;**342**(25):1913–6.
6. Stonawski M, Skirbekk V, Potančoková M. *The future of world religions: population growth projections, 2010–2050*. Pew Research Center; 2015. Assessed in May 16, 2021.https://assets.pewresearch.org/wp-content/uploads/sites/11/2015/03/PF_15.04.02_ProjectionsFullReport.pdf
7. Banin LB, Suzart NB, Guimaraes FA, Lucchetti AL, de Jesus MA, Lucchetti G. Religious beliefs or physicians' behavior: what makes a patient more prone to accept a physician to address his/her spiritual issues? *Journal of Religion and Health*. 2014;**53**(3):917–28.
8. Ehman JW, Ott BB, Short TH, Ciampa RC, Hansen-Flaschen J. Do patients want physicians to inquire about their spiritual or religious beliefs if they become gravely ill? *Archives of Internal Medicine*. 1999;**159**(15):1803–6.
9. King DE, Bushwick B. Beliefs and attitudes of hospital inpatients about faith healing and prayer. *Journal of Family Practice*. 1994;**39**(4):349–52.
10. MacLean CD, Susi B, Phifer N, Schultz L, Bynum D, Franco M, et al. Patient preference for physician discussion and practice of spirituality. *Journal of General Internal Medicine*. 2003;**18**(1):38–43.

11. **Williams JA, Meltzer D, Arora V, Chung G, Curlin FA.** Attention to inpatients' religious and spiritual concerns: predictors and association with patient satisfaction. *Journal of General Internal Medicine.* 2011;**26**(11):1265–71.

12. **Moreira-Almeida A, Koenig HG, Lucchetti G.** Clinical implications of spirituality to mental health: review of evidence and practical guidelines. *Brazilian Journal of Psychiatry.* 2014;**36**(2):176–82.

13. **Silva AF, Junior DI, Gonçalves LM, Ribeiro MRC, Damiano RF.** *Uma nova medicina para um novo milênio: a humanização do ensino médico.* São Paulo, Brazil: AME-Brasil; 2016.

14. **Lucchetti G, Lucchetti AGL, Badan-Neto AM, Peres PT, Peres MFP, Moreira-Almeida A, et al.** Religiousness affects mental health, pain and quality of life in older people in an outpatient rehabilitation setting. *Journal of Rehabilitation Medicine.* 2011;**43**(4):316–22.

15. **Balboni T, Balboni M, Paulk ME, Phelps A, Wright A, Peteet J, et al.** Support of cancer patients' spiritual needs and associations with medical care costs at the end of life. *Cancer.* 2011;**117**(23):5383–91.

16. **Lucchetti G, Lucchetti AL.** Spirituality, religion, and health: over the last 15 years of field research (1999–2013). *International Journal of Psychiatry in Medicine.* 2014;**48**(3):199–215.

17. Colleges AoAM. Report III: Contemporary issues in medicine: communication in medicine. Washington, DC: Association of American Medical Colleges (AAMC), 1999, 29 p. Assessed in May 16, 2021.

18. **Group WS.** A cross-cultural study of spirituality, religion, and personal beliefs as components of quality of life. *Social Science & Medicine.* 2006;**62**(6):1486–97.

19. **World Psychiatry Association (WPA)** [Internet]. 2016. WPA position statement on spirituality and religion in psychiatry; April [cited 15 December 2019]. WPA, Geneva, Switzerland. Available from: https://onlinelibrary.wiley.com/doi/full/10.1002/wps.20304.

20. **Internacional N.** *Diagnósticos de enfermagem da NANDA-I: definições e classificação 2018–2020.* Eleventh edition. Porto Alegre: Artmed; 2018.

21. **American Psychological Association. Society for the psychology of religion and spirituality–division 36** [Internet]. United States: APA; 2019 [cited 2019 December 15]. Available from: https://www.apadivisions.org/division-36.

22. **Kleinman A.** Caregiving as moral experience. *Lancet.* 2012;**380**(9853):1550–1.

23. **Van Slyke JA.** Understanding the moral dimension of spirituality: insights from virtue ethics and moral exemplars. *Journal of Psychology and Christianity.* 2015;**34**(3):205–15.

24. **Porter J.** Virtue ethics and its significance for spirituality. *The Way Supplement.* 1997;**88**:26–35.

25. **Antoniou SA, Antoniou GA, Granderath FA, Mavroforou A, Giannoukas AD, Antoniou AI.** Reflections of the Hippocratic Oath in modern medicine. *World Journal of Surgery.* 2010;**34**(12):3075–9.

26. **Korup AK, Sondergaard J, Lucchetti G, Ramakrishnan P, Baumann K, Lee E, et al.** Religious values of physicians affect their clinical practice: a meta-analysis of individual participant data from 7 countries. *Medicine.* 2019;**98**(38):e17265.

27. **Koenig HG.** Religion, spirituality, and health: the research and clinical implications. *ISRN Psychiatry.* 2012;**2012**:278730.

28. **Lucchese FA, Koenig HG.** Religion, spirituality and cardiovascular disease: research, clinical implications, and opportunities in Brazil. *Brazilian Journal of Cardiovascular Surgery.* 2013;**28**:103–28.

29. **Bonelli RM, Koenig HG.** Mental disorders, religion and spirituality 1990 to 2010: a systematic evidence-based review. *Journal of Religion and Health.* 2013;**52**(2):657–73.

30. **Smith TB, McCullough ME, Poll J.** Religiousness and depression: evidence for a main effect and the moderating influence of stressful life events. *Psychological Bulletin.* 2003;**129**(4):614.

31. **McCullough ME, Larson DB.** Religion and depression: a review of the literature. *Twin Research and Human Genetics.* 1999;**2**(2):126–36.

32. **Moreira-Almeida A, Neto FL, Koenig HG.** Religiousness and mental health: a review. *Revista Brasileira de Psiquiatria* (Sao Paulo, Brazil: 1999). 2006;**28**(3):242–50.

33. **Allamani A, Godlaski TM, Einstein SS.** Spirituality, religion, and addiction: a possible epilogue. *Subst Use Misuse.* 2013;**48**(12):1262–6.

34. **Borras L, Khazaal Y, Khan R, Mohr S, Kaufmann YA, Zullino D,** et al. The relationship between addiction and religion and its possible implication for care. *Substance Use and Misuse.* 2010;**45**(14):2357–410.

35. **Nadeem M, Buzdar MA, Shakir M, Naseer S.** The association Between Muslim religiosity and internet addiction among young adult college students. *Journal of Religion and Health.* 2019; **58**(6):1953–60.

36. **Testoni I, Russotto S, Zamperini A, Leo D.** Addiction and religiosity in facing suicide: a qualitative study on meaning of life and death among homeless people. *Mental Illness.* 2018;**10**(1):7420.

37. **Lawrence RE, Oquendo MA, Stanley B.** Religion and suicide risk: a systematic review. *Archives of Suicide Research: Official Journal of the International Academy for Suicide Research.* 2016;**20**(1):1–21.

38. **Wu A, Wang JY, Jia CX.** Religion and completed suicide: a meta-analysis. *PloS One.* 2015;**10**(6):e0131715.

39. **Kino S, Jang SN, Gero K, Kato S, Kawachi I.** Age, period, cohort trends of suicide in Japan and Korea (1986–2015): a tale of two countries. *Social Science & Medicine* 2019;**235**:112385.

40. **Kanwal S, Perveen S, Sumbla Y.** Causes and severity of suicide in developed nations of East Asia. *Journal of Pakistan Medical Association.* 2017;**67**(10):1588–92.

41. **Pierre JM.** Culturally sanctioned suicide: euthanasia, seppuku, and terrorist martyrdom. *World Journal of Psychiatry.* 2015;**5**(1):4–14.

42. **Leurent B, Nazareth I, Bellon-Saameno J, Geerlings MI, Maaroos H, Saldivia S,** et al. Spiritual and religious beliefs as risk factors for the onset of major depression: an international cohort study. *Psychological Medicine.* 2013;**43**(10):2109–20.

43. **King M, Marston L, McManus S, Brugha T, Meltzer H, Bebbington P.** Religion, spirituality and mental health: results from a national study of English households. *The British Journal of Psychiatry.* 2013;**202**(1):68–73.

44. **Farias M, Underwood R, Claridge G.** Unusual but sound minds: mental health indicators in spiritual individuals. *British Journal of Psychology.* 2013;**104**(3):364–81.

45. **Peres MFP, Kamei HH, Tobo PR, Lucchetti G.** Mechanisms behind religiosity and spirituality's effect on mental health, quality of life and well-being. *Journal of Religion and Health.* 2018;**57**(5):1842–55.

46. **Pargament KI.** *The psychology of religion and coping: theory, research, practice.* New York: Guilford Press; 1997. pp. xii, 548–xii.

47. **Gall TL, Guirguis-Younger M.** Religious and spiritual coping: current theory and research. In: *APA handbook of psychology, religion, and spirituality. Volume 1: Context, theory, and research.* APA handbooks in psychology. Washington, DC: American Psychological Association; 2013. pp. 349–64.

48. **Pargament KI, Koenig HG, Perez LM.** The many methods of religious coping: development and initial validation of the RCOPE. *Journal of Clinical Psychology.* 2000;**56**(4):519–43.

49. **Panzini RG, Bandeira DR.** Escala de coping religioso-espiritual (Escala CRE): elaboração e validação de construto. *Psicologia em Estudo.* 2005;**10**:507–16.

50. **Kremer H, Ironson G.** Longitudinal spiritual coping with trauma in people with HIV: implications for health care. *AIDS Patient Care and STDs.* 2014;**28**(3):144–54.

51. **Woods TE, Antoni MH, Ironson GH, Kling DW.** Religiosity is associated with affective and immune status in symptomatic HIV-infected gay men. *Journal of Psychosomatic Research.* 1999;**46**(2):165–76.

52. **Koenig HG, Cohen HJ, Blazer DG, Kudler HS, Krishnan KR, Sibert TE.** Religious coping and cognitive symptoms of depression in elderly medical patients. *Psychosomatics.* 1995;**36**(4):369–75.

53. **Tix AP, Frazier PA.** The use of religious coping during stressful life events: main effects, moderation, and mediation. *Journal of Consulting and Clinical Psychology.* 1998;**66**(2):411–22.

54. **Panzini RG, Bandeira DR.** Coping (enfrentamento) religioso/espiritual. *Archives of Clinical Psychiatry* (São Paulo). 2007;**34**:126–35.

55. **Gall TL, Bilodeau C.** The role of positive and negative religious/spiritual coping in women's adjustment to breast cancer: A longitudinal study. *Journal of Psychosocial Oncology.* 2019;**38**(1):103–7.

56. **Park CL, Smith PH, Lee SY, Mazure CM, McKee SA, Hoff R.** Positive and Negative Religious/Spiritual Coping and Combat Exposure as Predictors of Posttraumatic Stress and Perceived Growth in Iraq and Afghanistan Veterans. *Psychology of Religion and Spirituality.* 2017;**9**(1):13–20.

57. **de Campos R, Lucchetti G, Lucchetti ALG, da Rocha Ribeiro TC, Chebli LA, Malaguti C, et al.** The impact of spirituality and religiosity on mental health and quality of life of patients with active Crohn's disease. *Journal of Religion and Health.* 2019; Mar 25. doi: 10.1007/s10943-019-00801-1. [Epub ahead of print].

58. **Vitorino LM, Lopes-Junior LC, de Oliveira GH, Tenaglia M, Brunheroto A, Cortez PJO, et al.** Spiritual and religious coping and depression among family caregivers of pediatric cancer patients in Latin America. *Psycho-Oncology.* 2018;**27**(8):1900–7.

59. **Gall TL, Malette J, Guirguis-Younger M.** Spirituality and Religiousness: A Diversity of Definitions. *Journal of Spirituality in Mental Health.* 2011;**13**(3):158–81.

60. **Hill PC, Pargament KI, Hood RW, McCullough J, Michael E., Swyers JP, Larson DB, et al.** Conceptualizing religion and spirituality: points of commonality, points of departure. *Journal for the Theory of Social Behaviour.* 2000;**30**(1):51–77.

61. **Gonçalves JP, Lucchetti G, Menezes PR, Vallada H.** Religious and spiritual interventions in mental health care: a systematic review and meta-analysis of randomized controlled clinical trials. *Psychological Medicine.* 2015;**45**(14):2937–49.

62. **McCullough ME.** Research on religion-accommodative counseling: review and meta-analysis. *Journal of Counseling Psychology.* 1999;**46**(1):92–8.

63. **Oh PJ, Kim YH.** Meta-analysis of spiritual intervention studies on biological, psychological, and spiritual outcomes. *Journal of Korean Academy of Nursing.* 2012;**42**(6):833–42.

64. **Smith TB, Bartz J, Scott Richards P.** Outcomes of religious and spiritual adaptations to psychotherapy: a meta-analytic review. *Psychotherapy Research.* 2007;**17**(6):643–55.

65. **Oh PJ, Kim SH.** The effects of spiritual interventions in patients with cancer: a meta-analysis. *Oncology Nursing Forum.* 2014;**41**(5):E290–301.

66. **Xing L, Guo X, Bai L, Qian J, Chen J.** Are spiritual interventions beneficial to patients with cancer? A meta-analysis of randomized controlled trials following PRISMA. *Medicine* (Baltimore). 2018;**97**(35):e11948.

67. **Oman D, Hedberg J, Thoresen CE.** Passage meditation reduces perceived stress in health professionals: a randomized, controlled trial. *Journal of Consulting and Clinical Psychology* 2006;**74**(4):714–9.

68. **Wachholtz AB, Pargament KI.** Is spirituality a critical ingredient of meditation? Comparing the effects of spiritual meditation, secular meditation, and relaxation on spiritual, psychological, cardiac, and pain outcomes. *Journal of Behavioral Medicine* 2005;**28**(4):369–84.

69. **Kelly JF, Stout RL, Magill M, Tonigan JS, Pagano ME.** Spirituality in recovery: a lagged mediational analysis of Alcoholics Anonymous' principal theoretical mechanism of behavior change. *Alcoholism: Clinical and Experimental Research.* 2011;**35**(3):454–63.

70. **Bormann JE, Thorp S, Wetherell JL, Golshan S.** A spiritually based group intervention for combat veterans with posttraumatic stress disorder: feasibility study. *Journal of Holistic Nursing.* 2008;**26**(2):109–16.

71. **Bowland S, Edmond T, Fallot RD.** Evaluation of a spiritually focused intervention with older trauma survivors. *Social Work.* 2012;**57**(1):73–82.

72. **Huguelet P, Mohr S, Betrisey C, Borras L, Gillieron C, Marie AM,** et al. A randomized trial of spiritual assessment of outpatients with schizophrenia: patients' and clinicians' experience. *Psychiatric Services* (Washington, DC). 2011;**62**(1):79–86.

73. **Wachholtz AB, Pargament KI.** Migraines and meditation: does spirituality matter? *Journal of Behavioral Medicine.* 2008;**31**(4):351–66.

74. **Koenig H, King D, Carson V.** *Handbook of religion and health.* USA: Oxford University Press; 2012. 1169 p.

75. **Anyfantakis D, Symvoulakis EK, Panagiotakos DB, Tsetis D, Castanas E, Shea S,** et al. Impact of religiosity/spirituality on biological and preclinical markers related to cardiovascular disease. Results from the SPILI III study. *Hormones* (Athens). 2013;**12**(3):386–96.

76. **King DE, Mainous AG 3rd, Steyer TE, Pearson W.** The relationship between attendance at religious services and cardiovascular inflammatory markers. *International Journal of Psychiatry in Medicine.* 2001;**31**(4):415–25.

77. **Loucks EB, Berkman LF, Gruenewald TL, Seeman TE.** Social integration is associated with fibrinogen concentration in elderly men. *Psychosomatic Medicine.* 2005;**67**(3):353–8.

78. **Lutgendorf SK, Russell D, Ullrich P, Harris TB, Wallace R.** Religious participation, interleukin-6, and mortality in older adults. *Health Psychology: Official Journal of the Division of Health Psychology*, American Psychological Association. 2004;**23**(5):465–75.

79. **Dalmida SG, Holstad MM, Diiorio C, Laderman G.** Spiritual well-being, depressive symptoms, and immune status among women living with HIV/AIDS. *Women Health.* 2009;**49**(2–3):119–43.

80. **Berntson GG, Norman GJ, Hawkley LC, Cacioppo JT.** Spirituality and autonomic cardiac control. *Annals of Behavioral Medicine.* 2008;**35**(2):198–208.

81. **Mosqueiro BP, Fleck MP, da Rocha NS.** Increased levels of brain-derived neurotrophic factor are associated with high intrinsic religiosity among depressed inpatients. *Frontiers in Psychiatry.* 2019;**10**:671.

82. **Anderson MR, Miller L, Wickramaratne P, Svob C, Odgerel Z, Zhao R,** et al. Genetic correlates of spirituality/religion and depression: a study in offspring and grandchildren at high and low familial risk for depression. *Spirituality in Clinical Practice* (Washington, DC). 2017;**4**(1):43–63.

83. **Clark PA, Drain M, Malone MP.** Addressing patients' emotional and spiritual needs. *Joint Commission Journal on Quality and Safety.* 2003;**29**(12):659–70.

Chapter 8

Mechanisms: Religion's impact on mental health

Harold G. Koenig

Introduction

Research has gradually accumulated, over the past 30 years in particular, that has examined the impact of religion/spirituality (R/S) on mental health. Much of that research indicates positive effects, although not all. R/S can and often is utilized in a neurotic manner to adversely affect a person's mental health and relationships with others. A number of authors have emphasized this side of religion (1–3). Like it or not, religions are composed of people, and people have issues that drive them to manipulate others and their sacred belief systems for self-gain. But, for the vast majority of humanity, the research when examined objectively seems to indicate that religion affects mental health in ways that promote healthy attitudes, increase self-control and positive health behaviours, enhance interpersonal relationships, improve coping with stress, and increase ability to function in the face of adversity.

There are now many descriptive studies, innumerable cross-sectional studies, a number of very large, well-designed prospective studies, and several carefully conducted randomized clinical trials that document the positive impact that religion can have (4–6). For example, depending on the particular part of the world that one examines, rates of religious coping (the use of religion to adapt to stressful life experiences) exceed 90% (7, 8–11). Not only do many people around the world report that religious faith helps them to deal with difficult life circumstances, but when objectively assessing mental health through the use of quantitative methodology, those who are more religious and more engaged in religious practice generally appear to have better mental health—especially in the face of chronic disabling medical illness, loss, and unwanted change (7, 12, 13). Recent prospective studies report that frequency of religious attendance or importance of R/S in life predicts a lower likelihood of developing depression (14, 15) and of committing suicide (16, 17). Likewise, many observational studies (both cross-sectional and longitudinal) now show that religious involvement predicts greater well-being, happiness, life satisfaction, sense of purpose, optimism and hope, social support, and marital and family stability (5), including a number of recent studies (18–20).

These findings from observational studies are supported by results from randomized clinical trials that report benefits from religiously integrated forms of cognitive behavioural therapy (21, 22) and other R/S approaches to mental health problems such as depression or anxiety (23–25). These treatments produce large effect sizes in terms of reducing symptoms (26). For example, Koenig and colleagues found that 10 sessions of religiously integrated psychotherapy delivered remotely by telephone for major depression achieved an effect size (d) from baseline to follow-up of exceeding 3.0, where effect sizes of 0.80 or higher are considered large (27, 5, p. 270). Thus, taken together, qualitative studies reporting the frequent use of and benefits from religion when coping with stress, numerous prospective studies demonstrating that R/S predicts fewer negative and more positive emotions over time, and randomized clinical trials demonstrating the effectiveness of R/S interventions for emotional disorders provide evidence of positive effects on mental health.

This evidence base is now large enough for academic institutions such as Emory University (28), University of California at Berkeley School of Public Health (29), and the Harvard School of Public Health (30) to initiate courses to train graduate students in public health about the importance of religious involvement for preserving the health and well-being of populations. Medical schools in the United States (31), the United Kingdom (32), and South America (33) have long had courses teaching future doctors about this research and training them on how to identify and address the spiritual needs of patients. The same holds true for mental health professionals out in practice (34, 35).

But, the question remains, how does religious involvement have an impact on mental health? What are the underlying genetic, psychological, social, behavioural, environmental, and physiological mechanisms that might help to explain this effect? In this chapter, I will describe a number of mechanisms that may help to explain how religion enhances mental health. As the reader will see, if one or more of these mechanisms are correct, the research findings thus far supporting a connection between R/S and mental health may only be 'the tip of the iceberg'. As research advances and becomes more accurate in its measurement of R/S involvement, adopts research designs that examine exposure to religion across the lifespan (religious history), and uses new statistical methods to more sensitively identify and more fully capture such effects, the benefits of religious faith and practice may become more evident than they have heretofore (potentially dwarfing many other pathways to good mental health and greater well-being). Yes, I understand that this is quite an extraordinary claim and its objective documentation will be a tall task for researchers in the future. For now, though, let us explore seven possible mechanisms by which religious beliefs, devout commitment to those beliefs, and regular religious practice might help to uncover that iceberg.

Religious determinants of mental health

Religion's effects on mental health likely begin before birth (through genetic influences passed down from parents and grandparents), continue after implantation of the embryo in the womb, and then persist after the infant is born and from then on. Intrauterine development is when the mother's religious involvement is affecting the brain, central nervous system, and endocrine system development of the growing fetus, possibly even affecting weight at birth (36). That influence will continue to affect mental health and resiliency throughout the life course, from early infancy through childhood, adolescence, young adulthood, middle age, old age, all the way to the end of life (or at least as long as the person is conscious and aware, and maybe even after that through the influence of those who care for them, who may be influenced by their own religious beliefs). Fig. 8.1 describes seven pathways through which religion may

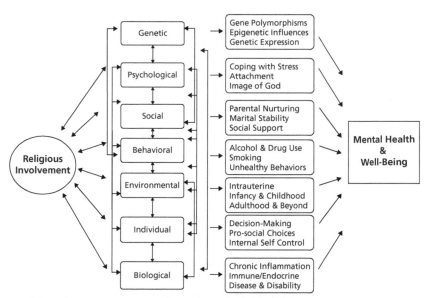

Fig. 8.1 Mechanisms by which religious or spiritual involvement may have an impact on mental health

Adapted with permission from Koenig, H.G. (2018). *Religion on Mental Health: Research and Applications.* Cambridge, UK: Elsevier.

have an impact on mental health. Taking the lifespan approach just described, I begin with genetic determinants.

Genetic pathways

Admittedly, research in this areas barely in its infancy, and there are no firm conclusions that can be made at this time. However, there is some evidence that genes transmit tendencies toward or away from R/S involvement, and those genes may also be associated with vulnerability to mental disorders and substance abuse. These studies indicate a link between religiosity and certain forms (or genotypes) of the serotonin transporter gene (SLCA4), serotonin receptor gene (HTR1A), alcohol dehydrogenase (ADH) gene, and dopamine gene (SNP rs1800497).

For example, the SS/SL genotypes of the SLCA4 gene are known to confer increased risk for drug use/abuse and depression; this genotype has also been shown to be less common in highly religious individuals, who are more likely to have the LL genotype (37, 22 or 27). Genetic factors have also been known to affect responsiveness to mental health treatments, both medications (38) and psychotherapy (39). We have found that medically ill patients with major depression who have the C/C genotype of the HTR1A [5-Hydroxytryptamine Receptor 1A; serotonin receptor gene] appear to be more responsive to religiously integrated CBT [cognitive behavioral therapy] than to conventional CBT, especially those who are less religious—as surprising as that may seem (22 or 27).

Research also suggests that the inverse relationship between R/S and drug or alcohol use/abuse may in part be explained by genetic factors that protect those who are more religious. For example, Chartier et al. (2016; 40) found that R/S modifies the relationship between high-risk alcohol dehydrogenase genotypes and alcohol use/dependence, finding that the relationship between the two is weaker among those who are more religious.

In a third study, researchers at Columbia University examined associations between the importance of R/S and the presence of single nucleotide polymorphisms of serotonin, dopamine, oxytocin, and monoamine vesicular transporter genes in those at high risk for depression (i.e. had a family history of major depression [MD] and those at low risk (41). Results indicated that among those at low risk (LR) for depression, R/S was significantly and inversely related to the minor allele of the serotonin gene, but was significantly and positively associated with the major allele of the oxytocin gene, monoamine vesicular transporter gene, and, most importantly, the major allele of the dopamine gene (SNP rs1800497). The minor allele (A) of the dopamine gene (SNP rs1800497) was also related to greater lifetime risk of MD. Thus, among those at LR for

MD, those high on R/S were less likely to have the minor allele (A) of the dopamine gene. The minor allele (A) is known to produce reduced brain dopamine binding and reduced receptor density, increasing risk for mood disorders. This could explain why those at low risk for MD who were also high on R/S were protected from MD.

Psychological

The primary way R/S influences mental health more directly is likely through psychological, social, and behavioural pathways, perhaps through psychological mechanisms more so than either social or behavioural. Religious beliefs and practices represent powerful coping behaviors for dealing with change, loss, trauma, and difficult life circumstances. The ability to adapt to the 'slings and arrows of outrageous fortune' that typify daily life for most humans is key to resilience and maintenance of good mental health. Such adaptation is often facilitated by religion, based on what is known from systematic research.

Many people in both developed and developing regions of the world continue to report in literally hundreds of qualitative studies that religion helps them to cope. Religious beliefs give meaning to life events, both traumatic and non-traumatic, provide a sense of control over uncontrollable events, and help to establish life priorities that often foster mental health. In the aftermath of September 11, which killed nearly 3,000 Americans, nearly 9 out of 10 people in the United States turned to religion to cope with the anxiety and trauma stirred up by these terrorist attacks (9). Likewise, when traumatized people in Afghanistan were asked how they coped with war and their devastating losses, 98% indicated 'Allah' (even more often than they mentioned family—that is, 81%) (10). In a study of Tibetan refugees in India, more than 90% indicated that their religious practices were key to their resilience (42); in a study of women with breast cancer in Chile, South America, 96% indicated that they depended on their religious beliefs to cope (43); and in a study of parents of children with cancer in the United Arab Emirates, 100% reported that they coped through religious faith (44). These are just a few examples of the widespread use of religion to cope with stress by many people throughout the world. This does not mean, however, that people everywhere turn to religion in response to life's trials. Indeed, in places like northern Europe and east Asia, religious coping is much less frequent (10% or less, even among those with terminal cancer) (5, p 60).

With regard to establishing priorities, monotheistic religions uniformly maintain that a connection with God should be most important in life. This is the First Commandment in Judaism, the first of the two great commandments in Christianity, and the primary teaching in Islam (the word 'Islam' means 'submission to God'). This preference is to be followed by family and community. This primary 'attachment' to God in monotheism has the same effect as that described by the Buddha for non-attachment in the Eightfold Path—an ordering of life that reduces pain, anxiety, and depression over losses, and instead increases peace and happiness. As long as the connection to the Divine remains intact, the loss of other attachment objects is less important and produces less suffering. Although suffering may not be eliminated, it is at least reduced down to a size and magnitude that is more manageable. Rather than bearing the entire burden of the loss, believers say God helps and accompanies them through their pain. Indeed, there is growing research showing that mental health is better when a person's attachment to God is 'secure', and, when that is present, religious activity is even more helpful in preserving well-being in the face of adversity (see 45, 46, 20, 47).

Of course, the mental health consequences of attachment to God may depend on what the person believes about the nature and intentions of the Divine. Does the person believe in a powerful and strong but loving and caring God, or a God that is powerful, controlling, and judgemental, or perhaps a God that is distant, impersonal, or uncaring? These beliefs are likely to affect the individual's interpretation of negative life events. Are the losses and traumas in life due to an extraordinary (but often poorly understood) tapestry that is being woven by a good God who has a person's (and others') best interests in mind, or are they a result of punishment from a police-like God trying to catch people in their mistakes? There has been considerable research now examining the relationship between 'image of God' and mental health that supports such observations (48, 45, 49, 50). The person who believes in and feels loved, accepted, and cared for by God is much more likely to experience mental health benefits from such a relationship, particularly in the face of stressful life circumstances, than the individual who views the Divine as punishing, vengeful, or distant (51–53).

Social

There is no doubt that many of the effects of religion on mental health are conveyed by social influences (social support, social integration). Some researchers, in fact, have claimed that the effect of religion on mental health is entirely due to social factors (54). Other investigators, however, have reported that social influences make up less than 25% of the total effect of religious involvement on mental health and health more generally (55, 16, 56). Not only has this been reported by experts in public health and psychology, but the same has been found by sociologists of religion who report that social factors explain only a relatively small proportion of the effect of R/S on mental health (57). Besides social influences, other factors contribute as well—particularly psychological, behavioural, and environmental ones.

Although improved social pathways are unlikely to be the only way that R/S influences mental health, they are definitely one way—given the strong relationship between social support and mental health. Indeed, R/S involvement has been linked with greater social support in over 80% of studies examining this relationship (58, 5). Religiously motivated social support appears to be more resilient and long-lasting than secular forms of support that are based purely on transaction (you scratch my back and I'll scratch yours, but only as long as you scratch my back). The reason is because religion-driven social support is not only based on transaction but also on strong religious teachings that encourage care of neighbour, particularly the neighbour in distress.

Other social influences of religion include the emphasis placed by many religions on family, childbearing, and the nurturing of children, which is likely to have intergenerational effects as discussed earlier. Religious involvement is related to greater marital satisfaction, marital stability, less family member abuse, and better relationships with children. In our systematic review of research conducted prior to 2010, we found that 68 of 79 quantitative studies (86%) reported significantly greater marital satisfaction and stability among those who were more religious (58). Reduced rates of delinquency, crime, and substance abuse, and increased life satisfaction and well-being among youth raised in religious families provides further evidence for the benefits that R/S has on the mental health of children through supportive family relationships (5, 18).

Besides strengthening social support and family functioning, religion also influences human interactions that often adversely affect health such as discrimination and stigma that lead to social ostracization. There is growing evidence that R/S may help to buffer the negative mental health effects of such experiences, even while in some cases contributing to them (e.g. discrimination towards gays/lesbians). A number of investigators have now found that among minority populations (Blacks, Hispanics, Muslims, gay/lesbian/transsexuals, etc.) who are more religious, the positive relationship between discrimination and poor mental health is weaker—that I, R/S moderates the negative effects on mental health that such social interactions have (59–63). While not true in all cases, most of the world's major religions promote the support of and demonstration of compassion for outsider groups that are viewed as vulnerable, such as the intellectually disabled, the sick, the poor, victims of natural disasters, foreigners, and other excluded population groups. Faith-based delivery of mental health services and disaster relief are well known (Salvation Army, and many mainstream Protestant and Catholic organizations; see (64, 65), underscoring the prosocial attitudes of many religious groups.

Environment

Many environmental factors influence mental health, especially those that are present during infancy and childhood. Religious involvement of parents and peers is crucial in shaping the kind of environment in which an infant, child, and later teenager will either flourish or flounder. Environments in which alcohol and drugs are not used, children are valued, the marriage of parents is stable and loving, and role models with solid character are available, will increase the likelihood that a child grows up mentally stable, happy, and productive. All these factors, as noted earlier, have been associated with greater religious involvement (58, 5, 18).

The environment provided by peers is also an important one, especially for adolescents and teenagers. When involved in religious activities and youth groups with others who must abide by the same standards as themselves, these youth have a better chance of developing habits and attitudes that foster mental health and well-being. The presence of positive role models in religious teachers, clergy, and members of the congregation also provide a positive environment for emotional growth, maturation, and the development of healthy coping behaviors in response to life stressors.

Finally, as an adult, membership in a religious community, attendance at religious functions, and engagement in religious volunteer activities provide an environment where individuals are surrounded by those with common positive values. The religious subculture often puts pressure on members to behave in a prosocial manner, places a priority on marriage and the raising of children, and emphasizes the need to be honest, hard-working, and responsible. Such pressures reduce the likelihood of crime and imprisonment, sexual promiscuity, divorce, auto accidents (from substance use or reckless driving), and being fired from one's job. Fewer stressful events of this nature will likely have an impact on mental health and functioning. The traits encouraged by most religions increase the likelihood that a person will have the resources to enable them to live in a safe neighborhood away from drugs and crime, and have a support network of friends and neighbours who share their values. Remember, though, that religious involvement is often greatest in poverty-stricken high-crime neighborhoods because it may be the only safe haven that people can turn to in order to survive.

Behaviours

The discouragement of alcohol/drug use and sex outside marriage, and the encouragement of behaviours that promote character building and development of moral values are all high priorities of religious organizations as part of religious education. Less alcohol use and abuse, drug addiction, and smoking, and more self-discipline, ability to handle responsibility, honesty, and prosocial behaviors, as noted earlier, are known to be associated with mental health and well-being, academic success, better job performance, and the presence of health insurance for medical and psychiatric care if needed.

Individual level

Closely related to behaviour are the daily decisions that people make, decisions about how to spend time, decisions related to pursuing goals in life, decisions on how to respond to others at work, and how to treat family members and friends. These decisions will be guided by moral values and religious beliefs day by day, hour by hour, minute by minute. Religious beliefs promote decisions that are prosocial and less self-centered, leading to both the person's own well-being and the well-being of others. Of course, this does not apply to radicalized forms of religion that emphasize doing harm to those who believe differently.

As indicated repeatedly earlier in this chapter, religion promotes prosocial decisions. In fact, religious involvement is one of the strongest predictors of what is called 'social capital'. Social capital is a measure of a community's 'culture of trust and tolerance' (66, p. 188) and is reflected by frequent volunteering, community and political involvement, and the degree to which people work with one another to solve problems that are common to all. In our systematic review of the literature, of 14 studies that quantitatively examined the relationship between community religious involvement and social capital, close to 80% (11 of 14) found a significant positive relationship (4). In that review, 33 of 47 studies found that religious people were more likely to volunteer and engage in altruistic kinds of activities. Furthermore, already discussed is the lower rate of crime and delinquency linked with religious involvement in over 80% of studies (82 of 104 studies identified in our review).

Religious beliefs serve as a form of internal social control that moderates powerful human drives for pleasure and self-gain. When this form of control is lessened or absent, *external* social control becomes necessary (i.e. law enforcement by the state). Because religious beliefs emphasize self-discipline and self-control, researchers have speculated that one of the most important mechanisms by which religious involvement affects mental health is through this pathway (67). Self-control and strong character result from repeatedly making good personal decisions that promote the well-being of others until it becomes a habit, and as noted above (67), religious teachings encourage that.

Biological factors

The psychological, social, behavioural, environmental, and individual level influences of religious involvement ultimately have their effects on biological

processes and physical health, operating in concert with genetic predisposi-
tions. Although genetic influences, as discussed earlier, are biological in nature, in this section I focus more on the impact that R/S has on physiological
processes that lead to physical disease and disability, and consequently affect
mental health.

One example of a physiological process that R/S may influence through
psychological and social pathways is the level of *inflammation* in the body.
Psychosocial stress is known to increase inflammation, which in turn
has a number of health consequences: coronary artery disease, stroke,
neurodegenerative diseases such as Alzheimer's and Parkinson's, rheumatoid
arthritis, asthma, other autoimmune disorders, diabetes, and obesity (68).
Inflammation may be a key mediator in the relationship between maternal
stress and infant risk of neuropsychiatric disorder (69). Chronic inflammation induced by psychological stress is also thought to contribute to the development of depression, which in turn may increase inflammation, leading
to a vicious cycle of greater inflammation leading to greater depression (70).
Religious involvement may help to break this vicious cycle by improved coping
with stress and increasing social support, both known to reduce inflammation
and decrease depression. In support of this hypothesis, an increasing number
of studies have found an inverse relationship between R/S and indicators of
inflammation such as C-reactive protein (71–76), pro-inflammatory cytokines
such as interleukin-6 (77–79), and Cystatin-C (76).

Likewise, consistent with the hypothesis that R/S may have an impact on biological functioning, are studies reporting an association between R/S and measures of immune and endocrine function, particularly those adversely affected
by stress. Several of these studies have been conducted in individuals with altered immune function due to HIV infection. These studies commonly report
that immune functions are better, viral load is lower, and disease progression
is slower among those who are more R/S (80–82). Improved immune function
among the religious has also been documented in other medical disorders as
well such as metastatic breast cancer (83). Rates of infection are likewise lower
among those who are more R/S, as found in those with periodontitis (84), men-
ingitis (85), sexually transmitted infections (86–88).

Religious involvement may also affect the structure of the brain, making it
less vulnerable to the development of depression and other mood disorders.
For example, Miller and colleagues (2014; 89) examined individuals at high
risk for major depression (MD) because they had a parent with MD, dividing
them into those for whom R/S was very important and those for whom religion
was not very important. Structural magnetic resonance imaging (MRI) scans

of the brain were conducted and brain structure compared between the two groups. In those who indicated that R/S was not very important, MRI scans revealed widespread areas of thinning of cerebral cortex regions, compared with the brains of those who indicated that R/S was very important. Similar findings were reported for frequency of religious attendance, although these did not meet the significance threshold when controlling for multiple comparisons. There are physiological mechanisms to help explain these findings. Depression is often associated with increased levels of serum cortisol, which has been shown to destroy large pyramidal cell neurons that make up the cerebral cortex, resulting in a reduced cortical volume. Those who have R/S resources, however, have ways to cope with depression and stressful life events that might bring it on, thus reducing the amount of circulating cortisol that would otherwise have negative effects on brain cells. A number of studies have now reported cortisol levels or healthier diurnal cortisol secretion rhythms in the more religious or in response to R/S interventions (90–92).

The findings above between R/S and basic physiological functions helps to explain the large and growing evidence base indicating an inverse relationship between stress-related medical illness, physical disability, cognitive dysfunction, and overall and disease-specific mortality, explained by effects through psychological and social pathways (4, 55, 93). Improved physical health has an impact on mental health given that one of the strongest predictors of depression/anxiety is the presence of medical illness and physical disability.

Interactions

It should now be clear from our discussion that the genetic, psychological, social, behavioural, environmental, individual, and biological pathways by which R/S influences mental health often overlap and interact with one another as part of a complex web of causation extending from in-utero development to birth and infancy and throughout the lifespan. Human beings are not simply conscious biological machines operating in a material and social environment, but also spiritual beings with hopes and dreams and the need for purpose and meaning in their lives. All influence one another, and when one of these is weak or lacking (i.e. whether that be poor physical health, impaired social relationships, difficulty coping with environmental circumstances, or poor decision making and lack of self-discipline), all the others are adversely affected in one way or another. Emotional healing requires healing of the whole person and mental health involves stability and continued growth in all these areas.

Conclusions

We still have a long way to go and much to learn before we fully understand the mechanisms by which religious involvement affects mental health, or what level of religious involvement is necessary to have such an impact. I have suggested in this chapter that we have only thus far detected the 'tip of the iceberg' with regard to the degree to which religious beliefs and practices influence mental health, and the same applies to pathways that may explain that effect. I have described seven pathways by which religious involvement might enhance mental health, decrease, or lessen the impact of emotional and other mental disorders, and improve life satisfaction and well-being.

In the majority of cases (although maybe not all), religious beliefs and practices have an enormous potential to influence mental health and well-being through a range of different pathways, each interacting with and affecting one another. Understanding how religion improves mental health, and in what circumstances it has the opposite effect, will be a high priority for future researchers. This will likely be accomplished by more qualitative studies conducted in different religions and different locations throughout the world that explore these questions in depth, the development of methods and analytic techniques to more accurately identify the direction of causation in these relationships (through quantitative longitudinal studies), and the development of interventions to take advantage of the power of religion to heal emotional problems and improve well-being.

References

1. Freud, S. (1907). Obsessive acts and religious practices. *The standard edition of the complete psychological works of Sigmund Freud*, Vol. 9 (J Strachey, ed. and trans., pp. 115–27, 1959).
2. Ellis A, Murray, JG. *The case against religion: a psychotherapist's view and the case against religiosity*. Cranford, NJ: American Atheist Press;1985.
3. Sloan RP. *Blind faith: the unholy alliance of religion and medicine*. London: Macmillan; 2006.
4. Koenig HG, King DE, Carson VB. *Handbook of religion and health*. Second edition. New York: Oxford University Press; 2012.
5. Koenig HG. *Religion on mental health: research and applications*. Cambridge, MA: Academic Press (Elsevier); 2018.
6. Koenig HG, VanderWeele TJ, Peteet JR. *Handbook of Religion and Health*. Third edition. New York: Oxford University Press; in preparation.
7. Koenig HG, Cohen HJ, Blazer DG, Pieper C, Meador KG, Shelp F, et al. Religious coping and depression in elderly hospitalized medically ill men. *American Journal of Psychiatry*. 1992;**149**:1693–700.

8. **Koenig HG.** Religious beliefs and practices of hospitalized medically ill older adults. *International Journal of Geriatric Psychiatry.* 1998;**13**:213–24.

9. **Schuster MA, Stein BD, Jaycox L, Collins RL, Marshall GN, Elliott MN, et al.** A national survey of stress reactions after the September 11, 2001, terrorist attacks. *New England Journal of Medicine.* 2001;**345**(20):1507–12.

10. **Scholte WF, Olff M, Ventevogel P, de Vries G-J, Jansveld E, Lopes Cardozo B, et al.** Mental health symptoms following war and repression in Eastern Afghanistan. *Journal of the American Medical Association.* 2004;**292**(5):585–93.

11. **Sharma M, Fine SL, Brennan RT, Betancourt TS.** Coping and mental health outcomes among Sierra Leonean war-affected youth: results from a longitudinal study. *Development and Psychopathology.* 2017;**29**(1):11–23.

12. **Kremer H, Ironson G.** Longitudinal spiritual coping with trauma in people with HIV: Implications for health care. *AIDS Patient Care and STDs.* 2014;**28**(3):144–54.

13. **Hawthorne DM, Youngblut JM, Brooten D.** Parent spirituality, grief, and mental health at 1 and 3 months after their infant's/child's death in an intensive care unit. *Journal of Pediatric Nursing.* 2016;**31**:73–80.

14. **Li S, Okereke OI, Chang SC, Kawachi I, VanderWeele TJ.** Religious service attendance and lower depression among women—a prospective cohort study. *Annals of Behavioral Medicine.* 2016a;**50**(6):876–84.

15. **Tomita A, Ramlall S.** A nationwide panel study on religious involvement and depression in South Africa: evidence from the South African National Income Dynamics Study. *Journal of Religion and Health.* 2018;**57**(6):2279–89.

16. **VanderWeele TJ, Li S, Tsai AC, Kawachi, I.** Association between religious service attendance and lower suicide rates among US women. *JAMA Psychiatry.* 2016; **73**(8):845–51.

17. **Koenig HG.** Association of religious involvement and suicide. *JAMA Psychiatry.* 2016a;**73**(8):775–6.

18 **Chen, Y., & VanderWeele, T. J.** (2018). Associations of religious upbringing with subsequent health and well-being from adolescence to young adulthood: an outcome-wide analysis. *American Journal of Epidemiology, 187*(11), 2355–54. Available from: https://doi.org/10.1093/aje/kwy142 OK

19. **Jung JH.** Childhood adversity, religion, and change in adult mental health. *Research on Aging.* 2018;**40**(2):155–79.

20. **Bradshaw M, Kent BV.** Prayer, attachment to God, and changes in psychological well-being in later life. *Journal of Aging and Health.* 2018;**30**(5):667–91.

21. **Propst LR, Ostrom R, Watkins P, Dean T, Mashburn, D.** Comparative efficacy of religious and nonreligious cognitive-behavior therapy for the treatment of clinical depression in religious individuals. *Journal of Consulting and Clinical Psychology.* 1992;**60**:94–103.

22. **Koenig HG, Gutiérrez B, Cervilla J, Pearce MJ, Daher N, Nelson B, et al.** Genes, religion, and response to religious *vs* conventional psychotherapy: a randomized clinical trial in medically ill patients with major depression. *Austin Journal of Psychiatry & Behavioral Sciences.* 2015a;**2**(1):1036.

23. **Rosmarin DH, Pargament KI, Pirutinsky S, Mahoney A.** A randomized controlled evaluation of a spiritually integrated treatment for subclinical anxiety in the Jewish community, delivered via the Internet. *Journal of Anxiety Disorders.* 2010; **24**(7):799–808.

24. **Hosseini M, Salehi A, Fallahi Khoshknab M, Rokofian A, Davidson PM.** The effect of a preoperative spiritual/religious intervention on anxiety in Shia Muslim patients undergoing coronary artery bypass graft surgery: a randomized controlled trial. *Journal of Holistic Nursing.* 2013;**31**(3):164–72.

25. **Babamohamadi H, Sotodehasl N, Koenig HG, Jahani C, Ghorbani R.** The effect of Holy Qur'an recitation on anxiety in hemodialysis patients: a randomized clinical trial. *Journal of Religion and Health.* 2015;**54**(5):1921–30.

26. **Anderson N, Heywood-Everett S, Siddiqi N, Wright J, Meredith J, McMillan D.** Faith-adapted psychological therapies for depression and anxiety: systematic review and meta-analysis. *Journal of Affective Disorders.* 2015;**176**:183–96.

27. **Koenig HG, Pearce MJ, Nelson B, Shaw SF, Robins CJ, Daher N,** et al. Religious vs. conventional cognitive-behavioral therapy for major depression in persons with chronic medical illness. Journal of Nervous and Mental Disease. 2015b;**203**(4):243–51.

28. **Idler E, Oman D, Kiser M, Hogue C.** Courses in religion and public health. *American Journal of Public Health.* 2017;**107**(6):E1.

29. **Oman, D.** (ed.). *Why religion and spirituality matter for public health: evidence, implications, and resources* (vol. 2). NY: Springer; 2018.

30. **VanderWeele TJ, Koenig HG.** A course on religion and public health at Harvard. *American Journal of Public Health.* 2017;**107**(1):47–8.

31. **Koenig HG, Hooten EG, Lindsay-Calkins E, Meador KG.** Spirituality in medical school curricula: findings from a national survey. *International Journal of Psychiatry in Medicine.* 2010;**40**(4):391–8.

32. **Culatto A, Sumerton CB.** Spirituality and health education: a national survey of academic leaders UK. *Journal of Religion and Health.* 2015;**54**:2269–75.

33. **Lucchetti G, de Oliveira LR, Koenig HG, Leite JR, Lucchetti AL.** Medical students, spirituality and religiosity-results from the multicenter study SBRAME. *BMC Medical Education.* 2013;**13**(1):162.

34. **Moreira-Almeida A, Sharma A, van Rensburg BJ, Verhagen PJ, Cook, CC.** WPA position statement on spirituality and religion in psychiatry. *World Psychiatry.* 2016;**15**(1):87–8.

35. **Peteet, JR, Al Zaben F, Koenig, HG** (2018). Integrating spirituality into the care of older adults. *International Psychogeriatrics,* **31**(1), 31–38. Available from: https://doi.org/10.1017/S1041610218000716 OK

36. **Burdette AM, Weeks J, Hill TD, Eberstein IW.** Maternal religious attendance and low birth weight. *Social Science & Medicine.* 2012;**74**:1961–7.

37. **Dew RE, Koenig HG.** Religious involvement, the serotonin transporter promoter polymorphism, and drug use in young adults. *International Journal of Social Sciences Studies.* 2014;**2**(1):98–104.

38. **Lin JY, Jiang MY, Kan ZM, Chu Y.** Influence of 5-HTR2A genetic polymorphisms on the efficacy of antidepressants in the treatment of major depressive disorder: a meta-analysis. *Journal of Affective Disorders.* 2014;**168**: 430–8.

39. **Bockting CLH, Mocking RJ, Lok A, Koeter MWJ, Schene, AH.** Therapygenetics: the 5HTTLPR as a biomarker for response to psychological therapy? *Molecular Psychiatry.* 2013;**18**(7):744.

40. **Chartier KG, Dick DM, Almasy L, Chan G, Aliev F, Schuckit MA.,** . . . **& Nurnberger Jr J.** Interactions between alcohol metabolism genes and religious involvement in

association with maximum drinks and alcohol dependence symptoms. *Journal of Studies on Alcohol and Drugs.* 2016;**77**(3):393–404.

41. **Anderson, MR, Miller L, Wickramaratne P, Svob C, Odgerel Z, Zhao R, Weissman MM.** Genetic correlates of spirituality/religion and depression: a study in offspring and grandchildren at high and low familial risk for depression. *Spirituality in Clinical Practice.* 2017;**4**(1):43–63.

42. **Sachs E, Rosenfeld B, Lhewa D, Rasmussen A, Keller A.** Entering exile: trauma, mental health, and coping among Tibetan refugees arriving in Dharamsala, India. *Journal of Traumatic Stres.* 2008;**21**(2):199–208.

43. **Choumanova I, Wanat S, Barrett R, Koopman C.** Religion and spirituality in coping with breast cancer: perspectives of Chilean women. *Breast Journal.* 2006;**12**(4):349–52.

44. **Eapen V, Revesz T.** Psychosocial correlates of paediatric cancer in the United Arab Emirates. *Supportive Care in Cancer.* 2003;**11**(3), 185–9.

45. **Bradshaw M, Ellison CG, Marcum JP.** Attachment to God, images of God, and psychological distress in a nationwide sample of Presbyterians. *International Journal for the Psychology of Religion.* 2010;**20**(2):130–47.

46. **Ellison CG, Bradshaw M, Flannelly KJ, Galek KC.** Prayer, attachment to God, and symptoms of anxiety-related disorders among U.S. adults. *Sociology of Religion.* 2014;**75**:208–33.

47. **Kent BV, Bradshaw M, Uecker JE.** Forgiveness, attachment to God, and mental health outcomes in older US adults: a longitudinal study. *Research on Aging.* 2018;**40**(5):456–79.

48. **Bradshaw M, Ellison CG, Flannelly KJ.** Prayer, God imagery, and symptoms of psychopathology. *Journal for the Scientific Study of Religion.* 2008;**47**:644–59.

49. **Krause N, Emmons RA, Ironson G.** Benevolent images of God, gratitude, and physical health status. *Journal of Religion & Health.* 2015;**54**(4):1503–19.

50. **Fider, C. R., Lee, J. W., Gleason, P. C., & Jones, P.** (2017). Influence of religion on later burden and health of new black and white caregivers. *Journal of Applied Gerontology,* E-pub ahead of press. Available from: https://doi.org/10.1177/0733464817703017

51. **Koenig HG.** *You are my beloved. Really?* Amazon: CreateSpace Publishing Platform; 2016b.

52. **Krauss SW, Hood Jr, RW.** *A new approach to religious orientation: the commitment reflectivity circumplex* (International Series in the Psychology of Religion (Book 16). Amsterdam, Netherlands: Rodopi; 2013.

53. **Exline JJ, Grubbs JB, Homolka, SJ.** Seeing God as cruel or distant: links with divine struggles involving anger, doubt, and fear of God's disapproval. *International Journal for the Psychology of Religion.* 2015;**25**(1):29–41.

54. **Stavrova O, Fetchenhauer D, Schlösser T.** Why are religious people happy? The effect of the social norm of religiosity across countries. *Social Science Research.* 2013;**42**(1):90–105.

55. **Li S, Stampfer MJ, Williams DR, VanderWeele TJ.** Association of religious service attendance with mortality among women. *JAMA Internal Medicine.* 2016b;**176**(6):777–85.

56. **Steffen PR, Masters KS, Baldwin S.** What mediates the relationship between religious service attendance and aspects of well-being? *Journal of Religion and Health.* 2017;**56**(1):158–70.

57. **Acevedo GA, Ellison CG, Xu X.** Is it really religion? Comparing the main and stress-buffering effects of religious and secular civic engagement on psychological distress. *Society and Mental Health*. 2014;4(2):111–28.

58. **Koenig HG, King DE, Carson VB.** *Handbook of religion and health*. Second edition. New York: Oxford University Press; 2012.

59. **Ojeda L, Pina-Watson B.** Day laborers' life satisfaction: the role of familismo, spirituality, work, health, and discrimination. *Cultural Diversity and Ethnic Minority Psychology*. 2013;**19**(3):270–8.

60. **Battle J, DeFreece, A.** The impact of community involvement, religion, and spirituality on happiness and health among a national sample of Black lesbians. *Women, Gender, and Families of Color*. 2014;**2**(1):1–31.

61. **Hodge DR, Zidan T, Husain A.** Modeling the relationships between discrimination, depression, substance use, and spirituality with Muslims in the United States. *Social Work Research*. 2015;**39**(4):223–33.

62. **Porter KE, Brennan-Ing M, Burr JA, Dugan E, Karpiak SE.** Stigma and psychological well-being among older adults with HIV: the impact of spirituality and integrative health approaches. *The Gerontologist*. 2017;**57**(2), 219–28.

63. **Butler-Barnes ST, Martin PP, Copeland-Linder N, Seaton EK, Matusko N, Caldwell CH, Jackson JS.** The protective role of religious involvement in African American and Caribbean Black adolescents' experiences of racial discrimination. *Youth & Society*, 2018;**50**(5):659–87.

64. **Koenig HG.** *Faith and mental health: religious resources for healing*. Philadelphia, PA: Templeton Foundation Press; 2005.

65. **Koenig HG.** *In the wake of disaster: religious responses to terrorism and catastrophe*. Philadelphia, PA: Templeton Foundation Press; 2006c.

66. **Inglehart R.** *Modernization and post-modernization: cultural, economic and political change in 43 societies*. Princeton: Princeton University Press; 1997.

67. **McCullough ME, Willoughby BL.** Religion, self-regulation, and self-control: associations, explanations, and implications. *Psychological Bulletin*. 2009;**135**(1):69–93.

68. **Kotas ME, Medzhitov R.** Homeostasis, inflammation, and disease susceptibility. Cell, 2015;**160**(5):816–27.

69. **Hantsoo, L., Kornfield, S., Anguera, M. C., & Epperson, C. N.** (2018). Inflammation: A proposed intermediary between maternal stress and, offspring neuropsychiatric risk. *Biological Psychiatry*, 85(2), 97–106. Available from: https://doi.org/10.1016/j.biopsych.2018.08.018 OK

70. **Slavich GM, Irwin MR.** From stress to inflammation and major depressive disorder: a social signal transduction theory of depression. *Psychological Bulletin*. 2014;**140**(3):774–815.

71. **King DE, Mainous AG III, Steyer TE, Pearson WS.** The relationship between attendance at religious services and cardiovascular inflammatory markers. *International Journal of Psychiatry in Medicine*. 2001;**31**(4):415–25.

72. **King DE, Mainous AG III, Pearson WS.** C-reactive protein, diabetes, and attendance at religious services. *Diabetes Care*. 2002;**25**(7), 1172–6.

73. **Ford ES, Loucks EB, Berkman LF.** Social integration and concentrations of C-reactive protein among US adults. *Annals of Epidemiology*. 2006;**16**(2):78–84.

74. **Hill TD, Rote SM. Ellison CG.** Religious participation and biological functioning in Mexico. *Journal of Aging and Health.* 2017;**29**(6):951–72.

75. **Ironson G, Lucette, A, Hylton E, Pargament KI, Krause N.** The relationship between religious and psychospiritual measures and an inflammation marker (CRP) in older adults experiencing life event stress. *Journal of Religion and Health.* 2018; **57**(4):1554–66.

76. **Suh H, Hill TD, Koenig, HG.** (2019). Religious attendance and biological risk: A national longitudinal study of older adults. *Journal of Religion and Health.* 2019;**58**(4):1188–1202 (https://doi.org/10.1007/s10943-018-0721-0)

77. **Koenig HG, Cohen HJ, George LK, Hays JC, Larson DB, Blazer DG.** Attendance at religious services, interleukin-6, and other biological indicators of immune function in older adults. *International Journal of Psychiatry in Medicine.* 1997;**27**:233–50.

78. **Lutgendorf SK, Russell D, Ullrich P, Harris TB, Wallace R.** Religious participation, interleukin-6, and mortality in older adults. *Health Psychology.* 2004;**23**(5):465–75.

79. **Ai, AL, Seymour, EM, Tice N, Kronfol Z, Appel H, Bolling SF.** Spiritual struggle related to plasma interleukin-6 prior to cardiac surgery. *Psychology of Religion and Spirituality.* 2009;**1**(2):112–28.

80. **Ironson G, Stuetzle R, Ironson D, Balbin E, Kremer H, George A, … & Fletcher MA.** View of God as benevolent and forgiving or punishing and judgmental predicts HIV disease progression. *Journal of Behavioral Medicine.* 2011;**34**(6),414–25.

81. **Kremer H, Ironson G, Kaplan L, Stuetzele R, Baker N, Fletcher MA.** Spiritual coping predicts CD4-cell preservation and undetectable viral load over four years. *AIDS Care.* 2014; **27**(1):71–9.

82. **Ironson G, Kremer H, Lucette A.** Relationship between spiritual coping and survival in patients with HIV. *Journal of General Internal Medicine.* 2016;**31**(9):1068–76.

83. **Sephton SE, Koopman C, Schaal M, Thoresen C, Spiegel D.** Spiritual expression and immune status in women with metastatic breast cancer: an exploratory study. *Breast Journal.* 2001;**7**(5):345–53.

84. **Merchant AT, Pitiphat W, Ahmed B, Kawachi I, Joshipura K.** A prospective study of social support, anger expression and risk of periodontitis in men. *Journal of the American Dental Association.* 2003;**134**(12):1591–6.

85. **Tully J, Viner RM, Coen PG, Stuart JM, Zambon M, Peckham C.** et al. Risk and protective factors for meningococcal disease in adolescents: matched cohort study. *British Medical Journal.* 2006;**332**(7539):445–50.

86. **Trinitapoli J, Regnerus MD.** Religion and HIV risk behaviors among married men: initial results from a study in rural sub-Saharan Africa. *Journal for the Scientific Study of Religion.* 2006;**45**(4):505–28.

87. **Gillum, RF, Holt CL.** Religious involvement and seroprevalence of six infectious diseases in US adults. *Southern Medical Journal.* 2010;**103**:403–8.

88. **Raghavan R, Ferlic-Stark L, Clarke C, Rungta M, Goodgame R.** The role of patient religiosity in the evaluation and treatment outcomes from chronic HCV infection. *Journal of Religion and Health.* 2013;**52**:79–90.

89. **Miller LR, Bansal R, Wickramaratne P, Hao Z, Tenke C, Weissman MM, Peterson BS.** Neuroanatomical correlates of religiosity and spirituality: a study in adults at high and low familial risk for depression. *JAMA Psychiatry.* 2014;**71**(2):128–35.

90. **Bormann JE, Aschbacher K, Wetherell JL, Roesch S, Redwine L.** Effects of faith/ assurance on cortisol levels are enhanced by a spiritual mantram intervention in adults with HIV: a randomized trial. *Journal of Psychosomatic Research.* 2009; **66**:161–71.

91. **Assari S, Lankarani MM, Caldwell C, Zimmerman M, Malekahmadi MR.** Baseline religion involvement predicts subsequent salivary cortisol levels among male but not female Black youth. *International Journal of Endocrinology & Metabolism.* 2015;**13**(4):e31790.

92. **Tobin ET, Slatcher RB.** Religious participation predicts diurnal cortisol profiles 10 years later via lower levels of religious struggle. *Health Psychology.* 2016;**35**(12):1356–63.

93. **VanderWeele TJ, Yu J, Cozier, YC, Wise L, Argentieri MA, Rosenberg L.,** . . . & **Shields AE.** Attendance at religious services, prayer, religious coping, and religious/ spiritual identity as predictors of all-cause mortality in the Black Women's Health Study. *American Journal of Epidemiology.* 2017;**185**(7);515–22.

Chapter 9

Sexual Minorities and Spirituality

Dinesh Bhugra, Cameron Watson, and
Susham Gupta

Introduction

To many individuals in cultures around the world, religion and spirituality
are very important aspects of their life, in part because religion offers a micro-
identity. Micro-identities relate to a number of factors such as religion, sexual
orientation, and gender, among others. An individual's identity is formed of
multiple micro-identities and at any given time one micro-identity may over-
ride others. For example, in some settings, religion will be of more relevance
than individual's sexual orientation. The distinction between spirituality and
organized religion has been discussed elsewhere in this volume, so will not be
described at any length here. The response of organized religion to alternate
sexualities also seen as sexual minorities often depends upon how specific religious tenets are interpreted, mostly by the religious leaders who act as commu-
nicators for the community in which an individual is born. Being brought up
in a particular (organized) religion helps formulate an individual's world view.
However, for LGB individuals, this view may clash with their own voyage of
self-discovery. The psychological impact of organizations on an individual's development cannot be overestimated whether such an organization is a school,
a university, a place of work or worship, or an institution like family. Messages
from cultures are imbibed quietly and subtly. Under these circumstances, pressures to conform and anti-alternate sexuality views may become negative and
all-pervasive. Not all organized religions are necessarily anti-LGBT, but their
emphasis and negative interpretations can be very pervasive and destructive.
The psychological impact of negative religious attitudes and responses on
identity development and perception of psychopathology can be extremely
powerful. Furthermore, these negative attitudes, if pervasive in society, can
affect policy development and further negative, alienating, stigmatizing, and
discriminatory attitudes and laws. These negative feelings can go on to contribute to further alienation from that particular aspect of society and a search

for acceptance elsewhere. These feelings can be particularly profound in LGBT individuals. It must be recognized that often feelings and participation in religious activities are not clearly binary and individuals, as well as religious institutions, can be extremely fluid in their attitudes and responses.

In this chapter the focus is largely on sexual identity and orientation rather than gender identity simply because there is more research evidence available. Although often LGBT terms are used to define one community there is marked heterogeneity and this variation needs to be remembered. Issues related to transgender individuals are not discussed in any detail in this chapter. Psychiatry itself has reflected social responses in negative attitudes to sexual identity variations.

It must be emphasized that the research in relationship between religion/spirituality and sexual orientation has been often cross-sectional. A recent systematic review found only 10 papers (1) published in a decade that studied relationships between LGBT+ youth and religion and spirituality. These authors concluded that discriminatory attitudes, shame related to disclosure, spirituality as a positive supportive resource and internalized conflict and external factors all played a role. Thus, mental health professionals, irrespective of their religious/spiritual beliefs and sexual orientation need to be objective in their approach.

Given the scarcity of high-quality studies, it is important to recognize the provisional nature of the current knowledge on the topic.

There is clear research evidence that religion can lead to negative attitudes to same-sex activities and sexual variations (see 2, 3). Although ten years old, it is worth recalling the introduction to a special issue of the *Journal of LGBT Issues in Counselling*, Kocet and Curry (2011; 4). The authors remind us that, for many LGBT individuals, issues related to spirituality and religion remind them of shame, stigma, and alienation by their religious leaders. These interpretations and attacks can take many forms from selective interpretation of scriptures and religious teachings to personal abuse. These negative attitudes may also affect therapists and counsellors, spilling over into therapy or counselling sessions. Furthermore, LGBT individuals may have felt abused and thus find it difficult to integrate their own personal identity.

In many cultures around the globe same gender relations were considered acceptable and normative whereas in others there is strong sense of disapproval. Herdt (1987; 5) points out that, in sex-negative cultures, sexual variations are disapproved of. Heterosexualism and power hierarchies, of all kinds, derive at least some of their force from organized religion (5, 6). As has been noted, sex has been worshipped, criticized, vulgarized, ignored, and vilified at various times during the history of mankind (7) as has sexuality and thus sexual orientation and same sex behaviours. In this context, we use the term 'sexuality' to reflect on sexual orientation. A distinction between sexual behaviour, sexual orientation and sexual fantasy needs to eb remembered. It is entirely possible that a male with heterosexual orientation with heterosexual fantasies may involve himself in same-sex behaviour if he is unable to find a female partner for any number of reasons.

In modern times, a stereotypical homosexual has been created, perhaps in order to fulfil the needs of the society to provide a despised and punished target in order to keep the said society pure (8); religion through religious texts and scriptures is one way of achieving such. On the other hand, interesting contrasts have emerged between male and female homosexuality because often the latter has been acknowledged less and often ignored.

In this chapter, we attempt to highlight the role organized religion can play in the lives of LGB individuals and how it differs from spirituality. Furthermore, creation of stigma and discrimination can be traced to religion through various religious texts and scriptures, and we develop this theme in the context of identity and processes of coming out to friends, family, and society in general. The role of religion in influencing attitudes in society which then also go on to affect psychiatric practice is important to recognize.

Definitions

It is important for clinicians and researchers alike to be fully aware of sensitivities—both cultural and legal—in ascertaining the identity of sexual minority individuals, but also how spirituality and religiosity are addressed and assessed in a particular group or society. It will be important to explore stages of coming out, and how people's religious and spiritual upbringing and values have played a role in the formation and development of their identity and different meanings attributed to both their sexuality and religious/spiritual values. Bhugra (1997) (9) reported that religion and family played a major role in getting gay individuals to come out.

Clinicians need to be open-minded in exploring similarities and differences across religions and must make sure that they do not have any unconscious bias towards a particular religion or sexual practice. In addition, if further information is needed to explore and understand sexual orientation, they should acknowledge this and go on to seek it, because there are plenty of resources for unbiased information available that they must apply and explore in assessment. Religion and spirituality are defined at length elsewhere in this volume. Suffice it to say, spirituality proceeds from the soul, which is defined as 'the repository of all that I feel my appetites and ambitions, sadness and joy. It is the place where inspiration germinates and from which vitality grows' (10). He goes on, 'somewhere in this great container of ceaseless death and rebirth, lies too the mystery of my being gay'. Thus, concepts of the self, how it is defined whether it is egocentric or sociocentric are thus very strongly influenced by cultures in which individuals are born and brought up. Cultures also influence development of identity and functioning and resulting acceptance by self in the first instance and then others. This is particularly relevant to minority sexual orientation.

Development of identity

Individual identity for a person is extremely important and relates to not only how they see themselves but, more importantly, how they see others seeing them. The concepts and definitions of self vary across cultures. The Western self is more likely to be egocentric whereas, from other or traditional societies, it may be more socio-centric (11). This notion and the development of the self may be further complicated and perhaps overshadowed by other dimensions of a culture and society.

Identity formation is an interactive process between the individual and society, and is highly influenced by the norms and values of family and society at large (12). The role that organized religion plays thus becomes a major one. The rituals as part of the organized religion can be both helpful and soothing on the one hand but potentially troublesome on the other.

The spiritual components of the identity and identity development need deeper exploration in both clinical practice and research. Another key question worth addressing is whether sexuality is a primary identity or a secondary one—for example, whether an individual sees themselves as a gay person or a person who is gay. It is also entirely possible that, during development of identity, different micro-identities may take precedence and at varying times other micro-identities may well emerge. For example, an individual may choose to hide their sexuality or religion in different situations and contexts. It is crucial that clinicians are aware of some of these aspects while assessing individuals.

Erikson (1950; 13) suggested eight stages in development of identity and notes that five of these occur below the age of 18, which in terms of sexual orientation and coming out can be extremely important and relevant. These stages are trust versus mistrust, autonomy versus shame, initiative versus quiet, industry versus inferiority, identity versus role confusion and then, after the age of 18, intimacy versus isolation, generality versus stagnation and ego-integrity versus despair. The latter two occur between 40 and 65+ years so clear parallels can be drawn with how gay identity develops and is sustained. These descriptive stages are not dissimilar to those that have been described in Hindu scriptures, although these are stages of life and only four in total. Within such a process, micro-identities form an important integral part of the self. Wachter et al. (2015; 14) note that micro-identities need to be managed by individuals in order to manage stigma based on religion, sex, or sexual orientation. For example, a gay, Indian, male, Hindu psychiatrist with a disability may see himself as a disabled Hindu psychiatrist who is male and gay or a male psychiatrist who is gay, Hindu, or disabled. Such personal identification depends upon both internal choices and decisions, and external circumstances such as place of work, place of worship, a gay club, etc. Thus, identity is about how one sees one's self and it can be argued that there is a core identity that is perhaps more difficult to change, and peripheral aspects of identity that are prone to change. Within this identity, for some individuals the religious/spirituality dimension may play a major role. However, the individual response to religious values and attitudes to homosexuality are likely to affect their acknowledgement of their own identity to others, especially in the process of coming out. Gay identity may be clear and readily accepted by some individuals, and they may feel confident with this at an early stage in their life whereas in others it may become clear at a particular late stage in life.

Monotheistic religions are much more likely to hold negative attitudes to sexual variations and they may, therefore, reject or exclude individuals who are also likely to be vulnerable. This rejection may lead for them to leave their religion and embrace gay lifestyle with great enthusiasm, whereas others may wish to conform and thus may look towards conversion therapies. These variations in responses need to be remembered in clinical settings so that the notion of a homogenous community can be dispelled.

Gay identity

The development of homosexual identity depends upon the meaning attached to the concepts of homosexuality and being a homosexual. These meanings and interpretations are important. The commitment to a homosexual identity cannot occur in an environment where the cognitive category of homosexuality does not exist (15). This creates tensions in many cultures where it may then be seen as an 'imported' disease as evidenced in many cultures where it is seen as a Western disease or condition.

Cass (1979; 16) described a six-stage model of homosexual identity formation based on two assumptions. First, that identity is developmental and, second, focus of stability and changes in behaviour are related to interaction between individuals and their environments. Identity is, of course, both personal and interactional, thus attributed characteristics to the self and self-perception of their own behaviour and that of another person's characteristics. These six stages are identity confusion, identity comparison, identity tolerance, identity acceptance, identity pride, and identity synthesis are all affected by various factors. In a small sample of LGBT individuals, Beagan and Hattie (2015; 17) found that, although not all had negative experiences with religion, the psychological and emotional damage was extensive in those who had experienced religious conflict. Many had left their formal religion, but among those who stayed in the religion in which they were brought up, a distinction between religion and spirituality was clearly identified. Dahl and Galliher (2012; 18) found that some LGBT youths felt alienated from the religion they were brought up in as their sexual identity emerged. Bhugra (1997; 9), in his sample of gay Asians, found that, in comparison with Hindus, Muslims found it difficult to combine their religion with their sexual orientation and also were more likely to experience homophobia from other Muslims. Reygan and Moane (2014; 19) reported from Eire that individuals experienced and responded to religious homophobia in different ways. Not surprisingly, in some individuals, it led to an intrapsychic tension, which resulted in them abandoning their religion altogether.

Fox (1984; 20) describes a fourfold path of spiritual development for gay men and lesbians. These include (i) creation when the gay self is truly embraced, (ii) letting go when the pain of rejection is acknowledged and then released, (iii) creativity (leading to the rebirth of the soul), and (iv) transformation when the individual is at ease and able to extend a sense of compassion and celebration. There is no doubt that many individuals will develop internalized homophobia and thus struggle in their personal and spiritual development. This devaluing and following structural discrimination can damage the individual's identity development. Haldeman (1996; 21) points out that similar stages can be gone through in gay supportive psychotherapy to enable the person to develop a stronger individual identity. Using religious or spiritual pathways can lead to similar emotionally meaningful conclusions. Even though organized religion can cause wounds in the individual (22), it can also be used to heal these wounds (21, 23, 20) as well. Thus, the therapist needs to be aware of the potential healing powers of religion/spirituality.

Coming out and religion/spirituality

In recent decades, coming out has become a common term and has been used for various phenomena—for example, public acknowledgement of one's minority sexual identity or same sex orientation but also for admitting publicly about having had psychiatric problems. This process of coming out is seen as a (complex) complicated process that involves, at a psychological level, a person's awareness and acknowledgement of homosexual thoughts and feelings (24). Coleman (1985; 25) described five stages in coming out and argued that each of these stages needs to be resolved before subsequent stages can be completed. It is obvious that such a resolution of sexual identity must mean that the individual feels comfortable not only with themselves but also with those around them who may be holding negative attitudes. This degree of being at ease will be affected by social factors as well as concepts of the self and other variables (26). These stages in the coming out process are pre-coming out (when the individual may be trying to identify their sexual feelings and struggling with their identity), coming out, exploration (of their sexuality), first relationships, and identity integration (25). It is possible that the last four stages can be easily amalgamated with a parallel development all ending up in a strong sense of the self. The first stage is parallel to gender identity development. This stage in coming out is the developmental task when the individual acknowledges to themselves their same-sex attraction and feelings. This has also been called by various names such as awareness (27), identification (28), and acknowledgement or signification (29, 30). Median age for this stage is generally around puberty, around 13 (31) but undoubtedly this will be affected by personal, family, and cultural factors. An individual may acknowledge these same-sex feelings and attraction to a friend first—often it is a female friend. In this period, they may be developing their social skills and reaching out to others who are similarly inclined. Support and acceptance from the family are still an exception rather than the norm across cultures and more so if their adherence to organized religion is strong. Exploration of one's feelings and same-sex behaviour may be experimental initially and encourages the person to develop social and interpersonal skills that may contribute to sexual competence. In addition, as Dank (28) notes, there is a primary stage where individual in rule-breaking behaviour regards this as normal, but the secondary stage (perhaps as a response to external social and cultural factors) may be interpreted deviant by themselves. Coming out should be seen as a search for a gay identity. Often, as mentioned above, an individual comes out to friends and then makes links with other similar individuals and then comes out to family and often lastly to people at workplace or employers (32). After disclosure to the family, there may be a period of turmoil and religion may play a major role in acceptance or rejection. If parents or families have negative attitudes to same-sex behaviour, a gay person may not come out to them or may rebel against them, again depending upon a number of external factors. Religion and spirituality play a major role as Gold and Stewart (2012; 33) reported. These authors found that their sample described spirituality as acceptance (of their sexuality) and managed multiple identities in intersectional way with irreconciliation, progressive development, arrested development, completed development, and reconciliation. There is no doubt that places of worship in different religions can also play different roles in offering positive or accepting, and negative or rejecting, attitudes. Some churches may offer recognition and reconciliation, whereas others, such as some but not all Roman Catholic churches, continue to be broadly hostile. Perhaps the underlying notion is that sexual orientation is a choice, therefore against the tenets of a particular religion, and hence sinful. This unproven hypothesis has become perceived truism creating further stigma and rejection thereby recommending 'conversion'.

So-called Conversion therapies

In many parts of the world, churches encourage conversion therapies (to change sexual orientation from homosexuality to heterosexuality) and many psychologists and psychiatrists continue to offer these. For many individuals, the role of the churches and other religious places in their lives and a sense of belonging or wanting to belong is such that they would undergo 'conversion therapies'. These seem to be based on spurious conclusions that innate sexual orientation can be changed. Haldeman (1996; 21) observes 'that an institution could hold such sway over a person's psyche is explicable when the institution performs a surrogate parental function'. Thus, seeking broader approval from the community in the context of organized religion may be seen as more important thereby seeking or accepting conversion therapies. Haldeman (1996; 21) also notes that many gay and lesbians discover after coming out that the external 'gay' environment may be hostile to religion, and therefore they retreat into church and seek conversion in order to belong. These conflicts are important and can play a major role in the process of coming out itself. A major problem with this approach is that very often sexual orientation gets confused with sexual behaviour. For any sexual act to take place, sexual fantasy leads to arousal and the person with whom the act is performed may well be the most available person. As seen in prisons or boarding schools, men may have sex with other men without homosexual fantasies or homosexual orientation, and without identifying themselves as homosexual.

Haldeman (1996) and Weinberg and Williams (1974; 34) observe that gay men are likely to be more inclined towards doctrinaire religious practice, are also likely to have low self-image, see homosexuality as sinful and to be more depressed as a consequence, thereby seeking support in churches and conversion. Many of these church ministers have themselves subsequently come out as gay, thereby proving a degree of low self-image and high self-loathing. Conversion therapies are not successful, do not create conversion and actually may cause harm to vulnerable individuals. It is apparent that focus in these therapies is on behaviour and not orientation.

Relationship between identities

A major challenge in research and clinical settings alike has been in exploring the relationship between sexual and religious/spiritual identities, which can be very subtle and intricate. These are complexly intertwined and, for many, the distinction between spirituality and religion is not clear. Halkitis et al. (2009; 35), through a survey of 498 LGBT individuals, found that spirituality was seen in relational terms whereas religion was defined in terms of communal worship and in terms of its negative influence on individuals as well as communities. Perhaps, not surprisingly, this sample saw spiritual identities more pronounced in the context of prosocial engagement and interconnectedness. Religious identity in this sample depended upon religion in which the individual was raised, but also educational attainment and stage of personal development. This social engagement therefore becomes important in individuals who may be getting ready to leave home and individuate. For many, this support may well be offered by religious organizations, whereas for others it will be through gay/lesbian subcultures and, of course, occasionally these will be in conflict with each other. This tension between religious/spiritual identity and sexual identity may lead towards full-blown conflict with one or other identity. The long-term outcome of such a conflict may well prove to be very destructive for the vulnerable individual. As Blumenfeld and Raymond (1988; 36) have noted, many branches of Protestantism see homosexuality as imperfect, thereby devaluing sexuality and injecting a dose of inferiority, and by seeking help the individual is no longer sinful. Schuck and Liddle (2001; 37), in a qualitative study of 66 lesbian, gay and bisexual individuals reported that nearly two-thirds had acknowledged a conflict between religion and sexual orientation. They identified factors such as scriptures, religious teaching, and congregational prejudice as contributing to this conflict and, interestingly, they were in favour of spiritual resolution rather than a religious one. There is every likelihood that, due to unconscious bias or prejudice, individuals may well read some passages in the scriptures but with different interpretations and varying perspectives. This is not dissimilar to right-wing or left-wing historians interpreting historical events according to their personal political views. Sexual orientation and sexual behaviour often get confused, and it is the sexual behaviour that is often illegal in many countries and also seen as a problem. Some who see sexual orientation as choice would interpret it as sinful, thereby urging them to seek redemption through cure. Others may see it as a disease that requires treatment, as was done in the past through androgen-suppressing drugs. These are based on subjective interpretations. They are influenced by social attitudes according to the social climate.

It is the social context that identifies behaviour as deviant and how it should be dealt with.

Recent scandals of priests in Roman Catholic churches abusing young boys has again changed the social perspective. Until recently, in countries such as Ireland and Australia, these were, if not actually accepted, at least tolerated and the amount of religious abuse continued unabated for decades. Religious abuse occurs when a religious leader intentionally or unintentionally uses coercion, threats, rejection, condemnation, or manipulation to force an individual into submission of religious views about sexuality (38), which may lead the individual to shame, alienation, and even suicide. Gibbs and Goldbach (2015; 39) suggest that suicidality among LGBT individuals in their sample was associated with internalized homophobia and religious contexts, and had led to chronic suicidal thoughts. Irwin et al. (2014; 40), in an online survey, found that virtually all of their LGBT sample had thoughts of suicide due to age, gender, and discrimination among other factors.

Religion and attitudes

In the following section, we shall very briefly describe the tenets of main religions around the world and their attitudes to same-sex behaviour. These are not comprehensive summaries so interested readers are directed to main sources.

Hinduism

Hinduism is one of the oldest religions in the world, is often described as a philosophy, and is polytheistic. It has no single guru or leader, and teaches that love and sex are of divine origin with strong approval of sex early in Hindu history (also see Vanita and Kidwai 2008; 41, 7, 6). The emphasis on reincarnation and nirvana in Hinduism indicates that salvation can be achieved through different paths and each is followed depending upon individual abilities (42). Bullough (1976; 6) notes that, in Hinduism, women are seen to enjoy sexual activity more than men. In many scriptures, women are seen as more subservient, but this changed following very many invasions (6) and colonisation.

Shiva, also described as the Lord of destruction among the trinity of Gods in Hindu pantheon, is represented in temples by lingam (the phallus) and the base and phallus are believed to depict the union necessary to sustain the universe (42). Hinduism taught that there is a third sex which can be classified into four categories: Kliba (the waterless or desiccated testes); mushka-sunya (testicle voided), shandha (neuter) or mastrikam (female eunuch) all of whom provided alternative sexual gratification (43). Tantric texts describe detailed patterns of oral sex with most important chakra (centre of psychic energy) along with anal potential. Yogic beliefs of concentrating on anus, anal sphincters and stimulation of this region during mystic poses have been well described (43, 44).

Masturbation has been shown to be a religious ceremony with use of various gadgets with prescriptions for enlarging the size of penis (45, 46).

Dualism in the body was described as sexual and is said to reside in two nerve channels running along the two sides of the spinal cord. Men can take on feminine roles. Bullough (1976; 6) reminds us that Hindus embraced sex with a mystical connotation and almost anything in the sexual field received approval from some segment of Hindu society. Although some texts decry homosexuality, Basham (1967; 47, p. 172) notes that homosexuality was not unknown. In this context it would appear that ancient India was far healthier than most other ancient cultures. At that point in time, the laws against homosexuality were not rigid and generally local customs were accommodated (48, 49). However, sexual relationships across castes were frowned upon. There is no doubt that homosexual behaviour existed in ancient India, the concept of ardhnarishwar (half man/half woman) exists, and Bullough (1976; 6) sees Hinduism as a sex-positive religion.

Islam

On a similar basis that Islamic tenets about sex are derived from pre-Islamic Arabic attitudes towards marriage and sexual behaviour, initially it was a sex-positive religion (6). Clearly a male-oriented religion, women have specific roles and Burton (1886/1934; 50) saw Islam as more tolerant of same-sex behaviour than Christianity. Homosexual behaviour may have been a natural outgrowth of sexually segregating religion as shown in a sample of Arab students who were much more likely to report same-sex experiences than their American counterparts (51, 52). Like Hinduism, over millennia, Islam became sex-negative, but attitudes to same-sex behaviour have continued to be very mixed. Muslim rulers often had young male lovers (53, 54, 55) and male brothels flourished (50, pp. 205, 237). There was advice that the spring season is best for sexual intercourse (56) and that one should not confine one's inclination to either sex, and the summer season was seen as more suitable for same-sex experiences. Subsequent changes in attitudes with a palpable shift to more negative attitudes, reflect changes in society and social norms, undoubtedly in response to invasions over the millennia.

Christianity

Early Roman Catholic churches did not oppose homosexuality or regard it as unnatural, though some authorities take a different view (6). Herdt (5) notes that certainly early Roman Catholic church did not go out of its way to punish anyone because of their sexual practices. This appears to have changed after the eleventh century when lasting negative attitudes started to emerge, though the reasons for this change are not entirely clear. One possible assumption is that this may have been due to increasing visibility of the minorities of the time or to changes in the power of the Church, and, therefore, religious tenets were used to 'control' people. Religion most certainly played a major role in Western attitudes towards homosexuality (57), but the persistence of these negative attitudes may be explained by the attitudes of religious leaders wanting to hang on to their power and control through continuing discrimination and creation of 'the other'.

Crompton (2003; 58) asserts that, although Christianity was the child of Judaism and inherited much from the earlier faith, it might have reflected undercurrents of same-sex attraction in that era as a follow-on from the Roman attitudes (p. 111). (For detailed account and explanation, see (58)). Walsh (1978; 59) and Boswell (1980; 60) both attack the idea perpetrated and perpetuated by the Western cultures that homosexuality is unnatural. Walsh, in particular, links many of these negative attitudes to the body, to sex and sexuality by the Judeo-Christian tenets. One of the major psychoanalysts, Carl Gustav Jung, studied religions and applied these to the study and application of psychoanalysis. In his writings although he paid little attention to homosexuality but noted in one of his early writings that the legal postion in Germany against these behaviours was harmful to homosexual individuals (61). His linking of spirituality, religion and analysis offers an interesting overview

Cultural competence

Broad principles of cultural competence can be applied to therapeutic assessment and engagement if the individual's and therapist's sexual orientations do not match. Cultural competence is about understanding one's own cultural strengths and weaknesses, including unconscious biases and prejudices on behalf of the therapist. At the same time, the therapist also needs to understand the cultural background of the individual in front of them, both in a broader sense but also a narrower one, especially related to both religion and sexual orientation in terms of micro-identities. Exploring rituals, taboos, role of religion, and role of spirituality are at the core of any cultural competence training. Additional problems in some cases seeking help may be internalized homophobia and/or lack of family support. The 'world- view' of an individual is formed by their cultures, cultural up-bringing, peer support, and other factors if all these are absorbed subconsciously or unconsciously. Wynn and West-Olatunji (2009; 62) recommend that non-Eurocentric and non-heterosexual world views are needed along with an awareness of the socio-political realities about lesbian, gay, bisexual, and transgender life. In an interesting paper, Wagner et al. (1994; 63) suggest that internalized homophobia can be managed by integrating religious views and sexual orientations. They give an example of a Catholic group of gay men who have managed to achieve this. These models can provide a degree of leadership and support. In many settings, spirituality augmented cognitive behaviour therapies can be offered and used successfully. Some other therapeutic approaches are described below.

Buchanan et al. (2001; 64) recommend that narrative perspectives can offer a way to engage with gays and lesbians who are confronted with spiritual or religious identity. Spiritually based sexual orientation programmes can be made available. Gay ministries have also played a role in many cities. Gay affirmative theologians can work with mental health professionals in providing therapies and support. Challenging institutional and ecclesiastical homophobia can help gays and lesbians overcome their internalized homophobia (also see Goss 1993; 65). Within specific churches and religions, specific support groups for LGBT members have been set up. For some individuals, a potential solution may be to follow the atheist path and ignore the religion. Of course, a minority of individuals may choose to change their religion, which is their choice and the therapist should not get involved in that.

Using spirituality in therapy

The purpose of psychotherapy has to be seen as integration of different identities in the individual. Incorporating spirituality into any treatment plan, especially if the individual sees it as clearly important to them, has to be based on careful assessment. Often mental health professionals feel very uncomfortable in exploring spirituality, so they actively choose not to do so. On the other hand, due to so-called differentiation between religion and science, the individual may choose not to disclose their religious or spiritual needs to the clinician. Exploring and understanding spirituality, and how it is used by the individual to make sense of their world and experience, is a key first step. This is likely to improve therapeutic engagement and collaboration. Exploring spiritual concerns and degrees of religious attachment are important. Depending upon the context of therapy, couple or family attitudes to religion and spirituality may need to be explored. Ganzevoort et al. (2011; 66) reported that, among gay individuals growing up in religious communities, negotiating the identities can result in a Christian lifestyle, gay lifestyle, commuting, (compartmentalization) and integration. So, the key question the therapist may need to ask is what does the individual sitting in front of them want as their preferred outcome? Levy and Reeves (2011; 67) in a qualitative study found that any discord between religions and sexual identity can be resolved in a staged process and is affected by parental, personal and contextual factors that may play a role. They conclude that faith and identity development are intertwined. Thus again, the expected outcome of therapy must be identified fairly early on. Cultural competence related to sexual orientation has been described in detail in 68. It is critical that mental health professionals irrespective of their specialism are aware of the individual needs of sexual minority individuals and are open to exploring this and not imposing their own values.

Conclusions

Historically, as psychiatry emerged from the influence of religion and moved towards a more 'scientific' path, psychiatrists have often felt very uncomfortable in exploring religiosity and spirituality. All our patients tend to be brought up in some formal or organized religion, and their world -view is formed by the culture they are brought up in and the religion they follow. Sometimes this is the religion they were brought up in and at other times it is something they may discover or change. Their religious identity may be twinned with their sexual orientation, thereby creating a complex scenario. Exploring sexual orientation and religious identity in non-judgemental ways is important for successful therapeutic engagement and negotiation of the care pathway. External and internal homophobias can play a role in managing personalized individual pathways. Profound personal meaning of spirituality and organized religion for many gay, lesbian, bisexual, and transgender people are to be taken seriously. Therapists' or mental health professionals' own religious views or sexual orientation may create personal prejudices and unconscious bias, and these must be recognized and taken into account. Spirituality is complex and requires careful attention by the therapist on its cognitive, affective, and existential features, and to explore the individual's religious values, rituals, and taboos, if indicated. Therapists need not be fully au fait with every religious nuance or complex pattern of spirituality, but they have to be open-minded and willing to consider other options and explore subtle nuances as well as broad frameworks. Certain religious doctrines are homophobic and, under these circumstances, the therapist must explore the desired outcomes as preferred by the individual. Being gay and religious can be double jeopardy and isolating. Therefore, the therapist must take each individual's personal pathways into account. Spirituality can offer a certain supportive way. In many settings, religious leaders can become effective partners in dealing with issues of sexual pressures on the individual because of this tension orientation.

References

1. **McCann E, Donohue G, Timmins, F.** An exploration of the relationship between spirituality, religion and mental health among youth who identify as LGBT+: a systematic literature review. *Journal of Religion and Health.* 2020;59:828–44. Available at: https://doi.org/10.1007/s10943-020-00989-7

2. Jackle S, Wenzelburger G. Religion, religiosity and the attitudes towards homosexuality—a multilevel analysis of 79 countries. *Journal of Homosexuality.* 2015:**62**:207–41.

3. Janssen D-J, Scheepers P. How religiosity shapes rejection of homosexuality across the globe. *Journal of Homosexuality.* 2019;**66**:1974–2001.

4. Kocet M, Curry J. Introduction to special issue: finding the spirit within: spirituality issues in the LGBT community. *Journal of LGBT Issues in Counseling.* 2011;5:160–2.

5. Herdt G. (1987): Homosexuality. In: *The encyclopaedia of religion.* New York: Macmillanpp. 445–52.

6. Greenberg DF. *The construction of homosexuality.* Chicago: University of Chicago Press; 1988.

7. Bullough V. *Sexual variance in society and history.* Chicago: University of Chicago Press: 1976.

8. Becker HA. *The outsiders.* New York: Free Press; 1963. p. 9.

9. Bhugra D. Coming out in South Asian gay men in the United Kingdom. *Archives of Sexual Behaviour.* 1997;**26**:547–57.

10. Thompson M. *Gay soul: finding the heart of the gay spirit and nature.* San Francisco, CA: Harper; 1994.

11. Morris B. *Anthropology of the self: the individual in cultural perspective.* London: Pluto Press; 1994.

12. Erickson E. Ego development and historical change. *The Psychoanalytic Study of the Child.* 1946;**2**:359–86.

13. Erickson E. *Childhood and society.* New York: Norton; 1950.

14. Wachter M, Ventriglio A, Bhugra D (2015): Micro-identities, adjustment and stigma. *International Journal of Social Psychiatry.* 2015;**61**:436–7.

15. Davenport-Hines R. *Sex, death and punishment.* London: Collins; 1990, pp. 114–16.

16. Cass VC. Homosexual identity formation. *Journal of Homosexuality.* 1979;4: 219–35.

17. Beagan BL, Hattie B. Religion, spirituality and LGBTQ identity integration. *Journal of LGBT Issues in Counseling.* 2015;**9**:92–117.

18. Dahl A, Galliher RV. The interplay of sexual and religious identity development in LGBTQ adolescents and young adults: a qualitative enquiry. *Identity.* 2012;**12**:217–46.

19. Reygan F, Moane G. Religious homophobia: the experience of a sample of lesbian, gay, bisexual and transgender people in Ireland. *Cult & Religion.* 2014;**15**:298–312.

20. Fox M. (1984): The spiritual journey of the homosexual ... and just about everyone else. In: R Nugent, (ed.), *A challenge to love: gay and lesbian Catholics in the church.* New York: Crossroad, pp. 189–204.

21. Haldeman D. Spirituality and religion in the lives of lesbians and gay men. In: RP Cabaj, TS Stein, (eds), *Textbook of homosexuality and mental health.* Washington, DC: APPI; 1996, pp. 881–96.

22. Harvey A. *Hidden journey: a spiritual awakening.* New York: Penguin; 1992.

23. Boyd M. Survival with grace. In: M Thompson, (ed.), *Gay soul: finding the heart of gay spirit and nature.* San Francisco, CA: Harper; 1994, pp. 233–45.

24. Cohen C, Stein T. Reconceptualising individual psychotherapy with gay men and lesbians. In: J Gonsiorek, (ed.), *A guide to psychotherapy with gay and lesbian clients.* New York: Plenum; 1986, pp. 105–13.

25. **Coleman E.** Developmental stages of coming out process. In: **W Paul** et al., (eds), *Homosexuality, social, psychological and biological issues*. Beverley Hills, CA: Sage; 1985, pp. 149–58.

26. **Hanley-Hackenbruck P.** Psychotherapy and coming out process. *Journal of Gay and Lesbian Psychotherapy*. 1989;1:21–40.

27. **Hencken JD, O'Dowd WT.** Coming out as an aspect of identity formation. *Gay Academy Union Journal*. 1977;1:18–22.

28. **Dank B.** Coming out in the gay world. *Psychiatry*. 1971;**34**:180–97.

29. **Lee JA.** Going public: a study in the sociology of homosexual liberation. *Journal of Homosexuality*. 1977;**3**:49–78.

30. **Plummer K.** Homosexual categories. In: **K: Plummer**, (ed.), *The making of a modern homosexual*. London: Hutchinson; 1975, pp. 53–75.

31. **Jay K, Young Y.** *The gay report*. New York: Summit; 1979.

32. **Trenchard L, Warren H.** *Something to tell you*. London: London Gay Teenage Group; 1984.

33. **Gold SP, Stewart DL.** Lesbian, gay and bisexual students coming out at the intersection of spirituality and sexual identity. *Journal of LGBT Issues in Counseling*. 2012;**5**:237–58.

34. **Weinberg M, Williams C.** *Male homosexuals: their problems and adaptations*. New York: Penguin; 1974.

35. **Halkitis PN, Mattis JS, Sahadath JK, Massie D, Ladyzhenskaya L, Pitrelli K, et al.** The meanings and manifestations of religion and spirituality among lesbian, gay, bisexual and transgender adults. *Journal of Adult Development*. 2009;**16**: 250–62.

36. **Blumenfeld W, Raymond D.** *Looking at gay and lesbian life*. New York: Philosophical Press; 1988.

37. **Schuck KD, Liddle BJ.** Religious conflicts experienced by lesbian, gay and bisexual individuals. *Journal of Gay & Lesbian Psychotherapy*. 2001;**5**:63–82.

38. **Super JT, Jacobson L.** Religious abuse: implications for lesbian, gay, bisexual and transgender individuals. *Journal of LGBT Issues in Counseling*. 2011;**5**:180–96.

39. **Gibbs J, Goldbach J.** Religious conflict, sexual identity and suicidal behaviours among LGBT young adults. *Archives of Suicide Research*. 2015;**19**:472–88.

40. **Irwin JA, Coleman J, Fisher C, Marasco M.** Correlates of suicidal ideation among LGBT Nebraskans. *Journal of Homosexuality*. 2014;**61**:1172–91.

41. **Vanita R, Kidwai S.** Same-sex love in India: a literary history. New Delhi: Penguin; 2008.

42. **Wilkins WJ.** *Hindu mythology: Vedic and Puranic*. Calcutta: Rupa; 1989, orig. 1882.

43. **Walker B.** *The Hindu world: an encyclopaedic survey of Hinduism*. (2 vols). New York: Praeger; 1968, pp. 390–2.

44. **Woodroffe J.** *Sakti and Sakta*. Madras: Ganesh & Co; 1972, pp. 376–412.

45. **De SK.** Ancient Indian erotica. Cited in **VL Bullough**, *Sexual variance*. Chicago: University of Chicago Press; 1932, p. 276.

46. **Vatsyayna.** *Kamasutra*. R Burton, F Arbuthnot (trans.). Bombay: Jaico; 1963.

47. **Basham AL.** *The wonder that was India*. London: Fontana; 1967.

48. **Derrett JD.** *Dharmashastra and juridical literature*. Wiesbaden: Otto Harrassowitz; 1973, pp. 2–3.

49. **Trautman RH.** The real self: from institution to impulse. *American Journal of Sociology.* 1976;**81**:989–1016.

50. **Burton RF.** *Book of the thousand nights and a night.* New York: Heritage; 1934, orig. 1886.

51. **Finger F.** Sex beliefs and practices among male college students. *Journal of Abnormal and Social Psychology.* 1947;**42**:57–67.

52. **Melikian L, Prothro ET.** Sexual behaviour of university students in the Arabs near East. *Journal of Abnormal and Social Psychology.* 1954;**49**:63–4.

53. **Yasin M.** *A social history of Islamic India 1605–1748.* Lucknow: Upper India; 1958, p. 107.

54. **Henriques F.** *Stews and strumpets: a survey of prostitution* (vol. 1). London: Macgibbon & Kee; 1961, pp. 174, 355.

55. **Saletore RN.** *Sex life under Indian rulers.* Delhi: Hind; 1974.

56. **Iskander K.** *A mirror for princes (Qubus Nama),* R Levy (trans.). London: Gesset; 1951, orig. 1082, pp. 77–8.

57. **Young-Breuhl E.** *The anatomy of prejudice.* Cambridge, Mass: Harvard University Press; 1996.

58. **Crompton L.** *Homosexuality and civilisation.* Cambridge, MA: Belknap Press of Harvard University Press; 2003.

59. **Walsh D.** Homosexuality, rationality and Western culture. *Hawest.* 1978;**24**:79–100.

60. **Boswell J.** *Christianity, social tolerance and homosexuality.* Chicago: University of Chicago Press; 1980.

61. **Hopcke RH.** *Jung, Jungians and homosexuality.* Boston, MA: Shambhala; 1989.

62. **Wynn R, West-Olatunji C.** Use of culture centred counselling theory with ethnically diverse LGBT clients. *Journal of LGBT Issues in Counseling.* 2009;**3**:198–214.

63. **Wagner G, Serafini J, Rabkin J, Remien R, Williams J.** Integration of one's religion and homosexuality. *Journal of Homosexuality.* 1994;**26**:91–110.

64. **Buchanan M, Dzelme K, Harris D, Hecker L.** Challenges of being simultaneously gay or lesbian and spiritual and/or religious: a narrative perspective. *American Journal of Family Therapy.* 2001;**29**:435–49.

65. **Goss R.** *Jesus acted up: a gay and lesbian manifesto.* San Francisco, CA: Harper; 1993.

66. **Ganzevoort R, van der Laan M, Olsman E.** Growing up gay and religious. Conflict dialogue and religious identity strategies. *Mental Health, Religion and Culture.* 2011;**14**:209–22.

67. **Levy D, Reeves P.** Resolving identity conflict: gay, lesbian and queer individuals with a Christian upbringing. *Journal of Gay and Lesbian Social Services.* 2011;**23**:53–68.

68. **Bhugra D, Ventriglio A, Bhui K.** *Practical cultural psychiatry.* Oxford: Oxford University Press; 2018.

Section II

General principles of religions and relationship with mental health

Chapter 10

Christianity and mental health

Alison J. Gray and Christopher C.H. Cook

Introduction

Christianity is the largest religious tradition worldwide, with around 2.3 billion followers. Along with Islam and Judaism, Christianity is one of the three major monotheistic traditions in the world today. Christians believe in one God. However, Christianity is distinctive by virtue of the centrality that it accords to the life and teaching of Jesus of Nazareth, a prophet who arose within the Jewish tradition in first-century Palestine. Jesus, is also referred to by Christians as 'Christ' (a title meaning 'anointed', or 'sent', by God) or Jesus Christ. Jesus died by crucifixion, a common form of execution in the Roman Empire, probably around 30 CE. According to Christian tradition, on 'the third day' (that is, two days after the crucifixion), Jesus rose from the dead and appeared to his disciples. His tomb was found to be empty. The resurrection of Jesus became a central Christian belief and is closely linked to the further assertion that Jesus was in fact God incarnate. While this is not understood to negate in any way the full humanity of Jesus, the belief in his divinity remains the major point of division between Christians on the one hand, and Jews and Muslims on the other.

The present chapter seeks to provide a brief introduction to the beliefs and practices of Christians worldwide and to explore the relationship between Christianity and mental health. Any overview has to make generalizations in order to fit the available space. Any individual, or group, who would identify as Christian will emphasize different aspects of the faith and may therefore come to different conclusions about certain beliefs, practices, or ethical issues. For example, abortion and marriage for same-sex couples are currently contentious issues. In our brief summary, we highlight the things (almost) all Christians will have in common, but during any clinical assessment it remains important to ask the person in front of you how their religion works out in practice in their life.

Belief

Christianity began as a renewal movement within Judaism. Jesus and his first followers were all Jewish, hence Christianity shares much of the worldview of Judaism. Hebrew Scriptures, referred to by Christians as the 'Old Testament', are also Christian scripture. In addition, Christians identify 27 further books of scripture, which they refer to as the 'New Testament'. These include four accounts of the life, death, and resurrection of Jesus, all written in Greek within 80 years or so following his death. The remaining books, also in Greek, include a history of the early church (the 'Acts of the Apostles'), a book of apocalyptic literature (the 'Revelation to St John'), and a series of letters (epistles), written by leaders of the early church, notably St Paul. Together, these scriptures remain the primary source of authority for teaching the faith, and deriving doctrine, for all Christians worldwide. However, the relationship of this to other sources of authority, such as tradition, experience, or Church teaching, varies significantly among different Christian churches. Scripture is amenable to diverse interpretations, and there is much debate as to whose interpretations should be seen as authoritative.

The fundamentals of Orthodox Christian belief are expressed in a series of creeds that emerged through a process of debate and consensus in the early centuries of the Christian Church, notably the Nicene Creed from 325 CE. This statement of belief is recited by believers in worship every Sunday in many Christian churches (1). The creeds centrally affirm that there is one God in three persons, Father, Son, and Holy Spirit. Known as the 'doctrine of the Trinity', this has been one of the most complex and confusing of all Christian beliefs, with critics arguing that it is impossible to understand, or else that it amounts to tritheism, the belief in three gods. Christians have continued to affirm the mystery (after all, who can claim to understand God?) and have held steadfastly to the fundamental monotheism within which this doctrine is understood.

In many other respects, Christian beliefs are similar to those of Judaism. God created the world and everything in it. God created humankind in His own image. Humankind has a natural tendency to mess things up, traditionally called 'sin'. The first humans rebelled against God (often referred to as 'the fall') and the perfection of creation was destroyed. Illness is, at least indirectly, a consequence of this rebellion at a fundamental level. This is not to say that an individual's sin leads to them developing an illness, rather that disease, sickness, pain, and death were not part of God's original plan. What it might mean to talk of God's 'original plan' is contentious, and subject to different understanding by different Christians, especially in the light of Darwinian theories of evolution.

There is a tension within Christianity between an emphasis on the goodness of creation on the one hand, and its fallenness on the other.

Distinctively, the self-sacrificial death of Jesus is understood by Christians to have broken the power of sin and brought about atonement, or reconciliation, between God and human beings. Jesus taught about a new kingdom where God reigns supreme. This kingdom will reach its fulfilment at the end of time when Jesus will judge all humankind and there will be a new heaven and a new earth. Anyone who turns away from their wrongdoing and chooses to follow the Jesus way becomes part of the Kingdom as God reigns in their lives. God the Holy Spirit lives within them and helps them to grow more like Jesus, worshipping God in a community of believers. Within this scheme of belief, forgiveness occupies a central place of importance. Paradoxically, this has sometimes seemed (to Christians or others) to emphasize sin and guilt. If forgiveness is important, then the conversation easily turns to what needs to be forgiven. In mental illness, this can sometimes express itself as a preoccupation with guilt and sin. However, the proper emphasis has always been on the message of Jesus as 'good news', placing the focus on redemption, not on condemnation.

The central belief of Christians in the incarnation of God in Christ has a broad and complex outworking that takes a variety of forms in different Christian traditions. While Christians believe in a transcendent God (above and beyond all material things), the incarnation recognizes that God is also intimately present within his creation—not only in Christ, but also more widely. Sometimes, this can look very similar to pantheism although strictly it is closer to panentheism (the distinction being that all things are in God, rather than the other way around in pantheism). It is also the basis for Christian belief in sacraments, visible and outward signs (e.g. baptism) of inner spiritual grace imparted by God.

The Christian vision of human flourishing occurs in relationship to God, and is a process not an event. We will live a good life when we use our gifts and talents, through God's grace, to help other people and the whole of creation to flourish (2). Health of body and spirit is a good thing but not the primary good. According to the gospels, Jesus taught that loving God was the most important rule in life, closely followed by love of others. He also taught that we only find our lives when we are willing to lose them. The self-sacrificial element in Christianity has sometimes unhelpfully valorized suffering, but it has also properly recognized that human flourishing comes at a cost. The Christian belief that humans are made in God's image is the basis for considering all human life as sacred, and worthy of honour and dignity. Thus, all people are to be treated with honesty and integrity, faithful love and compassion (3). This has provided the basis for many Christians to find vocations in medicine and in the helping professions, as well as in campaigning for social justice.

Divisions and denominations

From earliest times, there have been dissensions and divisions within the Christian Church. In the earliest days of the Church, these were concerned with how Gentile believers should be received within a primarily Jewish community, and about matters such as the eating of meat offered to pagan idols. Later, there were doctrinal disputes concerning different views on the nature of Jesus, how his divinity and humanity hold together. There are still groups of Christians who do not hold to the wider orthodoxy on these matters, such as the Coptic Church of Egypt. However, the first major split occurred in the eleventh century. This 'Great Schism' led to separation between the Orthodox churches in the east, and the Catholic Church in the west. In the sixteenth century. the European Reformation led to a further split within the western Church between the Roman Catholic (RC) and the Protestant, or reformed, churches (e.g. Anglican, Lutheran).

While 'catholics' are usually understood to be RC, it is important to be aware that 'catholic' and 'RC' are not synonymous. Many Christians would consider themselves to be catholic in a broader sense of belonging to the universal Church. In the Nicene Creed, all Christians express their belief in 'one holy, catholic, and apostolic church'. It is a matter of sadness to many Christians that this spiritual unity, or catholicity, is marred by historical and traditional divisions. Catholic (with a small 'c') also has a somewhat different sense of implying a form of church tradition involving bishops and an emphasis on sacrament and ritual. Catholics (in this sense) understand their faith more as membership of the universal catholic Church than as an individual or local affair.

The RC Church, as a particular division or denomination within Christianity, emphasizes the authority of the Pope, the priesthood, and Church tradition. Protestant churches focus more on the individual's relationship with God and on the primary authority of scripture. There tends to be more emphasis on the local congregation than on the wider institutional Church (although this also varies). Protestant churches further vary in how fundamentalist, conservative, or liberal and progressive they are. Some denominations include a very wide breadth of belief and practice. The Church of England (CofE), for example, includes both catholic and reformed elements in its liturgy and doctrine. Some of its churches are very catholic in their traditions of belief and practice, whereas others look much more reformed (Protestant).

The rite of baptism is recognized by all Christian churches as the means of Christian initiation, although there are differences—for example, as to whether or not children may be baptised. Baptist churches do not recognize infant baptism and only baptise adults. Baptism always involves water, and is always in the name of God, the Father, Son and Holy Spirit. In some churches, and especially where infants are involved, it is usually by sprinkling of water over the head. In others, notably (but not only) in Baptist churches, it is by total immersion.

Some churches—for example, the RC Church and the CofE, have a written liturgy that is the same in all churches of that denomination; other churches have nothing written down. The Society of Friends (Quakers) spend most of their meetings in silence before members share what they believe God has said to them. RC and Orthodox Christians venerate Mary, Jesus' mother, and ask her (and other saints) for assistance in prayer, in a way that most Christians from reformed traditions do not.

Almost all Christian churches have a place for the Eucharist or Holy Communion (also called the 'Lord's Supper' or 'Mass') (4) but its importance is greater in Catholic churches than Protestant. In the Eucharist, members of the congregation share bread and wine together, remembering Jesus' last supper with his disciples before his death. One of the key historical differences between the RC and Protestant churches concerned understanding of what exactly happened to the bread and wine during the Eucharist. For the RC Church, they were understood as becoming in some way the actual body and blood of Christ. For Protestant Christians, Holy Communion was more a commemoration and a reminder of Jesus' death and resurrection, and the bread and wine were more symbolic.

If the Eucharist has been one major point of division, then scripture has been another. Some conservative Christians see the Bible as the inerrant and/or infallible word of God and take it more literally. Others see the Bible as needing careful unpacking and interpretation in terms of the literary form of the passage (poetry, law, or history need to be read differently), and taking into account the differences in original and contemporary historical/cultural contexts. Some see a greater role for interpreting scripture in the light of science, whereas others would emphasize the authority of scripture over science, even to the extent of believing that the world was created literally according to the account in Genesis, in six days, and denying scientific theories of evolution.

Spirituality

Within Christian worship, prayer, singing, and reading sacred scripture are ubiquitous. However, Christian prayer can take many different forms, and spirituality can vary within the same denomination or church. For example, within the CofE, social justice is more emphasized by some, and evangelism (telling people the good news about Jesus) in others. Some emphasize a more contemplative, or even mystical, approach to prayer, devoting more time to silence, whereas others emphasize the use of words. Some use a prescribed and written liturgy, whereas others prefer a more informal and extemporary approach.

Within the more mystical strands of Christian spirituality, practices of contemplative prayer may closely resemble mindfulness (and there is much debate as to exactly what the differences are—if any). Mystical experiences are to a large extent ineffable and impossible to fully describe. While much may be said about Christian mysticism as a distinctive phenomenon, it also shares many features in common with mystical experiences in other traditions, such as Islam, Judaism, and even Buddhism.

Within Pentecostal and charismatic Christianity, there is a stress on the direct action of God in people's experience, so called 'signs and wonders', and miraculous healing. In extreme cases (particularly in some parts of the world or in certain churches), this emphasis on healing through faith may lead to avoidance of contact with medical services. Many Pentecostal and charismatic churches emphasize forms of prayer within which one is expected to 'hear' God, and such experiences are easily misinterpreted by mental health professionals who are unfamiliar with them as psychopathology. In fact, hearing God is a completely normal religious experience for many Christians worldwide.

Christian care for people suffering from mental illness

In the Christian gospels, healing is presented as a major part of the work of Jesus. Jesus healed in different ways. Sometimes he prayed aloud, sometimes he didn't. Sometimes Jesus took the initiative, and in other cases he responded to the request of another. Sometimes he laid his hands on people, and other times he healed at a distance. On one occasion, he is recorded as having mixed spit into mud and put it on the sufferer's eyes. There was no uniform way in which Jesus healed people but, whenever he did he also restored them socially, enabling them to return to their community. Healing in the gospels is a sign of God's Kingdom breaking through.

When Jesus sent out his followers, his instructions included to heal the sick, so the Christian church has always been involved in health and healing.

> ... the gospel [good news about Jesus] is about healing, about telling effectively, powerfully and transformingly the story of how God inhabits this world, telling it in words and thoughts and theology, and telling it also in what we do in our work for justice in our arts, in our care and our pastoring (5).

It seems likely that one of the reasons for the rapid spread of Christianity in the Roman Empire was that Christians routinely looked after those who were suffering from a plague, and if the patients recovered they often joined the Christian community (6). This led naturally to the development of general hospitals throughout Christian areas by the fifth century (7).

The church and individual Christians have been involved in setting up many mental health services and projects. The first Christian mental hospital was in Jerusalem in AD 490 (8). In medieval Europe, there was very patchy support for those who were deemed insane (9); most of the care was provided by family and local community. The Bethlem Royal Hospital in London, which eventually became the first European mental health hospital, was founded in 1247 as a Priory, run by Christian monks, originally as a place of hospitality and alms collection for the needy. The first town to offer community care was Geel in Belgium; this was recorded in the thirteenth century but may be much older. Here, people with mental illnesses continued to board with families as a family member, often for decades. This form of care sprang from the church of St Dymphna, the patron saint of the mentally ill, and was organized by the church ministers until the last century when local government took over (10).

Christianity has not always treated the mentally ill so kindly. Over the centuries following the founding of the Inquisition in 1233, many mentally ill people were executed as heretics or witches. The mentally ill were not singled out for such treatment, and many other people with different kinds of misfortune also suffered a similar fate. From the late sixteenth century onwards, an increasing preoccupation with demon possession further increased this trend and, although this subsided, even today some churches misidentify signs of mental illness as related to demonic affliction.

The Society of Friends (Quakers), founded by George Fox in the mid-seventeenth century, broke away from the Church of England and has its origins within Christianity. Some Quakers today hold non-theistic beliefs, and Quakerism generally does not subscribe to the Christian creeds. They emphasize the possibility of accessing the light within all people and teach that God can be encountered directly through personal experience. Quakers are non-hierarchical, committed to simple living, and social justice, winning the Nobel peace prize in 1947 (a).

Moral treatment in the UK began at the York Retreat that was founded by the Quakers in 1796, following the death of a member in a local asylum. This approach emphasizes kindness, compassionate care, and the moral and spiritual development of those experiencing acute mental illness, and it underpins modern psychiatric approaches (11). Faith-based activism also drove the actions of many of those involved in the development of mental health services in the USA such as Dorothea Dix in the 1840s (12).

The international spread of Christian medical care was intertwined with the broader colonial expansion of European influence. While many injustices were perpetrated around the world in the name of Christianity, the routes of travel that facilitated colonialism also facilitated mission, including medical mission. Medical missionaries abounded in the developing world in the nineteenth century, opening clinics and building general hospitals where such were not available. In 1910, Protestant churches ran 2,100 mission hospitals, and twice that number of clinics. The RC Church ran many mission hospitals and continue to do so in many countries. The Orthodox churches are generally not involved in direct medical provision. Although many facilities have been handed over to local governments, Christian missionaries continue to serve in hard-to reach-areas and unattractive specialities e.g. inner-city London (b), Mercy Ships (c), Ebola care (d), and leprosy missions (e). Such hospitals contribute to physical health and human flourishing. However, very few of these mission hospitals or clinics deal directly with mental illness (13).

Alcoholics Anonymous (AA) began in 1935 from the friendship of two men who had each experienced a Christian conversion as a significant part of their escape from alcohol addiction (f). The AA 12-step programme, although no longer specifically Christian, is explicit about the need for a spiritual awakening. It continues to be a highly successful programme of recovery from addiction (14), as attested to by its spread and continuing popularity. Prospective research is hampered by the anonymous nature of the groups (g). The 12 steps have been adapted for many issues including narcotic addiction, gambling, overeating, and sex addiction.

In the UK, mental hospitals were incorporated into the National Health Service after the Second World War. In other European countries (e.g. Germany), many such institutions continue to be administered by Christian groups. In the USA, Pine Rest (founded as the Christian Psychopathic Hospital in 1910) is the fourth largest behavioural health provider and holds to explicitly Christian standards (h).

The Samaritans telephone support line was begun in 1953 by Revd Chad Varah, an English priest, to listen to those contemplating suicide. As 'Befrienders worldwide', the group has a presence in 32 countries serving 7 million people per year (i). Like AA, it is no longer an explicitly Christian programme, but it provides a continuing legacy of Christian compassion for those who experience despair and contemplate the possibility of ending their lives.

L'Arche International is a network of homes for people with learning disabilities. In 1964, Jean Vanier, a Roman Catholic philosopher, welcomed two men with learning disabilities to live with him. The L'Arche philosophy is that those with disabilities live as equals with assistants, and all are valued as individuals made in God's image. The model has been adapted to work effectively in different cultures and has brought much to our understanding of how to care for those with learning disability (15).

CHRISTIANITY AND MENTAL HEALTH | **175**

There are multiple initiatives to educate Christians about mental health at national and regional levels. For example, The Episcopal Church in the USA has the Episcopal Mental Illness Network (j), and the RC Church is actively addressing mental health issues in the UK, USA, and elsewhere (k, l). Christian professionals in the UK started the Mind and Soul Foundation (m), and Saddleback churches in the USA (n) have begun to address mental health issues in the language of Evangelical and conservative Christianity.

Churches as healing communities

At its best, a Christian congregation is a healthy family, a gathering of people from all backgrounds and walks of life who accept, love, help, and support each other, and where all can belong. Mental illness can limit people's ability to relate to themselves, to others, and to God, both directly (because of the tendency to isolate oneself and the distortion of experience) and indirectly, through the effects of stigma. A mental health aware, tolerant, Christian congregation can provide listening; understanding; and spiritual, practical, and emotional care; and support people on their recovery journey:

> The call of Jesus is to hear the cries for love and to move forwards in friendship and in perseverant love; a mode of friendship which destroys stigma and opens up space for all of us together to be fully human even in the midst of our wildest storms (16).

Churches pray for the healing of both physical and mental health issues within services in most denominations. Evangelical and Pentecostal churches practise healing through faith, prayer, and the laying on of hands. Orthodox and Catholic churches identify the Eucharist as enabling an encounter with the living Christ that will result in healing. Christian healing is understood at multiple levels. For some, it may be associated with complete freedom from illness, understood to be an answer to prayer, and viewed as miraculous. For others, it may be more concerned with adjustment and acceptance of limitations, and restoring of meaning and purpose to life, even while living with ongoing symptoms of mental illness.

Alongside healing, fundamental themes in the Bible include care for the poor, struggling and marginalized, and welcoming strangers. In a recent UK survey, '94% of Anglican churches are involved in helping people with loneliness, 86% with family breakdown, and 83% in supporting people with mental health problems 93% support a food bank' (o):

> Jane was 48 when she had her first psychotic depressive breakdown triggered by a sexual assault. She was legally detained and treated in hospital. On discharge she could not bear to go back to her flat, since that was where the assault happened. Jane ended up moving home, losing all her social contacts. She remained terrified that she was demon

possessed and came to a church service looking for an exorcism. She was listened to by a minister, reassured that there were no signs of possession, encouraged to take her medication and offered practical support. Three years on she has made a full recovery from the psychotic illness, is well integrated into the church and local community and has begun to help and support other people.

Mental illness and demon possession

The authors of the gospels provide a series of accounts of Jesus casting demons out of people. While some take these stories literally, believing in demonic entities that afflict and perhaps 'possess' human beings, others point out that Jesus worked within the framework of beliefs that prevailed in his time, and that most of these individuals would now be considered to have epilepsy or another neurological condition. Only in one case (the story of the Gerasene demoniac) is there any apparent similarity to what we would now call mental illness.

Some Christians believe Satan is a living spiritual entity with influence on earth. Others see spiritual warfare purely in terms of a fight for social justice against oppressive, evil systems of power (17). Sixty per cent of American Christians surveyed agreed that 'Satan is not a living being, but is a symbol of evil' (p). Those who described themselves as 'born again' (i.e. evangelical) were more likely to disagree. RC exorcists worldwide have reported a 'dramatic increase in demonic activity' (q). CofE policy requires the involvement of mental health professionals in the work of deliverance ministry and, in many such cases, mental health concerns are identified. Exorcisms are correspondingly rare (18, 19). In developing countries, and in Pentecostal churches worldwide, exorcisms are very frequent; demon possession is considered a cause of multiple issues, abnormal behaviour, recurrent sickness, and same-sex attraction. Many gay and lesbian Christians have been prayed for to release them from a 'spirit of homosexuality', and some now see this as a form of spiritual abuse (20).

In terms of clinical practice, mental health professionals need to be aware of the range of different views within the Christian tradition, and the potential for abuse by those who take an extreme stance, or who are simply ill informed about the nature of mental illness. Close working with chaplains and clergy, and an understanding of the nature of beliefs within church and family, are vital to good practice.

Evidence for the impact of Christian faith on mental health

The impact of any particular belief system on any individual's health and well-being will depend a lot on the society around them. The significance of being a

Christian in the bible-belt of America will be different from being a Christian in contemporary Syria. Hence, it is difficult to make general statements about the 'impact of Christianity on mental health'; it all depends on the form of Christianity, in the particular social context (21). Point prevalence studies can show, for example, the prevalence of depression within a congregation, but they cannot separate out whether Christianity causes or cures depression, or whether people turn back to church when they feel low in mood. Hence, we shall briefly focus here on the results of the few controlled long-term prospective studies.

Psychosis

In a study of 115 out-patients with schizophrenia or schizo-affective disorder, two-thirds of whom were Christians, Mohr et al (22) were able to follow up 92 over a three-year period. Eighty-three per cent of patients reported that religion was a helpful coping resource. Among these, but not among those who found religion unhelpful, importance of spirituality was predictive of better outcome. However, outcomes did not differ overall between those who found spirituality/religion to be a helpful coping resource and those who found it to be unhelpful.

Depression

In a cross-sectional retrospective study of major depression, RC mothers were at 80% lower risk of major depressive disorder (MDD) over the preceding 10 years as compared with non-RC mothers (23). The offspring of the cohort who indicated religion or spirituality as important to them were 76% less likely to develop MDD over the next 10 years (24).

A 14-year follow-up of non-depressed citizens from the Canadian National Population Health survey (25) showed that there was a 22% lower risk of MDD for those who attended church at least once a month compared with those who never attended, varying in a dose–response manner. Neither self-report of spiritual values or faith being important, nor identifying as very religious or spiritual, had any impact on depression rates.

In the US Nurses' Health Study, among 50,000 women, mostly white (Protestant or RC), rates of clinical depression were recorded over a 12-year follow-up. Comparing those who attended religious services frequently with those who never attended, there was a 30% lower risk of incipient depression. Women with depression were subsequently less likely to attend services (26).

Suicide

The Nurses' Health Study demonstrated that those who attended any weekly religious services were 84% less likely to complete suicide compared with the never-attenders. Among Roman Catholics, those who attended once or more per week were 95% less likely to complete suicide than those who attended less frequently. This is thought to be due to the traditional RC teaching that suicide is a mortal sin, leading to eternal damnation (27).

Substance abuse

Religious service attendance was associated with far lower usage of illicit substances in Canadian teenagers over a five-year period, compared with non-attenders. Those who attended other types of club showed no such protective effect (28).

Happiness

Looking at the children of those in the US Nurses' Health Study, with a follow-up duration of 8–14 years, those who attended weekly religious services in youth were 18% more likely to report greater happiness aged 23–30 years than those who never attended. They were 33% less likely to report illicit drug usage, and 29% more likely to be volunteers (29). Daily prayer or meditation in childhood and youth had a similar effect on later happiness.

Resilience

A longitudinal study began in Kauai, Hawaii, in 1955 and continued over three decades, concentrating on children experiencing factors expected to be predictive of future mental illness: premature birth, abuse, poverty, and parental low education, mental illness, or addiction. The researchers found that one-third of these high-risk children grew up to become 'competent, confident and caring' adults. These successful children tended to come from families that held religious beliefs (usually Christianity), which provided stability. They also commonly experienced a positive relationship in childhood with an adult, teacher, neighbour, minister, or member of a church group, or had a near-death or religious conversion experience as a young adult (30).

Negative impact

There are Christian churches, groups, and individual teachers who argue that God always wants to heal everybody immediately. In this context, failure to experience healing is often attributed to such factors as lack of faith, unconfessed sin, or wrong belief. Such teaching causes much distress to those with severe and enduring mental illness and their families, and alienates people from God and their Christian community. Often, the same churches encourage people not to take antidepressants and psychotropic medication, leading to repeated relapses.

In this context, some people end up moving to a more understanding church, or else abandoning their faith, or at least leaving institutionalized religion:

> David was brought in as an emergency by his Evangelical church pastor. David had been to a Christian festival where those praying with him had declared that he was healed and should throw away his medication as a sign of his trust in God. Three weeks later he was floridly manic, talking rapidly, and singing modern Christian worship songs. It was impossible to get his attention. He began to sing a song I recognized so I quietly joined in. This deepened our rapport, I acknowledged my faith, and was able to convince him that God works through tablets too. He accepted some mood-stabilizing medication and cooperated with the admission process.

Even when churches do not espouse such ill-informed and harmful beliefs, there are elements within Christian faith and ritual that easily become the focus of psychopathology. Belief in guilt and sin, unbalanced by an emphasis on forgiveness and redemption, easily becomes a focus of concern in affective disorders. Christian rituals can feed into, and perhaps even worsen, obsessive-compulsive disorder (OCD):

> Sarah was a church minister. She began to develop a depressive illness in the context of overwork and her own perfectionism. Along with low mood she developed OCD and scrupulosity—believing that she must confess every single sin and that failure to do so would result in a catastrophe. She spent many hours a day in prayer unable to stop, in case that was a sin. She then developed the belief that when she touched the bread and wine at communion it became poison, and she had harmed her congregation through this. She accepted admission to hospital and needed ECT to treat her depression. Within six months she was able to return to ministry and has not experienced a relapse in 15 years.

There can be a gap between the authoritative teaching of the church and how that is translated into the espoused beliefs of a particular congregation, and then into the actual things that happen day by day, week by week, in the life of the church community (31). Christians often have the same stigmatizing attitudes as the society around them. A young woman known to one of us (AJG) was informed that she could serve in her church by helping people to park safely, but that she couldn't serve in a visible role during the service, simply because of her eating disorder:

> John had several episodes of bipolar disorder in his early twenties. This has been under control, off medication, for twenty years. He has a job, family, and an important role in his churches musical worship. Talking to the minister he mentioned he had been legally detained and forced to have treatment three times whilst at university; they have not spoken to him since.

The gap between teaching, stated beliefs, and actions is most painfully seen in the multiple stories of abuse by ministers from all denominations of the church, and by the failure of central institutions to respond adequately to these crimes

(32). In liturgical church services in many traditions, there is a time of recognition and confession of wrongdoing, with God's forgiveness being pronounced over the congregation by the minister. Within the Catholic traditions, there is also a confidential practice of private confession to a priest and reconciliation. Unfortunately, these practices have been misused by some abusers so as to persuade themselves or others that they have really changed, and to prevent legal action being taken.

Summary

In the Christian world view, each individual is made in the image of God and is precious and valuable, whatever their mental health or cognitive status. The Christian churches have been involved in mental health care, both directly through running hospitals and clinics and indirectly in supporting staff and patients who attend these. Local Christian churches have members who have experienced mental illness and have provided sometimes extensive and compassionate care for them. Churches enhance community and individual well-being by providing groups and services for many outside the congregation. While the teaching of some churches can be unhelpful, particularly when it over-spiritualizes or discourages timely interaction with health care and consistent treatment concordance, the evidence suggests that Christianity is generally a positive influence on mental health.

References

1. *The Book of Common Prayer of the Episcopal Church*. New York: Church Publishing Incorporated; 2007, pp. 326–7.
2. **Pennington JA.** *The Sermon on the Mount and human flourishing*. Grand Rapids: Baker Academic; 2017.
3. *Catechism of the Catholic Church*, Chapter 1, Article 7: The virtues. Available from: http://www.vatican.va/archive/ccc_css/archive/catechism/ccc_toc.htm
4. **Williams R.** *Being Christian: Baptism, Bible, Eucharist, Prayer*. London: SPCK; 2014. The Quakers and the Salvation Army do not celebrate any form of the Eucharist.
5. **Williams R.** A theology of health for today. In: **Baxter J**, ed. *Wounds that heal: Theology, Imagination and Health*. London: SPCK; 2007: pp. 13–14.
6. **Bentley Hart D.** *Atheist delusions: the Christian revolution and its fashionable enemies*. Yale: Yale University Press; 2009.
7. **Nutton V.** *Ancient medicine*. London: Routledge; 2012, pp. 306–7.
8. **Alexander FG, Selesnik ST.** *The history of psychiatry: an evaluation of psychiatric thought and practice from prehistoric times to the present*. New York: New American Library Inc; 1966.
9. **Porter R.** *The greatest benefit to mankind: a medical history of humanity from antiquity to the present*. London: Fontana Press; 1997.

10. **Goldstein JL, Godemont ML.** The legend and lessons of Geel: a 1500-year-old legend, a 21st century model. *Community Mental Health Journal.* 2003;**39**(5):441–58. doi:10.1023/A:1025813003347.

11. **Borthwick A, Holman C, Kennard D, McFetridge M, Messruther K, Wilkes J.** The relevance of moral treatment to contemporary mental health care. *Journal of Mental Health.* 2001;**10**(4):427–39. doi:10.1080/09638230124277

12. **Brown Thomas J.** *Dorothea Dix: New England reformer.* Harvard: Harvard University Press; 1998.

13. **McGilvray JC.** *The quest for health and wholeness.* Tubingen: German Institute for Medical Missions; 1981.

14. **Vaillant GE.** A 60-year follow-up of alcoholic men, *Society for the Study of Addiction to Alcohol and Other Drugs Addiction.* 2003;**98**:1043–51.

15. **Thulberry SC, Thyer BA.** The L'Arche program for persons with disabilities. *Journal of Human Behavior in the Social Environment.* 2014;**24**(3):348–57.

16. **Vanier J, Swinton J.** *Mental health: the inclusive church resource.* London: Darton, Longman and Todd; 2014.

17. **Wink W.** *The powers that be: theology for a new millennium.* New York: Doubleday; 1999.

18. **Ashworth P.** Deliver us from evil. *Church Times.* 17 February 2017. Available from: https://www.churchtimes.co.uk/articles/2017/17-february/features/features/deliver-us-from-evil.

19. **Cook CCH,** *Christians hearing voices: Affirming experience and finding meaning.* London: Jessica Kingsley Publishers; 2020.

20. **Ozanne J,** *Just love: a journey of self-acceptance.* London: Darton, Longman & Todd; 2018.

21. **Gray AJ** Reflections on the WPA position statement on spirituality and religion. *Mental Health, Religion & Culture.* 2017;**20**(6):552–7. Available from: http://dx.doi.org/10.1080/13674676.2017.1377997

22. **Mohr S, Perroud N, Gillieron C, Brandt P-Y, Rieben I, Borras L, Huguelet, P.** Spirituality and religiousness as predictive factors of outcome in schizophrenia and schizo-affective disorders. *Psychiatry Research.* 2011;**186**:177–82.

23. **Miller L, Warner V, Wickramaratne P, Weissman M,** Religiosity and depression: ten-year follow-up of depressed mothers and offspring. *Journal of the American Academy of Child & Adolescent Psychiatry.* 1997;**36**:(10):1416–25. Available from: https://doi.org/10.1097/00004583-199710000-00024

24. **Miller L, Wickramaratne P, Gameroff MJ,** et al. Religiosity and major depression in adults at high risk: a ten-year prospective study. *American Journal of Psychiatry.* 2012;**169**(1):89–94.

25. **Balbuena L, Baetz M, Bowen R.** Religious attendance, spirituality, and major depression in Canada: a 14-year follow-up study. *Canadian Journal of Psychiatry.* 2013;**58**(4):225–32.

26. **Li S, Okereke OI, Chang SC, Kawachi I, VanderWeele TJ.** Religious service attendance and lower depression among women-a prospective cohort study. *Annals of Behavior Medicine.* December 2016;**50**(6):876–84.

27. **VanderWeele TJ, Li S, Tsai A, Kawachi I.** Association between religious service attendance and lower suicide rates among US women. *JAMA Psychiatry.* 2016;**73**(8):845–51.

28. **Good M, Willoughby T.** Evaluating the direction of effects in the relationship between religious versus non-religious activities, academic success, and substance use. *Journal of Youth and Adolescence.* 2011;40:680–93. doi:10.1007/s10964-010-9581-y

29. **Chen Y, VanderWeele TJ,** Associations of religious upbringing with subsequent health and well-being from adolescence to young adulthood: an outcome-wide analysis. *American Journal of Epidemiology.* Online 13 September 2018. doi:10.1093/aje/kwy142

30. **Werner, E.** Resilience and recovery: findings from the Kauai longitudinal study. 2005. Available from: https://www.pathwaysrtc.pdx.edu/pdf/fpS0504.pdf

31. **Cameron H, Duce C.** *Researching practice in ministry and mission: a companion.* London: SCM Press; 2014.

32. **Harper R, Wilson A.** *To heal and not to hurt: a fresh approach to safeguarding in church.* London: Darton, Longman and Todd; 2019.

Weblinks

a. https://www.nobelprize.org/prizes/peace/1947/ceremony-speech/

b. http://www.themissionpractice.nhs.uk/

c. https://www.mercyships.org/

d. https://www.samaritanspurse.org/article/
first-patient-receives-christ-at-ebola-treatment-center/

e. https://www.leprosymission.org/about-us/tlms-historyK

f. https://www.alcoholics-anonymous.org.uk/About-AA/Historical-Data

g. https://www.alcoholics-anonymous.org.uk/About-AA/The-12-Steps-of-AAAlcoholics
Anonymous the Twelve Steps of Alcoholics Anonymous

h. www.pinerest.org/about-us/

i. https://www.befrienders.org/what-we-do

j. http://www.eminnews.com/wp/

k. http://www.catholicmentalhealthproject.org.uk/

l. https://www.ncronline.org/news/parish/
catholic-church-can-aid-shift-treatment-mental-illness

m. https://www.mindandsoulfoundation.org/

n. http://hope4mentalhealth.com/

o. https://www.cuf.org.uk/learn-about/publications/church-in-action-2017

p. https://www.barna.com/research/
most-american-christians-do-not-believe-that-satan-or-the-holy-spirit-exist/

q. https://catholicherald.co.uk/magazine/
driving-out-the-devil-whats-behind-the-exorcism-boom/

Chapter 11

Islam and mental health

Ahmed Okasha and Tarek A. Okasha

Mental health in Islam

An increased awareness of religion or spirituality in contemporary societies has both positive and negative aspects. From a positive point of view, religious belief systems may provide understandable explanations for traumatic life events or provide meaning for the individual or groups. From a negative point of view, any religious fundamentalism, regardless of a belief system, can be damaging, not only to individual mental health and social adjustment, but also to peaceful coexistence among cultures (1).

Around the seventh century, a newly inspired and emboldened sect—Islam—spread its influence over much of the Middle East and Europe.

The Muslims were the cultural, literary, and scientific leaders of their time. They introduced not only their religion and culture, but also the windmill, fireworks (also claimed by the Chinese), windowpanes, street lights, and fruit cultivation. Islamic scholars were prodigious in philosophy, chemistry, astronomy, mathematics, and medicine.

The Arabic language gave us words like algebra, zero, syrup, algorithm, and alcohol, and Islamic scholars bequeathed the Arabic numeral system, the alphabet of mathematics (2,3).

The approach of Islam to mental illness can be traced to two main sources: the basic connotations in the Koran referring to the mad person (i.e. insane or psychotic) as 'majnoon', mentioned five times in the Koran to ascribe how prophets were perceived. It is sometimes coupled with being a magician or a poet or a teacher. The word 'majnoon' (insane) is originally derived from the word 'jinn', which in Arabic overlaps with different connotations and can refer to a shelter, screen, shield, paradise, embryo, and madness.

In Islam, the 'jinn' is not necessarily a demon (i.e. an evil spirit). It is a supernatural spirit lower than the angels that can be good or bad. There are three dimensions of the concept of mental illness in Islam; a) possession (darkness era), b) innovations and expansion of the self, and c) disharmony or constriction of consciousness (enlightenment era). The psyche (Elnafs) was mentioned

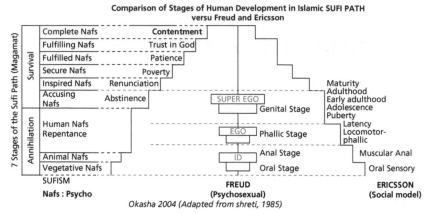

Fig. 11.1 This table is self-explanatory: it compares the Islamic view of personality development with the theories of Freud and Ericsson.
Reproduced with permission from Okasha, A. and Okasha, T. (eds.) (2018). *Contemporary Psychiatry*, 18th edition. Cairo, Egypt: Anglo-Egyptian Bookshop. Copyright © Authors.

185 times in the Koran as a broad meaning to the human existence as a body, behaviour, affect, conduct as a total psychosomatic unity. We find an interesting analogy between the seven stages of human development on the Sofi path and psychosexual Freudian and psychosocial Eriksonian development that lag behind the Sofi development (Fig. 11.1) (4).

Islamic physicians

The Egyptian historian Al-Maqrizi, who wrote in the early fifteenth century, gives a full description of the Bimristan al-Mansuri, sometimes called the 'Bimristan of Kalaoon' or simply Dar 'Ash-Shifa' (= house of healing). Al-Maqrizi says that the reason for the sultan's foundation was that in the year 1276, when he was a prince fighting the Byzantine, he was attacked by a severe colic in Damascus and the doctors treated him with medicines brought from the Nur ad-din hospital. AlMansuri recovered and went to inspect the hospital; he admired it and vowed that, if God made him King, he would build such a hospital. Soon after, he became Sultan of Egypt in 678/1279, and he began the construction of his hospital (6).

According to Al Maqrizi, 'When the building was finished, Al-Malik Al-Mansour endowed it with the revenue from several properties in Cairo and other places that amounted to about a million dirhams a year. He fixed the expenditures for the hospital, the mausoleum, the school and an orphanage. Afterward, the sultan secured the drugs, doctors, and everything that was necessary for the sick in the hospital. He appointed attendants of both sexes to serve the sick, male and female, and established their fees and he set up beds with mattresses and everything that was needed by the sick. He set apart a special place for each kind of illness. Thus, the four alcoves of the hospital were designated for those with fevers and similar illnesses. He assigned a hall for the oculist, a hall for the surgeon, a hall for those with diarrhea, a hall for women, and a place for those who had a cold temperament (i.e. the insane), who were divided into two sections, one for men and the other for women. He had flowing water installed in all parts of the hospital and places were designated for the kitchen, medications, potions, and preparing electuaries, eye powders, and similar things as well as places for storing these products and for distributing the drugs and drinks. He also made a place in the hospital for the head of the physicians for the reading of medical texts. The number of admissions to the hospital was not fixed; all had access to it, without distinction between rich and poor. Besides, the duration of treatment was not limited, and the sick received even at home the medications that they needed (7).'

By the ninth century, Muslim physicians were writing medical textbooks. The Arabic medical profession was cosmopolitan and sophisticated, open to members of all faiths. The illustrious Arab physician Rhazes was a brilliant clinician who gave excellent descriptions of illnesses, including mental ones. Apparently, he used psychotherapy in a primitive but dynamic way. Avicenna the most brilliant of Arab physicians, wrote the *Canon Medicine*, which was used as the main medical reference until the sixteenth century. The eleventh-century physician Ibn Jazlah described melancholia with delusion, manic depression, and psychosis, although he attributed these disorders to humors.

Arab scientists produced a number of drugs. A thirteenth-century work listed 1,400 drugs. Avicenna used rauwolfia in the treatment of acute mental symptoms. The teaching of the great clinician Rhazes had a profound influence on Arab as well as European medicine. The two most important books of Rhazes are *El Mansuri* and *Al-Hawi*. The first book consist of 10 chapters and includes the definition and nature of temperaments, the dominant numerous and comprehensive guides to physiognomy. *Al-Hawi* is the greatest medical encyclopedia produced by a Moslem physician. It was translated into Latin in 1279 and published in 1486. It is the first clinical book presenting the complaints, signs, differential diagnoses and effective treatment of illnesses. One hundred years later, *El-Canoon in Medicine* (The Law in Medicine) by Avicenna was a monumental, educational, and scientific medical book with better classification (8).

After the fourteenth-century magic and superstition began to creep back into the medical works of Muslim writers, a time that some authors call the 'dark ages of Islam', when the scientific approach in thinking was replaced by magic, superstitious beliefs, and sorcery.

Religion plays an important role in symptom phenomenology, attribution (God's will), and management, and the explanatory models held by patients, their carers, and families often reflect this in clinical practice. Psychological symptoms are attributed to weakness of personality, lack of faith, lack of conformity, laziness, or other factors, hardly factors that entitle an individual to a right of choice. Statements such as 'if God is willing', 'I seek refuge in God from the accursed Satan', 'God is the healer', are widespread in the Muslim world, indicating a belief that the final decision is made where no human has control and, therefore, that human choice is a marginal variable in the determination of the final outcome (9).

Ali Abbas wrote the Royal book (*El-Maleki* or *Liber Regius*)—like 'the Continents', a monumental work on the theory and practice of medicine. Arab interpreters gave due emphasis to psycho-social factors. They realized the psychological importance of the hidden (maknun) part of the dream and of self.

Al-Ghazali's work not only predates Pavlov, but also exceeds the contemporary knowledge of conditioning. His books were burnt by Mediterranean bigots from Spain to Syria. Al-Ghazali's scientific, psychological discoveries, though widely appreciated by academics of all kinds, have not been given the attention they deserve because he specifically disclaims the knowledge or logical method as their origin. An examples of his writing explains his philosophy: 'He who does not doubt, does not investigate, and he who does not investigate, does not perceive, and he who does not perceive remains in blindness and error' (9).

Ibn Rushd made remarkable contributions in philosophy, logic, medicine, music, and jurisprudence. In medicine, his well-known book, *Kital al-Kulyat fi al-Tib* (The Totalities in Medicine) was written before 1162 AD (10).

Rights of women: Qur'anic ideals versus Muslim practice

Certainly, if by 'Islam' is meant 'Qur'anic Islam', the rights that it has given to women are, indeed, very impressive. Not only do women partake of all 'General Rights' for any individual, they are also the subject of much particular concern in the Qur'an. Underlying much of the Qur'an's legislation on women-related issues is the recognition that women have been disadvantaged persons in history to whom justice needs to be done by Muslim 'Ummah'. However, in practice, very little of these Qur'anic ideals were practised down the ages due to the patriarchal, male-biased nature of Muslim countries and cultures (11).

Islamic culture and mental health

In the Islamic culture, the humanitarian interaction with a doctor is valued as much, if not more, than their technical ability or scientific knowledge. The humanitarian nature of this interaction depends on the way the doctor deals with the patient and his or her family and the extent to which the doctor expresses respect for, and acceptance of, local cultural and spiritual norms (9).

In traditional cultures, social integration is emphasized more than autonomy—that is, the family, not the individual, is the unit of society, which clearly reflects the inter-dependence and socio-centric nature of the community and the people. Dependence is more natural and infirmity is less alien in these cultures. When affiliation is more important than achievement, how one appears to others becomes vital and shame, rather than guilt, becomes a driving force. In the same manner, physical illness and somatic manifestations of psychological distress become more understood and acceptable, and evoke a caring response; in contrast, a vague complaint of psychological symptoms may be disregarded or considered to indicate that the patient is 'soft' or, worse, 'insane', or lacks faith (9).

In some cultures, and we argue that Arab and Islamic culture is one of them, the collectivity of the community is valued rather than the individuality of its members. Decisions are made not at an individual level but at a familial, tribal, or communal level, in the best perceived collective interest.

These differences are the mainstream norm and not an absolute description of a stereotyped behaviour. Cultural diversity may influence the implementation of ethics in different societies. In traditional societies, the family is an extended one, decision making is group and family oriented, the Western attitude regarding individual autonomy does not exist. In traditional societies, the concept of external control, dependence on God with regard to health and disease, and attribution of illness and recovery to God's will all maintain a healthy doctor–patient relationship, which makes trust, confidence, and compliance characteristic in traditional societies (Table 11.1)(9).

Religion, spirituality and mental health

Religion can provide a source of explanation and understanding for questions such as the meaning of life and death (12).

Islam, in its true sense, is not simply a religion but also a way of life, and it gives a number of directions about leading life and sorting out the day-to-day problems. There are five pillars of Islam—that is, faith in oneness of Allah and prophet Mohammed being the last prophet, prayers five times a day, fasting in the month of Ramadan, Zakat (Alms) and Pilgrimage to Mecca at least once in

Table 11.1 Comparison between traditional societies and non-traditional societies

Traditional societies	Non-traditional Societies
Family and group oriented	Individual oriented
Extended family (not so geographical as before, but conceptual)	Nuclear family
Status determined by age and position in the family, care of elderly	Status achieved by own efforts
Relationship between kin obligatory	Determined by individual choice
Arranged marriages with an element of choice dependent on interfamilial relationship	Choice of marital partner, determined by interpersonal relationship
Extensive knowledge of distant relatives	Restricted to only close relatives
Decision making dependent on the family	Autonomy of individual
Locus of control external	Locus of control internal
Respect and holiness of the decision of the physician	doubt in doctor–patient relationship
Rarely malpractice suing	Common
Deference is God's will	Self-determined
Doctor–patient relationship is still healthy	Mistrust
Individual can be replaced; the family should continue and the pride is in the family tie	Irreplaceable, self-pride
Pride in family care for the mental patient	Community
Dependence on God in health and disease, attribution of illness and recovery to God's will	Self-determined

Reproduced with permission from Okasha, A. 'The Impact of Arab culture on Psychiatric Ethics', in Okasha, A. Arboleda- Florez, J. and Sartorius, N. (Eds.). (2000). *Ethics Culture and Psychiatry*, 15–23. Washington, USA: American Psychiatric Association.

a lifetime if one can afford it. These are the basic pillars and every Muslim has to believe and practise on these principles. In addition to the pillars of Islam, the Code of Conduct to lead day-to-day life has been explained in the religion with some approvals and disapprovals.

Mental illnesses are also recognized as disease entities and emphasis has been made about the care and the rights of the mentally ill. Islamic doctoring has dealt with a number of psycho-social issues including marital relationships, child rearing, family care, adoption, orphanages, women's rights, love, mercy, dutifulness, justice, and modesty, as well as topics that include well-defined guiding principles for normal and civic duties.

The role of Islam in coping behaviour can be expressed by what happened in the tsunami in Indonesia. Hundreds of children lost their parents in Achte in Indonesia and the World Health Organization (WHO) sent experts to deal with post-traumatic stress disorder (PTSD). However, because of their resilience and their coping behaviour following their fundamentalist Islamic upbringing that everything was attributed to God's will, there was no PTSD. Some experts stated that PTSD is a Western diagnosis because in some Islamic cultures it is infrequent (13).

The concept of mental illness in Islamic societies

Moslems attribute all events in life to God's will, and it can be understood that the concept of mental illness can be influenced by cultural and religious aspects. For example, negative symptoms can be attributed, in some sectors of Moslem societies, to deeper contemplation about God—that is, virtuousity and piety, to the extent that avolition, anhedonia, indifference, and blunting of affect secondary to psychiatric disorders, can be considered desirable social traits in certain religious cults, and so these conditions can be missed. Again, positive symptoms like auditory hallucinations can be attributed as gifted from God by extraordinary perception—that is, a special person. There may be religious interpretations to personality disorders—for example, schizotypal can be explained as being close to God, schizoid as a kind person, paranoid as careful, avoidant as religious, and anankastic as meticulous in following religious rituals (10).

Obsessive compulsive disorder and Islam

The role of religious upbringing has been evident in the phenomenology of obsessive compulsive disorder (OCD) among Muslims. The psycho-socio-cultural factors are so varied that they can affect the onset, phenomenology, treatment, and outcome of OCD. The emphasis on religious rituals and the warding off of blasphemous thoughts through repeated religious phrases could explain the high prevalence of religious obsessions and repeating compulsions among our Islamic sample. To elaborate further, Moslems are required to pray five times a day. Each prayer is preceded with a ritualistic cleansing process (Wuddu or ablution), which involves washing several parts of the body in a specific order, each three times.

The emphasis on cleanliness or ritual purity is the cornerstone of most of the compulsive rituals. The number of prayers and their verbal content can be the subject of scrupulousness, checking, and repetition. The ritualistic cleansing procedures can also be a source of obsessions and compulsions about religious purity. Other evidence of the religious connotation inherent in OCD in Moslem culture lies in the word 'weswas' in Arabic. This term is used in reference to the devil and at the same time is used as a name for obsessions. Blasphemous thoughts are common and, if the patient goes to the religious people, it is usually attributed to the weswas, which here means the devil, and not obsession, which aggravates the agony of the patient who considers himself sinful (5, 14–17).

Cultural values and mores play a very significant role in Egyptian society and particularly so in seeking help for various psychiatric disorders. The religious nature of upbringing and education in Egypt, the emphasis on religious rituals, especially related to ablution r lasting for hours, and the warding-off of blasphemous thoughts through repeated religious phrases, such as 'I seek refuge with the Lord from the accursed Satan', can explain the high prevalence of religious obsessions and repeating compulsions among our Egyptian sample, even if the subjects are not practising their religious duties (18,19).

To elaborate further, Moslems, who constitute almost 90% of the Egyptian population, are required to pray five times a day. The five daily prayer times are: dawn (2) genuflexion followed by prosternation; noon (4); afternoon (4); sunset (3); evening (4). Each prayer is preceded with a ritualistic cleansing process (El Wuddu or ablution), which involves the washing of several parts of the body in a specific order, each three times. Wuddu involves ritualistic washing of mouth, nose, face, ears, hands to elbow, and feet each three times, provided the person has not urinated or defecated between two prayers (he should wash the orifices after these physiological functions). The emphasis on cleanliness (In Arabic, Tahara; in Hebrew, Taharat) or ritual purity is the cornerstone of most of the compulsive rituals. The number of prayers and the verbal content can be subjects of scrupulous checking and repetition. A bath is necessary after ejaculation and excretion whatever its nature (19,20).

Women are not allowed to pray or touch the Koran during their menstruation, after which they should clean their bodies through a ritualistic bath. The prayers themselves are different in length and consist of certain phrases and 'souras' from the Holy Koran that have to be read in certain sequence (19).

The ritualistic cleansing procedures can also be a source of obsessions and compulsions about religious purity—for example, in some compulsives, the color red (reminder of menstruation) may trigger a compulsive washing. Further evidence of the religious connotation inherent in OCD in Moslem culture lies in the term 'El Weswas' (in Arabic). This term is used in reference to the devil, and at the same time as a name for obsessions.

It is also characteristic of a conservative society like that of Egypt to expect sexual obsessions to be among the most frequent in female patients. Although it is accepted socially (but prohibited religiously) for Egyptian males to have a wide range of sexual freedom in all stages of their lives, sexual matters remain an issue of prohibition, sin, impurity, and shame for Egyptian women. The female gender is surrounded by so many religious and sexual taboos that the issue becomes a rich pool for worries, ruminations, and cleansing compulsions in women susceptible to developing OCD (19).

Christians represent approximately one-tenth of the population in Egypt, which is equivalent to their number in this study sample (about 10%). The presenting symptoms were almost similar in terms of obsessions, where religious and sexual thoughts were predominant. However, there was a marked difference in rituals, which were more frequent among Moslems, and emphasized the role of ritualistic Islamic upbringing compared with Christian upbringing in our community (18).

A comparison in this context was also drawn between the most prevalent symptoms in the study sample and those of other studies performed in India, England, and Jerusalem (Table 1). Contamination obsessions were the most frequently occurring in all studies. However, the similarities of the contents of religious obsessions—for example, blasphemous between Moslems and Jews compared with Hindus and Christians—signify the role played by cultural and religious factors in the presentation of OCD. The obsessional contents of the samples from Egypt and Jerusalem were similar, dealing mainly with religious matters and matters related to cleanliness and dirt. Common themes between the Indian and British samples, on the other hand, were mostly related to orderliness and aggressive issues. It is interesting to note that the English sample had no religious obsessions (Table 11.2)(19).

Another cultural characteristic of Egyptian psychiatric patients is reflected in the Y-BOCS (Yale- Brown Obsessive Compulsive Scale) rating of the severity of OCD in our sample. The majority of patients were rated between moderate and severe, and the total Y-BOCS score was in the severe range in most of the cases (71.1%), indicating the high tolerance Egyptian patients have for their psychiatric morbidity before they decide to seek help. Native healers, religious people, friends, and family elderly are the primary caregivers for psychologically disordered individuals. When those lines of intervention fail, the general practitioner, followed by the psychiatrist, are the next resort (19, 21).

This delay in seeking help may also explain the fact that males outnumber females in our sample, which is in contrast to most of the literature concerning OCD. An explanation could be attributed to the reluctance of females to seek help for a complaint that could be managed within the household. Although

Table 11.2 Common themes of obsessions in Egypt, India, England, and Jerusalem

Country	No.	Contamination	Aggressive	Ordering	Sexual	Religious
Egypt (Okasha et al., 1994)	90	60%	41%	53%	47%	60%
India (Akhtar et al., 1975)	82	46%	29%	27%	10%	11%
England (Stern and Cobbs, 1978)	45	38%	23%	11%	9%	0
Jerusalem (Greenberg, 1984)	10	40%	20%	10%	10%	50%

Source: Data from Akhtar S, Wig NN, Varma VK, et al. A phenomenological analysis of symptoms in obsessive compulsive neurosis. *British Journal of Psychiatry*. 1975;127:342–8; Pollitt J. Natural history of obsessional states. *British Medical Journal*. 1957;1(5012):194–8; Okasha A, Saad A, Khalil AH, el Dawla AS, Yehia N. Phenomenology of obsessive-compulsive disorder: a transcultural study. *Comprehensive Psychiatry*. 1994;35(3)May/June:191–7;

Greenberg D. Are religious compulsions religious or compulsion. A phenomenological study. *American Journal of Psychotherapy*. 1984;38(4):524–32; Okasha A, Okasha T. Transcultural aspects of obsessive compulsive disorder: an Egyptian perspective. In: *Psiqiatria: situacion actual y perspectivas de futuro, libro homenaje al Profesour Juan Jose Lopez-Ibor*. Jose Antonio Gutierrez Fuentes, Maria Ines Lopez-Ibor Alcocer and Jose Antonio Sacristan, (eds.), Fundacion Juan Jose Lopez-Ibor, 2016, pp. 101–124.

males could have difficulty incorporating—for example, washing, repeating, or checking rituals—into their work life, these compulsions or related obsessions could be tolerated in the context of housework and a long day spent at home, away from exposure to public life. Also, local surveys on health-related behaviours in Egypt have shown that women meet their health needs only after children's' and husbands' needs have been fulfilled (22, 23) Therefore, this sex difference does not reflect the rate of morbidity in the population, but rather the socio-cultural variables that influence the pattern of referrals to psychiatric clinics (22).

Hysteria (dissociation) and possession

The perception of hysteria as a primitive mechanism of defence against frustration was previously mentioned by Tewfik and Okasha in the early 1960s. They reported hysterical spells to be related to sexual rivalry, jealousy, and domestic quarrels in the setting of closed, fervently religious communities where a belief in possession by external agencies exists, or where people are easily excitable and emotional, and have a high level of acceptance for each other's outbursts.

Another category that used to be diagnosed as hysteria is the belief that one is possessed and controlled by para-natural forces (jinns, devils, etc.). This possession can sometimes lead the individual to live a double life: one that is his and the other that belongs to the possessing agent (24,25,26).

The oldest of the papyri, Kahun Papyrus—dating back to about 1900 BC—deals specifically with the subject of hysteria. It is lamentably incomplete: only fragments having survived. The fragments were evidently part of a small treatise describing a series of morbid states, all attributed to the displacement of the uterus. Most of these diseases are defined clearly enough to be recognizable today as hysterical disorders: a woman 'who loves bed, she does not rise and does not shake it'; 'who is ill in seeing, who has pain in her neck'; 'pained in her teeth and jaws, she does not know how to open her mouth'; 'aching in all her limbs with pain in the sockets of her eyes, she cannot hear what is spoken' (27).

These and similar disturbances were believed to be caused by the 'starvation' of the uterus by its upward displacement with a consequent crowding of other organs. As treatment, the genital parts were fumigated with precious and sweet-smelling substances to attract the womb, or evil-tasting and foul-smelling substances were injected or inhaled to repel the organ and drive it away from the upper part of the body where it was thought to have wandered. As a final measure to cause the womb to go back to its place, an Ibis of wax was placed on charcoal and 'let the fumes thereof enter the vulva'. This merits a special comment because it introduces a magico-religious element to the otherwise entirely rational basis of treatment. The Ibis was the symbol of the God Thoth. The use of these ordeals to repel or attract the uterus would suggest their belief in uterine displacement as a cause of these ailments, contrary to the statement that the idea of the wandering womb did not originate from Egypt (27).

These methods were still carried out in recent times. Strong-smelling herbs such as Valerian and Asafoetida in the form of aromatics, sedatives, and anti-spasmodics were still recommended as specifically anti-hysterical remedies in medical textbooks as recently as the beginning of the twentieth century (28).

Perception of suicide in Islam

Following Christianity, Islam is the second most common religion in the world. In fact, one-fifth of the world's population is Muslim, forming the majority of inhabitants within 56 countries, predominantly in Asia and Africa (29).

In ancient Egypt, suicide was a disaster for both the body and the soul. By destroying the body, instead of having it embalmed, the soul would lose its home, because the soul must return every night to the body to be reborn, and the following morning at sunrise in order to live eternally. Not only the soul, but the whole body, is under the responsibility of the Gods. The subject of eternal reprobation and whether suicide was sinful is irrelevant: it makes no difference whether one reaches death by suicide or by waiting for it. Suicide was not an issue in ancient Egypt, except in the case of Cleopatra, who was originally Greek.

Suicide is one of those issues that exist in a twilight zone between religion and psychiatry. Historically, there was always an overlap between those who provided the spiritual and the health needs of people, mostly represented by the clergy. This overlap, although separated throughout the ages, has in some cultures still left its imprint on the medical profession. In many Islamic cultures, a doctor is still referred to as 'Hakim', which means 'the wise man'. When health concerns are psychological rather than physical ailments, the boundaries between medical and spiritual/religious healing may become even more blurred (30).

Few authors have investigated the influence of religion on suicide from a medical and suicidological perspective. Bertolote and Fleischmann (31) discussed the importance of the religious context and the prevalence of a religion in a country as major cultural factors in the determination of suicide. There are some indications that the religiousness of a person might serve as a protective factor against suicide.

Islam advocates preservation of life. Suicide or harming oneself is prohibited. There have been a number of reports that confirm that suicidal acts are less common in severely depressed Muslim patients: 'Nor take life which Allah has made sacred except for just cause. And if anyone is slain wrongfully, we have given his heir authority to demand Qisas or to forgive, but let him not exceed bounds in the matter of taking life, for his helped (by God).' The Holy Koran (Surat Al Isra'a 33).

Suicide in Islam is 'Haram', which means prohibited by religion because it manipulates something that is meant to be only God's concern—that is, life—and it indicates lack of trust in God. Making things better, however, 'haram' also means unjust to self, unjust to others, and, as mentioned in the holy Quraan, 'Take not life which Allah has made sacred, except by way of justice and law, thus does he command you, that you may learn wisdom' (Surat Al Anam 151).

Suicide as a leading cause of death comes number seventh in Europe, eighth in Western Pacific, sixteenth in South-East Asia, and twenty-fifth in East Mediterranean region (all Moslems) so it is not an urgent health problem (32).

There is extreme under-reporting in Moslem countries because it is a stigma to the family, especially in the case of female suicides that are usually taken to indicate breaking of moral codes and fear of police investigations.

Notably, Islamic countries tend to display lower suicide rates compared with other countries of the world (33, 34). Data from the WHO (35) highlighted that in 2012 the Eastern Mediterranean Region, which was the only Muslim-dominated region, had one of the lowest estimated rates of suicide. However, it had been previously noted in reference to earlier findings that many studies looking at the relationship between Islam and suicide had not focused on the underlying mechanisms, but instead had concentrated descriptively on the extent of the issue (27).

Islam means submitting to God. This submission entails that at the end it is God who decides everything. It follows that everything that happens carries with it a certain wisdom or rationale. Even if the individual fails to grasp that wisdom, Islam demands that a Muslim believe in their presence and in God's final judgement. Suicide is prohibited by Islam. It is haram—forbidden. The logic behind the prohibition is that it is an act that manipulates something, in this case life itself, which is meant to be only God's concern. Furthermore, it indicates lack of trust in God who is capable of making things better. However, haram also means acting in a way that is unjust to self and to others (28).

The Arab social historian Ibn Khaldoun (1332–1406) was the first author to give a clear description of the relationship between mental health and culture. He described the effects of urbanization on Islamic tribe warriors when they moved from nomadic life to live in towns. The movement was associated with an increase in the prevalence of psychological ailments—namely, jealousy, suspiciousness, self-indulgence, and fear of others. He viewed this behaviour as a reaction to the change of social structure. In his view, the tribal system failed to adjust to the process of urbanization. Such failure was, in Ibn Khaldoun's view, at the origin of decline of Islamic civilization. The prevailing concept of mental illness at a particular state in the Islamic world depends on the dominance of development or deterioration of genuine Islamic issues. For instance, during periods of deterioration, the negative concepts of the insane as being possessed by evil spirits dominate, whereas during periods of enlightenment and creative epochs, the disharmony concept dominates, and so forth (36).

In the West, an individual is brought up from an early age to appreciate separateness, freedom, and self-responsibility. Life, even within the family, is focused clearly on give and take, and dependence is not tolerated for long. The extended family has almost disappeared except among the very affluent, and the nuclear family is under serious challenge from a high rate of marriage breakdown. Individuals are presumably left to fend for themselves with a make it or break it philosophy. These general statements are often compounded in individuals who are less endowed or disabled in one or more ways. Society tends to impose a subtle form of isolation on those with physical illness, elderly people, and the mentally ill, among others, creating a state of defeat and alienation that becomes self-perpetuating and malignant towards the end. Research shows that in many traditional societies the social structure is different. The family retains a presence in the individual's life, and anomie is probably less frequently encountered or recognized (33).

Islam bans self-destructive behaviour as an act of violation of the will of God in taking away life. For example, the Koran states in one verse (4:29) 'you should not kill yourself because god has been merciful to you' (34). Even the widely debated issue of suicide bombing is denounced by high-ranking religious authorities in the region, refusing to describe the actors as martyrs. Those who contemplate suicide know of never-ending graphic descriptions of torture in hell awaiting the person who takes their own life. A depressed believer would argue when questioned that they have been unhappy in this life and would not want to suffer eternally as well after death. Suffering in our common life is taken by believers as a test from God that should be endured and promises even greater happiness in the afterlife. Suicidal behaviour drops markedly in frequency during the holy month of Ramadan (36, 37, 38). Ramadan is considered a holy month because the Koran was revealed during that month: it is a time of fasting and is dominated by religious rituals.

Drug abuse and intoxication in Islam

The five imperatives of Islam are the preservation of religion, mind, body, wealth, and honour. A Muslim is enjoined by texts in the Quran and in the Sunna to avoid anything that may cause their own death or bring about their own destruction, as God says: 'And cast not yourselves to ruin with your own hands' (2:195), 'And kill not yourselves' (4:29).

It has become clear that smoking and illicit drugs, in no matter which form or by which means, causes people a great deal of damage sooner or later, both to health and to wealth, as well as a variety of diseases. Consequently, and by virtue of these texts, the use of narcotics is forbidden. No Muslim is allowed to use psychoactive substance of any kind or in any form. A believer who is in a healthy condition is better and more dearer to God than a believer in a weak condition.

The starting point in forbidding wines and intoxicants was that Muslims were not allowed to offer their prayers when they were under the influence of drink. Hence, the final stage included a complete and full prohibition: 'Believers, intoxicants and gambling, (dedication of) stones and divination by arrows, are all an abomination of Satan's work. Refrain from such abomination so that you may prosper.'

In the absence of direct and clear-cut religious provisions classifying smoking under one of the five verdicts of Islamic law (inevitability, impermissibility, abominability, recommendability, and permissibility), it is quite understandable that the jurists were of diverse opinion with regard to smoking. Some of them ruled that smoking was haram, others were of the opinion that it was abominable, a third group judged it to be permissible, a fourth group did not wish to give a ruling one way or the other on account of the fact that physical and financial hazards and effects of smoking differ from one person to another.

A saying of the Prophet enjoins: 'Cause harm neither to yourself nor to others.' Since smoking is at the root of much harm, it is haram (10).

Other psychological aspects

Stress is considered a test of endurance and patience. It is accepted as God's will, calling for patience and then appealing to God to relieve stress. This is a very interesting concept because here there is no hopelessness: instead, there is hope and one approaches God to get guidance and help to overcome the stress. Looking from the religious perspectives, stress also elicits the support of others, limits personal responsibility towards events, and is based on forgiveness and generosity (18).

Mental hospitals

The first Islamic mental hospital (maybe in the whole world) appears to have been established by the early eighth century (705 AD) in Baghdad in Iraq and to have been modelled on the East Christian institutions, which would seem to have been mainly monastic infirmaries. Baghdad Hospital was followed by ones in Cairo (800 AD), Damascus then Aleppo (1270AD) (39).

Among the hospitals that appeared throughout the Islamic world, perhaps the most famous one was that created in Cairo by the Egyptian, Sultan al-Mansour Kalaoon in 683/1284.

The fourteenth-century 'Kalaoon Hospital' in Cairo had sections for surgery, ophthalmology, medical conditions, and mental illnesses. Contributions by the wealthy of Cairo in the form of paying Zakat (in Islam a way to purify one's income and wealth from sometimes worldly, impure ways of acquisition), endowment, and philanthropy allowed a high standard of medical care and provided for patients during convalescence until they were gainfully occupied. Two features were striking: the care of mental patients in a general hospital, and the involvement of the community in the welfare of the patient, which foreshadowed modern trends by six centuries.

The first mental hospitals built in Europe were influenced by the then prevalent Islamic culture in Spain : Seville (1409), Saragossa and Valencia (1410), Barcelona (1412), Toledo (1483), and from there mental hospitals started all over Europe (4,6).

Conclusion

Religion is a protective factor from vulnerability to many conditions including depression but can also contribute to other conditions as discussed in this chapter. Psychiatry has rarely used the multidimensional assessments of religion, including measures of religious beliefs, attitude, practices, and reasons: religion has remained on the periphery of professional interest. Psychiatrists have been unaware of the generally beneficial association religion and spirituality have with mental health status.

Although science and technology have made our lives easier, they did not teach us how to live: science has produced a vacuum in our spiritual life. It is expected that there will be a return to faith, spirituality, and religion for better mental health and for more harmony between the self and the environment, to enhance virtue and altruism and to give a meaning to our life.

References

1. **Boehnlein K James.** *Introduction in psychiatry and religion. The convergence of mind and spirit.* Washington, DC: American Psychiatric Press. Inc; 2000.
2. **Arnold T, Guillaume A.** The legacy of Islam. In: **A Zahoor** (ed.), *Muslim history.* Oxford University Press; 1997.
3. **Tan SY.** Medicine in stamps: Rhazes (835–925 AD) medical scholar of Islam. *Singapore Medical Journal.* 2002;**43**(7):331–2.
4. **Okasha A, Okasha T.** Notes on mental disorders in Pharaonic Egypt. *History of Psychiatry.* 2000;**11**(44, Part 4):413–24.
5. **Okasha A.** OCD in Egyptian adolescents: the effect of culture and religion. *Psychiatric Times.* 2004;**21**(5).
6. **Okasha A, Okasha T.** Mental health in Cairo (Al-Qahira). *International Journal of Mental Health.* 2000;**28**(4),winter 1999–2000:62–8.
7. **Dols MW.** *Majnun: the madman in medieval Islamic society.* **Diana E. Immisch** (ed.), Oxford: Clarendon Press; 1992.
8. **Tan SY.** Medicine in stamps: Avicenna (980–1037): prince of physicians. *Singapore Med J.* 2002;**43**(9):445–6.
9. **Okasha, A.** The impact of Arab culture on psychiatric ethics. In: *Ethics culture and psychiatry*, **A. Okasha, J. Arboleda- Florez** and **Sartorius, N.**, (eds), American Psychiatric Press, USA, 2000, pp. 15–23.
10. **Okasha A.** Focus on psychiatry in Egypt, *British Journal of Psychiatry.* 2004;**185**:266–72.

11. The Islamic Conference number 19 for Ministers of Foreign Affairs of Islamic States issued in August. In: *The Cairo Declaration of Human Rights in Islam*. Cairo; 1990.

12. **Peck DL.** Religious conviction, coping, and hope, *Case Analyses*. 1988;**2**: 201–19.

13. WHO Regional Office for Eastern Mediterranean- Alexandria—Egypt 2015. Openning address by Dr. Hussien El Gazzerli

14. **Akhtar S, Wig NN, Varma VK,** et al. A phenomenological analysis of symptoms in obsessive compulsive neurosis. *British Journal of Psychiatry*. 1975;**127**:342–8.

15. **Pollitt J.** Natural history of obsessional states. *British Medical Journal*. 1957;**1**(5012):194–8.

16. **Okasha A, Saad A, Khalil AH, el Dawla AS, Yehia N.** Phenomenology of obsessive-compulsive disorder: a transcultural study. *Comprehensive Psychiatry*. 1994;**35**(3)May/June:191–7.

17. **Greenberg D.** Are religious compulsions religious or compulsion. A phenomenological study. *American Journal of Psychotherapy*. 1984;**38**(4):524–32.

18. **Okasha A, Raafat M, el Dawla AS, Effat S.** Obsessive compulsive disorder in different cultures: an Egyptian perspective. *Egyptian Journal of Psychiatry*. 1991;**14**:15–30.

19. **Okasha A, Okasha T.** Transcultural aspects of obsessive compulsive disorder: an Egyptian perspective. In: *Psiqiatria: situacion actual y perspectivas de futuro, libro homenaje al Profesour Juan Jose Lopez-Ibor*. **Jose Antonio Gutierrez Fuentes, Maria Ines Lopez-Ibor Alcocer** and **Jose Antonio Sacristan,** (eds.), Fundacion Juan Jose Lopez-Ibor, 2016, pp. 101–124.

20. **Okasha, Tarek A.**:Religious perspectives in urban and rural mental health in the Moslem world. In: *mental health and illness in the city*, (eds), **Niels Okkels, Christina Blanner Kristiansen** and **Povl Munk-Jørgensen.** Springer, 2017, pp. 299–315.

21. **Okasha, T**: Psychosomatic medicine in Egypt and North Africa: development, research, education and practice. Chapter 21. In: **Hoyle Leigh** (ed.), *Global psychosomatic medicine and consultation-liaison psychiatry*. Springer Nature, Switzerland AG. 2019, pp. 451–70.

22. **Okasha A, Saad A, Khalil AH,** et al. Phenomenology of obsessive-compulsive disorder: a transcultural study. *Comprehensive Psychiatry*. 1994;**35**(3):191–7.

23. **Central Agency for Public Mobilization and Statistics (CAPMAS) and United Nations Children's Fund (UNICEF) Egypt.** *The situation of women in egypt*. Cairo: UNICEF; 1992, pp. 29–31.

24. **Tewfik GI, Okasha A.** Psychosis and immigration. *Postgrad Medical Journal*. 1965;**41**:603–12.

25. **Okasha A.** A cultural psychiatric study of El Zar cult in U.A.R. *British Journal of Psychiatry*. 1966;**112**(493):1217–21.

26. **Okasha A.** et al. Presentation of hysteria in a sample of Egyptian patients—an update. *Neurology, Psychiatry and Brain Research*. 1993;**1**:155–9.

27. **Okasha, T**: Major trends of Psychosomatic Medicine in North Africa and Middle East. Chapter 8. In: **Hoyle Leigh** (ed.), *Global psychosomatic medicine and consultation-liaison psychiatry*. Springer Nature, Switzerland AG. 2019, pp. 147–61.

28. **Gardiner AH.** *Chester Beaty Papyrus; Hieratic papyri in the British Museum* (vol. 1). London: British Museum: 1934.

29. **Rezaeian M.** Islam and suicide: a short personal communication. *Omega*. 2008;**58**:77–85.

30. **Okasha A, Okasha T.** *Suicide in Islam in Oxford textbook of suicidology and suicide prevention*. **Danuta Wasserman** and **Camilla Wasserman** (eds), Oxford University Press, 2009, pp. 49–56.

31. **Bertolote JM, Fleischmann A.** A global perspective in the epidemiology of suicide. *Suicidology*. 2002;**2**:6–8.

32. **Javed, A.** World Congress of Psychosocial Rehabilitation WAPR Regional meeting, Hungary 2006. Plennary lecture of the congress.

33. **Lester D.** Suicide and Islam. *Archives of Suicide Research*. 2006;**10**:77–97.

34. **Shah A, Chandia M.** The relationship between suicide and Islam: a cross-national study. *Journal of Injury and Violence Research*. 2010;**2**:93–7.

35. **World Health Organization (WHO).** *Preventing suicide: a global imperative*. Library Cataloguing-in-Publication Data. WHO. 2014, pp. 9–16.

36. **Okasha A.** Mental health in the Middle East: an Egyptian perspective. *Clinical Psychology Review*. 1999;**19**(8): 917–933.

37. **Al-Ansari EA, El-Hilu MA, Hassan KI.** Patterns of psychiatric consultations in Kuwait general hospitals. *General Hospital Psychiatry*. 1990;**12**:257–63.

38. **Bensmail B, Merdji Y, Touari M.** Reflections on detection and intervention in depression in Algeria. *Psicopatologia*. 1989;211–214.

39. **Okasha A, Okasha T.** (eds), *Contemporary psychiatry*. Eighteenth edition. (In Arabic). Cairo: Anglo Egyptian Bookshop; 2018.

Chapter 12

Hinduism

Matcheri S. Keshavan,
Bangalore N. Gangadhar, and
Ananda K. Pandurangi

Hinduism and psychotherapy: a general overview

The past century has witnessed the development of progressively refined approaches to psychotherapy mainly in the Western hemisphere, beginning with psychoanalysis in the early twentieth century, and followed by behavioural, existential, cognitive, and interpersonal approaches. Hindu thought, which arose more than three millennia ago in India, offers insights that differ in important ways from Western psychology. Although different aspects of Hindu thought have already influenced a number of well-known psychologists, such as Carl Jung (1999; 1) and Abraham Maslow (1943; 2), its implications for research on emotion and its afflictions have not been fully elucidated. Some convergences between Hindu thinking and current models of psychotherapy suggest the fruitfulness of integrating these diverse approaches.

Hinduism is the world's third largest and perhaps oldest religion, with over one billion people practising it, including over 60–70 million living outside India. Unlike many other religions, 'Hinduism' is not the original name for this religion. Ancient Persians referred to people living on the banks of the river Sindhu (Indus) as 'Hindus'. Since the ancient times, people in the Indian subcontinent simply called their way of life as 'Sanatana dharma', which simply means 'the eternal laws of living'. Hinduism encompasses numerous related traditions that share common elements but do not require a unified set of beliefs or practices. In fact, one can be an atheist or a naturalist etc., but still be a Hindu. Many Hindu scriptures have developed over its long history, including the Vedas. While dating Hindu scriptures has been a challenging and controversial enterprise among scholars, we can safely say that the Vedas were composed over centuries beginning around 1500 BC, and the Upanishads, which are the terminal portions of the Vedas may be dated to around 800 BC.

Around the time of the later Upanishads, Buddhist thought evolved as well (~ the fifth and sixth century BC), with many parallels to Hindu thought. There are four *Vedas (Rig Veda, Yajur Veda, Sama Veda, and Atharva Veda)*, which begin as largely religious hymns and incantations (Samhitas), proceed to more explanatory hymns (Brahmanas), then advance into introspective hymns (Aryanakas) that ultimately evolve into philosophical and metaphysical speculations (Upanishads), like the Old Testament. Upanishads (which are over hundred in number) are later stages of the Vedic thinking, and are more concise summaries and interpretations of Vedic thought. The most cryptic version of the Vedas and Upanishads is a work titled *Brahmasutras* by the Sage Badarayana, dated approximately to the fourth century BC. Both the Vedas and the Upanishads present their teaching in the form of hymns but also in the form of critical dialogues between Vedic personalities such as Yajnavalkya, Maithreyi, and others (3). The Upanishads, Brahmasutras, and the Gita (see next paragraph) together are referred to as the three foundational pillars of Hindu philosophy (*Prasthana Trayi*). The Vedic-Upanishadic bodies of knowledge, including the Gita, are more theistic and the rich psychological-spiritual framework for human life embedded in them is ultimately attributed to a unitary God Almighty. Other more clearly atheistic schools of thought, such as Samkhya, Nyaya, and Yoga, offer an even richer contribution to the understanding of the human psyche (4).

In this chapter, we rely primarily on the Bhagavad-Gita ((5); referred to hereafter as 'the Gita'), a 700-stanza poem, which is an even more concise summary of earlier Hindu scriptures (6), and on the psychology presented in the Samkhya-Yoga school of Hindu philosophy. The Gita is embedded within the Indian epic, Mahabharata, the world's longest poem of about 124,000 stanzas with an unknown date of origin but likely compiled around 200–500 BC). We discuss how models of Western psychology when applied to insights from centuries of Hindu thought can shed new light on approaches to positive mental health. The focus in this review is mainly on mental health. The abundant philosophical, theological, and spiritual insights in the Gita are beyond the scope of this chapter, and interested readers are referred to authoritative texts elsewhere (7, 8). We first discuss the concept of the mind and its workings as embodied in the Gita and other ancient Hindu scriptures. The definition of positive mental health, as outlined in the Gita, is then introduced. Steps outlined in these texts help cultivate positive mental well-being, focusing on an integrated psychobiological approach represented by the eight steps of Yoga. Finally, traditional Hindu theory is discussed in light of the relevant Western psychological research to demonstrate how dialogue and empirical study can enrich both traditions.

Historical and comparative psychotherapeutic perspectives in Hindu traditions

Nature of the mind and happiness

Topography of the mind

The Hindu scriptures provide a lucid description of the topography of the human mind as well as its ontology. The Katha Upanishad, dated around the fifth century BC (9), prior to the Gita, posited that the senses (*Indriyas*) are subservient to the mind (*manas*), and that the mind is in service of the intellect *(buddhi)*, which itself is the instrument of the spirit (soul/*aatman*). The body is likened to the chariot, and the horses are the senses; The intellect is the reins held by the spirit, the charioteer (Katha Upanishad 1.3.3–4). A similar chariot allegory was described by Plato (fifth–fourth centuries BC) to elucidate the relation between the soul, reason, and passion. In this uniquely non-dualistic view, the body, the mind, and the spirit are seen as three legs of a stool. Implicit in this hierarchical organization is the principle that mental well-being is achieved by unattached action (conation), regulation of the senses, and affect (emotion) by higher reasoning aspects of the mind and an accurate appraisal of the nature of the self and its relation to others (cognition), as will be discussed later.

Dimensions of the mind and their development

Hindu scriptures describe Gunas as the three 'tendencies, qualities, or temperaments': the three Gunas are *Sattva*, the quality of balance, harmony, and goodness; *Rajas*, which refers to passion, activity, self-centeredness, egoism, individualization, driven-ness, movement, and dynamism; and *Tamas*, which refers to imbalance, disorder, negativity, dullness or inactivity, apathy, inertia or lethargy, violence, viciousness, and ignorance. These qualities are not either-or categories: everyone has all three, only in different proportions and in different contexts. The individual's personality and character are viewed as the composite effect of these three qualities. Hinduism allows and encourages moving from the primitive tamasic traits towards Rajasic traits, and eventually developing more and more Sattvic traits, both within the current life and from one life to another. The former is somewhat similar to the goals of modern psychotherapy whereby the therapist assists the individual to replace primitive and unhealthy defences with healthier ones.

Developmentally, the operations of the human mind are thought to evolve from a focus on survival and physiological needs (*Tamasic*) to needs of power and domination and sensory pleasures (*Rajasic*), and toward altruistic and self-less service goals (*Sattvic*), in a manner somewhat similar to the hierarchy of needs outlined by the well-known psychologist Abraham Maslow (2). Maslow regarded the origins of human motivation as a pyramid, with the physiological needs of survival and safety at the bottom; the needs for love and belonging; and then the needs to be recognized for one's accomplishments represented one level higher. Finally, at the highest level, are the needs for self-fulfillment by pursuing creativity and moral ideals, which Maslow termed 'self-actualization'. The similarities between these *Gunas* and Maslow's hierarchy of needs is striking.

Concept of happiness and the stable mind

The concept of mental health is also well defined in the Hindu scriptures. The Gita outlines the characteristics of a person with positive mental health under the concept of *Sthithaprajna* (stable mind). 'The sage, whose mind remains unperturbed amid sorrows, whose thirst for pleasures and need for anger has altogether been overcome, is called as one with "stable mind". He who is un-attached to everything, and when meeting with good and evil, neither overly rejoices nor recoils, his mind is stable. He who has given up all desires, and is free from attachments, egoism and thirst for enjoyment attains peace' (the Gita, Chapter 2, Verses 54–55). As an important aside, the Gita clarifies that unattachment should not be confused with inaction. Thus, one is of stable mind even as one goes about performing one's assigned role in life. Again, the similarities in the end goals as taught by the Gita and the goals of modern psychotherapy of emphasizing role performance is evident.

Whereas Western cultures tend to associate positive hedonic experience of happiness with personal achievement, people in Eastern cultures such as the Japanese associate it with social harmony (10). While Eastern traditions focus on continuous excellence of 'being', signifying stable traits or character strengths, Western emphasis is on 'doing' or efforts (11), oriented toward rewards. The Hindu scriptures imply that episodic events (such as winning the lottery or succeeding in an athletic competition) may increase an individual's *state* of transient pleasure but will decrease the individual's long-term level of happiness. By contrast, happiness is defined as an enduring sense of being contented, and this 'trait' (sukha) and peace of mind (shanti) can be cultivated by specific yogic practices, especially the meditative aspects of yoga. It represents a deep sense of well-being, reduced vulnerability to outer circumstances, and recognition of the interconnectedness with people and other living beings in one's environment.

Pathways to happiness

The Gita and the earlier Hindu scriptures indicate three ways to achieve lasting happiness: the path of action (*Karma Yoga*), the path of knowledge (*Jnana Yoga*), and the path of contemplative meditation (*Dhyana Yoga*). Girding these pathways is faith (Bhakti). The *Karma* path entails action that is not contingent on reward, but is focused on the process itself (The Gita, Chapter II, Verse 47); Karma is not simply engaging in passive action, but is one of skilled action in which the person is fully involved with the goal of perfection (The Gita, Chapter II, Verse 50). *Jnana* refers to metacognitive awareness of the mind observing itself; *Dhyana* is contemplation both on internal reality and the external cosmos. *Bhakthi* refers to the devotional awareness of a personal God or Divine Power (12). Notably, Hinduism allows for such divine power to range from a totally abstract entity with no form whatsoever (*Nirguna Brahma*) to an omnipotent energy with a resplendent form (*Saguna Brahma*).

Concept of the self

According to the ancient Hindu scriptures including the Gita, there is no clear separation between the self and the object, and it is argued that the self is inextricably interdependent with other people and the environment. Nevertheless, people confound the real nature of the self by attributing to it the concepts of permanence and autonomy. The Upanishads were among the earliest to ask profound questions of 'Who am I?', 'Who or what is God?', 'What is reality?', 'What is the relation between these?', etc. Understanding these is fundamental to Jnana yoga. The sources of knowledge for such understanding are our perceptions, information provided by others, and internal deduction. Pertaining to the Self, the Hindu scriptures came to the conclusion that the self is not what it seems. The self we all know is the collection of our physical, mental, and social attributes that we create for ourselves with input from our perceptions, and input from our families and society. In reality, the '*self*' may well be a collection of atoms and energy that takes on a temporary definition, surely subject to change over time, a beginning and an end. The consequence of such a world view is the egoistic tendency to crave for the 'I' and for what is mine, and repulsion toward the other. The Upanishads and the Gita define the *Self (Atma)* or *soul* as the observer, and not the observed, one which may reflect pure consciousness, one that cannot be defined by space, time, or ego boundaries. In this view, which many Hindus believe in, the soul outlives the body and the mind after death. Similar views about the Self have been described in Buddhism though Buddhists deny the concept of self altogether (the No-self or *Anatma*). In Hindu thought, the realization of this *self*-illusion and the awareness of a universal *Self* ('I am Brahman'), leads to an understanding that there is no difference between 'I' and 'you', or 'I' and 'him'. This can be a source of liberation. More practically, this concept of the soul being permanent can provide much relief during mourning the loss of a loved one. The Gita says 'the wise do not lament the death of the body' (Gita, Chapter 2, Verse 11). (Also see Case report 2.)

Nature of psychopathology

The *Gita* is a dialogue between Krishna and Arjuna at the beginning of the *Mahabharata war* where the armies of two related families fight each other for territory. Arjuna, a great and brave warrior, finds himself suddenly over-whelmed with feelings of mental depression, grief, and fear when he realizes that he has to fight with close relatives—brothers, uncles, and teachers—as his enemies in the war. Arjuna is disturbed about the outcome of the war: destruction and death. He thinks it better to lay down his arms and retire. He seeks advice from his charioteer Krishna on what is the right thing to do. Arjuna's moral dilemma, and Krishna's answers, touch on many aspects of human emotions and reasoning, ethical dilemmas, philosophical issues, and life's choices (11). In this sense, the Mahabharata war is an allegory for a 'war within' for the human condition. Arjuna's emotions of love for the near ones, his concepts of duty and Dharma, all appeared to be confusing, and lead to severe existential anxiety, as eloquently described, thus:

> "Thinking of the tasks ahead, O Krishna, my hands holding the bow tremble, my mouth goes dry, my limbs are failing me, and my hair stands on end. My mind is beginning to waver and I am beginning to see unwelcome visions, and I am unable to stand upright" (The Gita, Chapter 1, Verses 28–29).

The Gita views attachment as one of the primary root causes of mental afflictions, such as today's neuroses and adjustment and personality disorders. Attachment involves the desire to acquire objects and situations for oneself. Excessive attachment disrupts the balance of the mind, giving rise to the negative emotions outlined above. All the negative emotions can thus be traced back to excessive attachment: *Kama* (Excessive attachment to the desired object), *Krodha* (Anger if approach to desired object is obstructed), *Lobha* (Greed for more of the desired object), *Moha* (Possessiveness and infatuation toward the desired object), *Mada* (Excessive attachment to ones' own positive qualities and arrogance), and *Maatsarya* (Resentment toward another who is the recipient of one's object of desire or jealousy).

The Gita clearly outlines the sequence by which negative emotions may have a cascading effect, a phenomenon well known to cognitive theorists. The root cause of such a cascade is excessive desire (*Kama*). Anger or hatred (*Krodha*) are driven by the wish to harm or destroy anything that blocks the pursuit of objects and situations desired by the self. Perception of the desired object, coloured by excessive desire, exaggerates the undesirable qualities of objects and de-emphasizes their positive qualities. Such a cognitive distortion leads the mind to be trapped in a deluded perception (*SamMoha*) that the source of its unhappiness stems from the external object (The Gita, Chapter 2, Verses 62, 63).

Attachment is based on the perceived distinction between self and others (between subject and object)—as being absolute. Attachment involves acquiring or preserving a desirable object or situation for 'me' and 'mine', which is thought to be threatened by 'the other' (faulty cognition). The individual exaggerates the desirable qualities that are inherent in the object desired (increased emotional valence or salience), while under-emphasizing that object's undesirable qualities (selective attention). Excessive attachment results from falsely displacing the source of one's well-being from one's own mind to objects. This then leads to an unhelpful way of engaging with the world (maladjustment), and can be harmful when it leads to negative emotions such as anxiety, anger, and depression.

The approach to cognitive change in the Hindu scriptures

The Gita's approach to addressing Arjuna's existential problems is to get to the root cause of the conflict. Krishna in the Gita provides his client Arjuna with a cognitive theory of origin of his conflict, as does the modern cognitive therapist. Krishna takes several steps: a) he encourages Arjuna to understand, and monitor himself; b) prescribes an approach to eliminate the negative emotions by focusing on the right action without attachment; c) encourages Arjuna to accentuate the positive by replacing negative and self-centered (*tamasic and rajasic*) thoughts by positive (*Sattvic*) attitudes; and d) teaches Arjuna the yogic steps needed to help him move toward self- realization and freedom from anxiety.

Yoga

The overall approach to healing Arjuna's existential anxiety is embodied in Yoga. Broadly defined, Yoga is a comprehensive approach for balancing the body, mind, and spirit. The word 'Yoga' means' 'yoke' and a stable yoke is critical in balancing the chariot. The eight steps of the *Ashtanga Yoga* outlined by Patañjali (around the second century BC) involve such integration (13). First, the individual's lifestyle and value system are addressed systematically by self-discipline, with a number of don'ts and do's (*Yamas and Niyamas*). *Yamas* include truth, non-violence, celibacy, non-stealing, and non-covetousness; *Niyamas* include purity, austerity, self-surrender, self-study, and the practice of contentment. Such discipline is expected to result in shifts of fleeting emotions and eventually to help develop an even temperament. For millennia, Yoga practitioners have developed and tested ways of gradually cultivating emotions that are conducive to the pursuit of lasting happiness and of freeing themselves from negative emotions. It is also important to withdraw senses from their sense objects (*Pratyahara*). Regulation of the somatic nervous system by physical training (*Asanas*) and of the autonomic nervous system by breath control (*Pranayama*) are the needed next-level steps that set the stage for bringing the mind under control. One of the characteristics of the undisciplined mind is its distractibility, allowing itself to be drawn by senses in myriad directions. This is remedied by cultivation of steady concentration (*Dharana*), which is defined in the Gita as sustained, voluntary attention continuously focused on a familiar object, without distraction. *Dhyana* is a further step in meditation wherein the meditator and the object of meditation become one. *Samadhi*, the final stage of consciousness, is considered an experience of blissful ego-lessness. These steps are similar to, though not identical with, the eightfold path of Buddhist cannon (14).

The four keys to peace are summarized by Patanjali in this well-known verse: 'By cultivating attitudes of friendliness toward the happy, compassion for the unhappy, delight in the virtuous, and disregard toward the wicked, the mind-stuff retains its undisturbed calmness' (Patanjali Yoga Surtra, Verse 133).This concept is also well captured in the Gita (the Gita, Chapter 12, Verses 13–14). The concept of friendliness and benevolence (*Maitri* in Sanskrit) is central to several forms of loving-kindness mediation practised in Hindu, Buddhist, and Jain traditions (15).

Insights from the Gita and comparison to Western psychotherapeutic models

It may be seen from the above that the Gita approach has some parallels with, as well as unique differences from, Western models of psychotherapy, when compared (Table 12.1). The insights in the Hindu scriptures, especially in the

Table 12.1 Comparison of a Western model (cognitive behavioural therapy) with Hindu models of psychotherapy

	Cognitive behaviour therapy	**Hindu insights in psychotherapy**
Theme	Worldly	Worldly and spiritual
Theory	Faulty cognitive schemas	Excessive salience to objects of attachment
Focus	Restructuring *content* of thoughts	Metacognitive observation and regulation of thought *process*
Subject of interest	Individuals with cognitive distortions	Promoting positive well-being in health as well as in disorder
Application	Therapeutic	Preventive as well as therapeutic
Strategies	Focused, confined to correcting faulty cognitive schemas	Comprehensive, involves lifestyle modification, physical as well as psychological and spiritual well-being

Bhagavad Gita, have been examined in the context of many contemporary psychotherapeutic approaches, as outlined below.

Psychoanalytic psychotherapy

The central premise of psychodynamic treatments is to help the individual develop insight into the links between unconscious conflicts and the conscious mind. Bhatia and colleagues (2013; 16) suggest that three *Gunas*, or character traits, may represent the three layers of the mind inherent to psychanalytic theory. Thus, the *Tamas Guna*, with its focus on self-centeredness without regard for consequences, may be akin to the Id, while the *Satvic Guna*, in which altruistic action and morality are central, might be similar to the superego. On the other hand, the *Rajas Guna*, which entails goal-directed action contingent on reward expectation, may resemble the functioning ego. It may be argued that the Gita involves a successful resolution of conflicts faced by Arjuna between the three *Gunas*. However, the Gita does not explicitly take the approach of linking current predicaments to past conflicts of current life, unlike psychoanalytic therapies. However, it should be noted that Hindu scriptures often relate current conflicts to events of previous lives, or the so-called Karma theory. Further, the Gita's approach is more directive than is typical for dynamic psychotherapy, and more in line with supportive psychotherapy.

Another school of Hindu philosophy closely related to Yoga is the atheistic *Samkhya* school mentioned earlier in this chapter. While a full presentation of this school is beyond the scope of this chapter, the early developers of *Samkhya* described the incorporation of external entities into internal objects, and transactions with the same (4), similar to the modern descriptions by Neo-Freudians.

Cognitive psychotherapies

There are some similarities to *here and now* approaches to psychotherapy such as rational emotive behaviour therapy (REBT; 17) and cognitive behavioural therapy (CBT; 18), psychotherapies based on the views that the way in which individuals perceive and interpret situations in their daily lives was a key to therapy (19). Aaron T. Beck who developed CBT argued that 'cognitive errors' in thinking could cause or maintain depression, such as arbitrary inference, selective abstraction, over-generalization, and magnification (of negatives) and minimization (of positives). Cognitive therapy seeks to identify and change 'distorted' or 'unrealistic' ways of thinking, and therefore to influence emotion and behaviour. Clearly, Krishna's approach in the Gita involves several of the above elements (20). Table 12.1 contrasts CBT and Hindu approaches to psychotherapy. It may be seen that, while there are some similarities, there are also interesting differences between these approaches; Hindu approaches have similarities to several more recent psychotherapeutic models developed in the west, as will be seen below.

Metacognitive therapies

By contrast to CBT, however, the Gita places a large emphasis on metacognition, which refers to thinking (appraising, monitoring, and controlling) about thinking (21). A recent approach to psychotherapy is metacognitive therapy (MCT), which focuses more on the process of thinking than on the content of thoughts (22). Most of us are able to deal flexibly with negative thoughts generated by our minds but some become trapped in emotional disturbance because of faulty metacognitions; an example is a pattern called the cognitive attentional syndrome consisting of worry, rumination, fixated attention, and faulty self-regulatory strategies. The problem isn't really negative thoughts but how the person reacts to them. This contrasts with the basic premise of CBT and REBT, which view biases in thinking as causing psychological disorder. MCT is similar in principle but emphasizes more the process of thinking not the cognitive distortions (e.g. black-and-white thinking). CBT deals with changing thought content; MCT is about changing the process of thinking. Thus, the patient who states 'I'm worthless', is addressed by the CBT therapist who asks 'What is the evidence?', while the MCT therapist questions, 'What is the point in evaluating your worth?' or 'Who is evaluating your worth?' (23). Mindful meditation involves metacognitive awareness, which helps the individual to shift their cognitive set away from a self-focused activity toward alternate appraisals of life events, thereby 'depersonalizing' the negative preoccupations and moving toward a positive or neutral reappraisal of events (24).

Mindfulness-based approaches

Several recent approaches to psychotherapy have evolved in the context of increasing appreciation of the positive benefits of mindfulness. Mindfulness refers to attention, non-judgemental acceptance and independence from thoughts. These principles are inherent to mindfulness-based stress reduction (25), Dialectical behaviour therapy (DBT; 26) and acceptance commitment therapy (27). While commonly viewed as a Zen Buddhist practice, the Hindu scriptures including the Patanjali Yoga Sutras and the Gita have several references to this concept as part of the comprehensive approach to yoga, as outlined earlier. Kabat-Zinn has developed a widely used approach to integrate mindfulness practices (including compassionate meditation) and yoga (28).

Although not for therapeutic purposes, dialecticism is also heavily emphasized in several Hindu philosophical approaches called Nyaya and its corollary called *Tatva Vaada* (rule-based argumentation). As in DBT, there is a thesis and an antithesis proposed in these metaphysical works with the winner of the debate pointing out the inaccuracies in perception and faulty logic. However, unlike in DBT, there is no validation of the affect nor any therapeutic synthesis.

Positive psychology

An important difference between Hindu and Western psychological approaches is the former's focus on enhancing happiness (*Sukha*), whereas several western psychotherapeutic models (e.g. CBT, psychoanalysis) focus largely on treating psychopathology. An increasing effort in Western psychology has aimed at cultivating positive attributes of mind in individuals without mental disorders (29). The Gita and other Hindu scriptures presciently provide insights into a number of aspects of modern positive psychology.

First, Western and Hindu traditions differ in their approaches to positive states: while Western approaches emphasize time-limited, peak performance states (e.g. *doing* extraordinarily well in sports and in the arts), Hindu traditions emphasize states of heightened experiences of *being* as character strengths or traits. Happiness, in Western positive psychology approaches, is focused on developing "flow" states (Csikszentmihaly 1990, 47) into everyday life. Mihaly Csikszentmihalyi discovered that the experience of being immersed in action itself rather than being focused on the finished work led to a state of happiness he called the "flow" state. This view is reminiscent of eastern traditions which seek to enhance a persistent state of effortless action and mastery (30).

Second, the Hindu traditions take a different perspective on the self. Western psychology treats the self as an enduring entity. A strong ego is viewed as critical to success in work and relationships. Therapy seeks to strengthen the ego and to correct low self-esteem. Hindu conceptualizations view the self as non-enduring, even illusory, as discussed earlier. According to the Gita, over-indulgence in the finite self leads to false perception and consequently to suffering (*Dukkha*). Replacing the notion of 'individual self' with that of the universal self with yoga, meditation, and mindfulness can be corrective.

Third, Hindu traditions place a major emphasis on intrinsic motivation. This refers to initiating an activity for its own sake because it is inherently interesting, satisfying in itself, and the right thing to do (*Nishkaama Karma*), as opposed to doing an activity to obtain an external goal (extrinsic motivation; 31). People who are intrinsically motivated tend to have a higher sense of competence at tasks and lesser affective responsivity to outcome as compared with those who are extrinsically motivated (32).

Fourth, an important component of Hindu thought on the self is to view one's experiences as part of a more collective human experience (*Loka Samgraha*) instead of seeing them as being separate. This allows the individual to mindfully hold one's thoughts in balanced awareness and avoid over-identifying them with the narcissistic individual self. This can counter self-centredness, increase focus on actions toward goals larger than one's own interests, and reduce interpersonal comparison (33).

Final is the concept of balance (*Samatwam*). The Gita explains that the essence of Yoga is the goal to balance the individual's mind, body, and intellect (the Gita, Chapter 2, Verse 48). Central to this is the synchronization between thought and perception (cognition), emotion and the senses (affect), and action (conation). This concept is also developed in Buddhism (34).

Clinical practice implications and evidence

Despite the rich wisdom inherent in Hindu spiritual traditions relevant to mental health, these insights have not been routinely embedded in psychotherapeutic practice. In part, this may be related to the practice models of psychiatrists themselves and their training. Reluctance to adopt these approaches in psychotherapy may also be related to the possibility that many clinicians in the mental health profession have an agnostic bent, or may hold beliefs that bringing up religious/spiritual beliefs may violate therapeutic boundaries.

It is well known that cultural background and spiritual beliefs contribute to both the manifestations and the presentation of psychopathology as well as determining their acceptance. For these reasons, major psychiatric organizations such as the World Psychiatric Association (WPA; 35), the Royal College of Psychiatrists (36) and the American Psychiatric Association (37) recommend integrating spiritually based assessment and treatment planning in routine psychiatric practice. The WPA has recommended spirituality as part of its 'Core Training Curriculum for Psychiatry'.

The principles of adapting psychotherapeutic approaches to Hindu patients are particularly relevant in the Indian context, though the large population of Hindus across the globe makes them relevant to mental health practitioners across different countries (38, 39). On the other hand, considerable cultural and religious diversity exists even within India, making it critical for treatments to be tailored at an individual level, taking into account the patients' unique individual, family, and cultural contexts. In general, certain characteristics of the Hindu psyche make it important for the Western models of individual psychotherapy to be remodelled while treating patients from the Hindu culture. First, Hindu patients typically prefer a more directive and authoritarian approach rather than the 'therapeutic neutrality' of Western-trained psychotherapists (40). The therapeutic relationship in the Indian context has been likened to a teacher–student (Guru-Chela) relationship (41). In the Gita too, Arjuna requests and submits to be a disciple of Krishna for 'therapy' (Chapter 2, Verse 7). Second, Hindus traditionally value dependability more than autonomy and independence. Hence, both the client and the therapist are vulnerable to frustration if working towards different goals. Third, Hindu patients often believe in the immortality of the soul and of re-birth, and fatalistic views are common; this can have an impact on how patients attribute causation to events in their lives, and how they choose to take personal responsibility for their actions. Fourth, confidentiality exercised by the therapist is often frowned upon by the families, in regard to decisions made for the patient (42). Therapists can benefit from using the psychotherapeutic paradigms depicted in the Hindu scriptures as outlined in this chapter, and also use anecdotes from the Hindu mythology and religious texts as a way to educate patients in regard to psychological concepts and defence mechanisms (43). The two cases below, both drawn from the first author's practice, illustrate the potential value of using Hindu religious principles and practices in addressing anxiety and depression. The cases have been partly fictionalized to protect anonymity.

Case report 1: Mr A

Mr A, a 23-year-old college student double majoring in biochemistry and neuroscience with a minor in art history, presented with 'constant internal angst and depression' for the previous few years of his life in college and studying abroad in a city. His parents, both of Indian origin, are successful doctors. Mr A reported inability to concentrate because of low self-esteem, worries of failure ('not living up to my parents' expectation'), and anxiety and depression as a consequence; he began experiencing panic attacks as term exams approached. He would always compare himself with others (such as his brother who was in medical school), leading to anger and jealousy. He reported not enjoying his studies (doodling in classes). He felt that he was 'straining my mind and body over the past five years to become something that I am inherently not ... ' He kept asking himself: What is my mission in life? What am I to do? Who am I? Should I drop out of school? All this interfered with him functioning well in school and he thought of dropping out.

Mr A's treatment involved regular discussion on principles in the Gita with the therapist. In particular, he benefited from the concept in the Gita that one should choose action that is inherently motivating, and is in congruence with one's own strengths. Such actions, when performed without the expectation of extrinsic rewards, is more likely to be effective. He took a semester off, and focused on regular exercise (Yoga) and meditation: initially one point (Vipassana) followed by an open source meditation using an app (Calm) helped, which helped him to focus more on the present moment. Family meetings with parents helped reduce perception of parental pressure on academic performance. Self-evaluation of his unique strengths and aspirations led A. to reevaluate what he most cared about: creativity as opposed to critical thinking (needed for his premedical courses). Back to school with a focus on art, and then to graduate school in design, he is now functioning well as a designer for a publishing company.

Case report 2: Mrs B

Mrs B is a 36-yearold married woman who works as an engineer. She has been generally in good health except for mild depression when she had been briefly laid off from work some years earlier. She has a strong family history of depression and bipolar disorder in several first-degree relatives. She was admitted to the psychiatry inpatient service with a severe depression for over three months. This episode had followed an unfortunate event in which her four-year-old daughter died after falling fell into her swimming pool in her backyard when Mrs B was hosting a party for several friends. Mrs B had severe guilt feelings, recurrent suicidal thoughts, hopelessness, and lacked a will to live and go on.

Following treatment with electroconvulsive therapy and fluoxetine up to 40 mg per day, Mrs B stabilized and was discharged. She was started on a course of cognitive behaviour therapy. Her depression persisted despite a higher dose of fluoxetine and a second antidepressant, with guilt feelings and beliefs that she deserved to be punished because of her sins in her past lives as well as this life. Though she was able to see the irrationality of her self-blame in regard to her daughter's death, she could not resist having recurrent automatic negative thoughts of remorse, which would snowball into preoccupations that she had sinned. CBT sessions did not seem to particularly help her take control of these ruminations. She took the position that she had to suffer the consequences of her past deeds (*Karmas*), and that any treatment would be futile.

The therapist enlisted the help of a family friend, who was well versed in the Hindu scriptures. This spiritual healer got Mrs B regularly reading the Bhagavad Gita, especially the section (Chapter 2, Verse 22) that refers to the transmigration of the soul. Mrs. B. began finding relief in the view that her daughter's body but not her soul was deceased (just like a change of clothes, as the Gita says), and that she must be reborn somewhere. Mrs B came to the conclusion that perhaps she might feel better if she and her husband adopted a child born around the same time as when her daughter passed away. The healer and the therapist concurred with her, and the family sought and adopted a girl from India. She was also advised to regularly practice yoga and one-point meditation, which helped her to reduce her ruminations. She gradually improved and, when seen two years later, she had maintained a remission from her depression.

Both these cases illustrate the potential value of using selected concepts from the Gita or other Hindu scriptures in addressing their sources of anxiety and depression. Mr A. benefited from understanding his own nature and matching it with appropriate, intrinsically motivating pursuit of work in his school, so that he could address his problem of performance anxiety, Mrs B. addressed her depression and intense grieving by taking recourse to the Hindu concept of the immortality of the soul, and the benefit of appropriate action (her adopting a girl was a good *Karma* counteracting her remorse about past karmic influences). In neither case did the therapist have to be directive in imposing his own views on the patient's approach to their choices. Rather, the therapist facilitated the patients to utilize their own spiritual beliefs in addressing their respective causes of psychological difficulties. Such an approach was integrated with conventional psychiatric treatment as needed, and also with Yoga and mindfulness practices.

Relatively few studies have investigated the effectiveness of integrated psychotherapy incorporating Hindu psychotherapeutic insights. One exception is Pearce and colleagues (2015; 44) who have developed a novel religiously integrated adaptation of (and elsewhere) CBT for individuals with depression in the context of chronic medical illness. Their manualized therapeutic approach incorporates principles from five major world religions (Christianity, Judaism, Islam, Buddhism, and Hinduism). Therapeutic elements include Scripture memorization, contemplative prayer, challenging thoughts using one's religious resources, religious practices (e.g. gratitude, altruism, forgiveness), and religious/spiritual resources involvement in the individual's religious community. There are several studies examining therapeutic benefits with religiously or spiritually integrated approaches to psychotherapy compared with their eclectic (or non-religious) counterparts (45, 46). This research is only beginning and the results are inconsistent. Further, these authors could not find any studies that have systematically investigated such psychotherapeutic interventions using Hindu religious/spirituality principles. Clearly, there is a need to develop, implement empirically validated, theory-driven spiritually and religiously integrated psychotherapy using Hindu traditions, and to test their effectiveness in practice.

Conclusions

There are several pearls of wisdom relevant to modern psychotherapeutic practice (Meeks and Jeste, 2009) (48) that may be unearthed by a careful review of Hindu scriptures. Some of these concepts have elements that appear to anticipate later emerging psychotherapeutic models, notably cognitive, meta-cognitive and positive psychology-based therapies. It is likely that using these spiritual and religious concepts can be of value in contemporary psychiatric practice. However, such integration of spiritual/ religious principles needs to be tailored to the specific patient characteristics as well as specific clinical needs. More work is needed to develop and implement psychotherapeutic approaches incorporating Hindu spiritual/ religious principle, as well to empirically test their effectiveness.

References

1. **Jung CG.** *The psychology of Kundalini Yoga. Notes of the seminar given in 1932.* S. Shamdasani (ed.), Princeton, NJ: Princeton University Press; 1999. Bollingen Series XCIX.

2. **Maslow AH.** A theory of human motivation. *Psychological Review.* 1943;**50**(4):370–96.

3. **Diwakar RR.** *Upanishads in story and dialogue.* Bombay: Bharatiya Vidya Bhavan; 1988.

4. **Ramachandra Rao SK.** *Development of psychological thought in India.* Bangalore: Surama Prakashana; 2012.

5. **Prabhupada AC** et al. *Bhagavad Gita as it is.* Bhaktivedanta Book Trust (1972 edition); 2015.

6. **Pandurangi AK, Shenoy S, Keshavan MS.** Psychotherapy in the Bhagavad Gita, the Hindu scriptural text. *American Journal of Psychiatry.* 2014 Aug;**171**(8):827–8.

7. **Easwaran E.** *The Upanishads.* Nilgiri Press; Tomales, California, 2007, pp. 38–9.

8. **Radhakrishnan S.** *The Bhagavad Gita.* New York: Harper Collins; 1948.

9. **Johnston, Charles.** *The Mukhya Upanishads.* Kshetra Books. Scotts Valley, CA: CreateSpace Independent Publishing Platform; 2014.

10. **Uchida Y, Kitayama S.** Happiness and unhappiness in east and west: themes and variations. *Emotion.* 2009 Aug;**9**(4):441–56.

11. **Flood G, Martin C.** *The Bhagavad Gita: a new translation.* New York: WW Norton & Company; 2013.

12. **Yogeshwar G.** Swami Vivekananda's concept of jnana yoga, raja yoga, karma yoga and bhakti yoga. *Ancient Science of Life.* 1994 Jan;**13**(3–4):261–5.

13. **Patañjali; James Haughton Woods (trans.)** *The Yoga Sutras of Patañjali.* Published for Harvard University by Ginn & Co.;1914.

14. **Brekke, Torkel.** The religious motivation of the early Buddhists. *Journal of the American Academy of Religion.* 1999 Dec;**67**(4):849–66.

15. **Dunne FP.** *The world religions speak on 'The relevance of religion in the modern world'.* New York: Springer; 2013, pp. 94–5.

16. **Bhatia SC, Madabushi J, Kolli V, Bhatia SK, Madaan V.** The Bhagavad Gita and contemporary psychotherapies. *Indian Journal of Psychiatry.* 2013 Jan;**55**(Suppl. 2):S315–21.

17. **Ellis A, Dryden W.** *The practice of rational emotive behavior therapy.* Second edition. New York: Springer; 2007.

18. **Beck AT.** The past and future of cognitive therapy. *Journal of Psychotherapy Practice and Research.* 1997 Fall;6(4):276–84.

19. **Teasdale JD, Segal ZV, Williams M.** How does cognitive therapy prevent relapse and why should attentional control (mindful-ness) training help? *Behaviour Research and Therapy.* 1995;33:25–39.

20. **Balodhi JP, Keshavan MS.** Bhagavadgita and psychotherapy. *Asian Journal of Psychiatry.* 2011 Dec;4(4):300–2.

21. **Flavell JH.** Metacognition and cognitive monitoring: a new area of cognitive development inquiry. *American Psychologist.* 1979;34: 906–11.

22. **Wells Adrian.** *Metacognitive therapy for anxiety and depression.* New York: Guilford Press; 2011.

23. **Wells A, Sembi S.** Metacognitive therapy for PTSD: a preliminary investigation of a new brief treatment. *Journal of Behavior Theraphy and Experimental Psychiatry.* 2004 Dec;35(4):307–18.

24. **Garland E, Gaylord S, Park J.** The role of mindfulness in positive reappraisal. *Explore (NY).* 2009;5(1):37–44. doi:10.1016/j.explore.2008.10.001

25. **Kabat-Zinn J, Massion AO, Kristeller J,** et al. Effectiveness of a meditation-based stress reduction program in the treatment of anxiety disorders. *American Journal of Psychiatry.* 1992;149(7):936–43.

26. **Linehan Marsha M.** *DBT skills training manual.* Second edition. New York: Guilford Press; 2014.

27. **Hayes Steven C, Strosahl Kirk D, Wilson Kelly G.** *Acceptance and commitment therapy: the process and practice of mindful change.* Second edition. New York: Guilford Press; 2012.

28. **Wilson Jeff.** *Mindful America: the mutual transformation of Buddhist meditation and American culture.* Oxford: Oxford University Press; 2014.

29. **Seligman ME, Csikszentmihalyi M.** Positive psychology. An introduction. *American Psychologist.* 2000 Jan;55(1):5–14.

30. **Brown D.** Mastery of the mind East and West: excellence in being and doing and everyday happiness. *Annals of the New York Academy of Sciences.* 2009 Aug;1172:231–51.

31. **Deci E, Ryan R,** (eds), *Handbook of self-determination research.* Rochester, NY: University of Rochester Press; 2002.

32. **Abuhamdeh S, Csikszentmihalyi M.** Intrinsic and extrinsic motivational orientations in the competitive context: an examination of person-situation interactions. *Journal of Personality.* 2009 Oct;77(5):1615–35.

33. **Kissen M, Kissen-Kohn DA.** Reducing addictions via the self-soothing effects of yoga. *Bulletin of the Menninger Clinic.* 2009;73(1):34–43.

34. **Wallace BA, Shapiro SL.** Mental balance and well-being: building bridges between Buddhism and Western psychology. *American Psychologist.* 2006 Oct;61(7):690–701.

35. **Moreira-Almeida A, Sharma A, Van Rensburg BJ, Verhagen PJ, Cook CCH.** WPA Position Statement on Spirituality and Religion in Psychiatry. *Actas Españolas de Psiquiatría.* 2018;46(6):242–8.

36. **Cook CH.** *Recommendations for psychiatrists on spirituality and religion.* Position Statement: PS03/2011. The Royal College of Psychiatrists; 2013.

37. **Lukoff D, Lu F, Turner R.** Toward a more culturally sensitive DSM-IV: psychoreligious and psychospiritual problems. *Journal of Nervous and Mental Disease.* 1992;**180**:673–82.

38. **Avasthi A, Kate N, Grover S.** Indianization of psychiatry utilizing Indian mental concepts. *Indian Journal of Psychiatry.* 2013;**55**(Suppl. 2):S136–44.

39. **Varma VK.** Present state of psychotherapy in India. *Indian Journal of Psychiatry.* 1982;**24**:209–26.

40. **Sethi BB, Trivedi JK.** Psychotherapy for the economically less privileged classes (with special reference to India) *Indian Journal of Psychiatry.* 1982;**24**:318–21.

41. **Neki JS.** Psychotherapy in India. *Indian Journal of Psychiatry.* 1977;**19**:1–10.

42. **Neki JS** Confidentiality, secrecy, and privacy in psychotherapy: sociodynamic considerations *Indian Journal of Psychiatry.* 1992 Jul; **34**(3):171–3.

43. **Sham Sundar C.** Therapeutic wisdom in Indian mythology, *Journal of Psychotherapy.* 1993;**47**:443–50.

44. **Pearce MJ, Koenig HG, Robins CJ, et al.** Religiously integrated cognitive behavioral therapy: a new method of treatment for major depression in patients with chronic medical illness. *Psychotherapy (Chic).* 2015;**52**(1):56–66.

45. **Lim C, Sim K, Renjan V, Sam HF, Quah SL.** Adapted cognitive-behavioral therapy for religious individuals with mental disorder: a systematic review. *Asian Journal of Psychiatry.* 2014;**9**:3–12.

46. **Koenig HG, Pearce MJ, Nelson B, Daher N.** Effects of religious versus standard cognitive-behavioral therapy on optimism in persons with major depression and chronic medical illness. *Depression and Anxiety.* 2015;**32**(11):835–42.

47. **Csikszentmihalyi, Mihaly.** *Flow: the psychology of optimal experience.* First edition. New York: Harper & Row; 1990.

48. **Meeks TW, Jeste DV.** Neurobiology of wisdom: a literature overview. *Archives of General Psychiatry.* 2009 Apr;**66**(4):355–65.

Chapter 13

Principles and practices of Buddhism in relationship to mental health

Malcolm Huxter and Leandro Pizutti

Introduction

The term 'Buddha' refers to an awakened one. It is derived from the Pali verb root 'budh', which means 'to understand' or 'to awaken'. Around 2560 years ago Siddhartha Gautama woke up to four realities and became the Buddha. These realities are also called the 'four noble truths' and they are essentially two cause–effect relationships: suffering (first) and its causes (second); freedom from suffering (third) and its causes (fourth). For 45 years, the Buddha taught a path where individuals could realize for themselves the nature of psychological freedom. He taught in a way that was adaptable to the individual and the culture within which the individual lived their life, spreading widely throughout Asia and to a range of cultures over the centuries. From culture to culture, the outward appearance and often the practices would vary, yet the liberating core principles of Buddhism would remain the same. Throughout the twentieth century, interest in Buddhism in Western cultures grew and accelerated in the 1960s and 1970s. Since then, Buddhism has flourished in Western cultures and it has been adapted in many different ways. One adaptation has been its application to psychotherapy and mental health services, and there is evidence of parallels with practices used in contemporary therapies and the teachings of the Buddha (1).

According to some Buddhist scholars, the four truths have two levels: noble and ennobling (2). The noble truths involve inclining towards waking up to complete freedom, or Nirvana (Sanskrit). The ennobling truths involve working towards the reduction of suffering in a way that is more basic and mundane than Nirvana. The ennobling or basic level of the four truths is evident in the adaption of Buddhism to psychotherapy and mental health (3).

At a personal level, both authors of this chapter have confidence in the teachings of the Buddha and adhere to a personal meditation practice that is Buddhist. As clinicians, we also adhere to scientifically valid, evidence-based practices in our roles as a clinical psychologist (MH) and a psychiatrist (LP). We both find that the teachings of the Buddha support and enhance our clinical understanding and professional skills, as well as interpersonal relationships with our patients, students, and colleagues.

The lotus is often a symbol of Buddhism because this flower is something beautiful that grows out of the slime and slush, compost and mud, at the bottom of a pond. Both personally and professionally, we have found that Buddhist principles and practices can transform anguish, despair, frustration, misery, and other forms of mental torment to a greater and more spacious sense of psychological freedom. I (MH) lived in Thailand as a Buddhist monk for two years in the late 1970s. A decade later, after returning to Australia and studying, I became a clinical psychologist. As a clinician and teacher, I have integrated the insights and strategies of scientifically based contemporary psychology with the wisdom, compassion, and meditation practices found in Buddhism. In our opinion, the Buddhist framework as a whole is too broad and comprehensive to be considered a single therapy. For us, it is more an umbrella paradigm under which one can understand the effectiveness of many mental health therapies. The Buddhist framework also provides contextual understanding of how to adapt and use specific practices, such as mindfulness and compassion, skilfully, effectively, and for specific clinical populations.

The aims of this chapter are to provide a general overview of the principles and practices related to Buddhism, and their implications for an individual's mental health. As mindfulness is possibly one of the main Buddhist practices evident in Western psychotherapies, there will be a brief, recent, historical account of this therapeutic practice. We will also refer to some theoretical and practice differences between the traditional Buddhist and contemporary approaches to mindfulness. Finally, we will reflect on the utility of Buddhism for mental health.

A Buddhist framework: principles and practices

As Buddhism has spread across the globe, the way it has been taught and practised has varied. However, what has been consistent across cultures, traditions, and sects are the four noble truths because they are the foundational framework of all Buddhist principles and practices. As mentioned earlier, the four truths are as follows:

1. The reality of suffering or un-satisfactoriness, in both its gross and subtle forms.
2. The reality of there being underlying psychological roots that cause and maintain our suffering.
3. The reality that it is possible to be free from suffering.
4. The reality of there being a path of practice that frees us and keeps us free from suffering.

In Pali, the language closest to that spoken by the Buddha, *dukkha* is the term used to describe the first truth. *Dukkha* is often translated as suffering, but it is better to consider it as un-satisfactoriness. It ranges from the gross, such as the struggles we have with severe mental and physical illness and death, to the subtle, such as not getting what we want exactly how and when we want it (4).

The Buddha's second truth is based on natural relationships and principles. *Dukkha* arises because of interdependent interactions between external (objective) events in the environment; internal events such as sensations, thoughts, and emotions; and internal (or subjective) responses or reactions to these events. The way we interpret and relate to experience influences the extent to which *dukkha* arises. From a Buddhist perspective, the extent of our *dukkha* is contextually dependent on tendencies that incline towards:

♦ Greed—craving, clinging, and addiction to pleasant feelings;
♦ Hatred—aversion, avoidance, rejection, condemnation, and struggle with unpleasant feelings; and
♦ Ignorance—not knowing, misunderstanding, misapprehension, and misperception (5).

The third truth, freedom, is the result of waking up to our patterns of *dukkha* and realizing the causes. Freedom results from reducing and eventually abandoning greed, ignorance, and hatred, and exiting unhelpful interdependent cycles that feed and reinforce *dukkha*.

The fourth truth consists of eight interdependent practices (or factors) in three groups: wisdom (view and intentions), ethics (wholesome speech, actions, and livelihood) and meditation (effort, mindfulness, and concentration). These groups and practices are interdependent, such that wisdom, ethics, and meditation are inseparably interconnected, because ethical behaviour provides the emotional composure required for meditation, while meditation allows the cultivation of wisdom.

The eight-fold path, often depicted as a wheel with self-sustaining momentum, is both a path to freedom and a path of practice. Each of the eight factors is prefixed by the Pali term '*samma*', usually translated as 'right'. Here 'right' means that the given factor is functioning in a wholesome way in that it directs the mind towards freedom from suffering. Within this framework, it is possible to have 'wrong' view, intention, speech, action, livelihood, effort, mindfulness, and concentration. Wrong mindfulness, as one example, is the type of mindfulness that does not lead toward psychological freedom. Wrong mindfulness and concentration could include the mental factors required to act out harmful plans, such as robbing a bank or murder.

The aim of practising the eight-fold path is freedom from *dukkha*. Psychological freedom emerges with the realization of the four noble truths and the three universal characteristics of existence, those of impermanence, un-satisfactoriness and interdependence (4). The four truths can be seen as sequential aspects of a single process (6). First, we understand *dukkha*, and thus see clearly the root causes of our distress. Then, as we would naturally let go of a hot potato because it is painful, we abandon the causes of our *dukkha*. This is the realization of the second truth. The third truth then emerges as we realize the cessation of *dukkha* after abandoning its causes. Now this psychological freedom is experienced, we endeavour to practise and live according to the eight-fold path, which is the fourth truth (6).

From a therapeutic perspective, the four truths could be described as follows:

1. We humans experience psychological problems. These problems, which include all the disorders we find in diagnostic manuals such the DSM–5 (7), are *dukkha*.

2. There are causative and maintaining factors in the arising and continuation of psychological problems, such as experiential avoidance, feeding into addictions, and denying as well as misunderstanding the way things are.

3. It is possible to reduce the severity of symptoms and, in some cases, to find freedom from the distress of psychological disorders.

4. There are healing and therapeutic pathways that access cognitive, behavioural, and affective strategies as well as human relationships based on benevolence, compassion, appreciation/gratitude, and equanimity (5).

Dependent arising

The four truths are an example of a principle called 'dependent arising'. This principle is the way the Buddha explained how things come into being and how they change and disappear. While dependent arising is complex and difficult to understand, it could be understood by considering that, if there is no cause for suffering, then suffering does not arise. Avoidance, for example, is a maintenance factor for anxiety disorders (8). In the language of the four truths, avoidance conditions and maintains anxiety. A general strategy for working with anxiety is to gradually and slowly reduce these patterns of avoidance, and this helps to reduce the suffering of anxiety (8).

Psychological freedom develops when we choose to not do the things that are keeping us bound in reactive cycles of suffering, and choose instead to do something that helps us break free. The choice to refrain from unhelpful actions and engage in helpful actions is represented in an acceptance and commitment therapy (ACT) saying that goes: 'If I continue to do what I've always done, then I'm going to get what I've always got.' (9).

The direction of the eight-fold path leads away from *dukkha* and towards psychological freedom. As mentioned earlier, the eight-fold path has three groups: wisdom, ethics, and meditation.

Wisdom

When I (MH) conduct groups, I often ask participants about what wisdom means to them. This question usually stimulates discussion and eventually a relevant rationale for why it is helpful to practise mindfulness and meditation. One time, aided by a Farsi interpreter, I was leading a group session in mindfulness (without mention of Buddhism) for about 50 Islamic Shi'ite men, women, and children asylum seekers. A girl who seemed about 9 years old shared her thoughts on wisdom. She said that wisdom was knowing what is good and what is bad. After some discussion, we collectively agreed that wisdom could refer to knowing what is helpful for well-being and happiness and actively cultivating it, as well as knowing what causes and feeds into unhappiness and discontent and actively trying to remove these causes.

The wisdom component of the eight-fold path has two aspects: view and intention. Traditionally, right view includes the understanding that actions have consequences and that all conditioned phenomena are impermanent, interdependent, unreliable, and thus unsatisfactory. The view aspect of wisdom usually relates to understanding the causes of *dukkha* and how to be free of it. The second aspect of wisdom, intention, is found in how we apply our understanding. Intentions to cease feeding the root causes of *dukkha* (greed, hatred, and ignorance) are helpful intentions. It is worth noting that, traditionally, liberating intentions are those that incline towards letting go, goodwill (including loving-kindness and compassion), and harmlessness. When we have a clear view and good intentions, we are more likely to act, with our speech, action, and livelihood, in ways that are consistent with our insights and best intentions. These behaviours constitute the ethical component of the path, which traditionally follows on from wisdom.

At a basic therapeutic level, for example, someone with agoraphobia who actively avoids shopping centres may begin to understand that their avoidance behaviour contributes to anxiety maintenance. With this insight, they could make the resolve to wisely embark on graduated exposure tasks. With firm commitment, it is then possible to courageously engage in the types of actions that reflect their understanding and intentions. These actions that eventually lead to the reduction of their anxieties and suffering could be called ethical.

Ethics

In groups, after we have engaged in discussions about wisdom, I (MH) will often pose questions about what wise and unwise action of body, speech, and mind could be. Most participants are usually able to make lists of behaviours that are helpful for the long-term well-being and happiness of themselves and others, as well as those types of behaviors that lead to misery, unhappiness, and discontent in the long run. The Buddhist understanding of ethics relates to the choice to act helpfully or wholesomely as distinct from the choice to act in ways that increase *dukkha*. When we are more aware of the cause–effect relationships of our choices and actions, we may be more likely to act ethically and less likely to act unethically. Traditionally, a commitment to ethical principles precedes training in meditation, and its ongoing adherence forms the basis and foundation of meditation.

In the literature, (10) the inclusion of overt reference to ethics in mindfulness training within a contemporary context is often considered as if it is imposing Buddhist values. A key feature of evidence-based contemporary psychology is for its practices and strategies to be value-neutral, which means that they are oriented against imposing the therapist's beliefs and values on the patient (10). Consequently, contemporary psychotherapists have ethics as a protective and not prescriptive tool in the clinical setting, which can be confused with an orientation contrary to the approach of ethics in patient behaviour. In addition, contemporary mindfulness-based programmes do not explicitly address the importance of ethics, and the ethical component of a programme relies only on the teacher's skills. As Buddhist therapists and group programme leaders we (MH and LP) feel that sidestepping consideration about ethics as an important factor in our well-being and happiness is a valuable therapeutic opportunity missed (11). From a Buddhist perspective, choices to act ethically are based on an individual's own maturing wisdom and not another's values.

When ethical awareness is part of a theoretical framework, programme leaders or therapists can skilfully weave opportunities for reflection and discussion into their programme or therapy session. In this way, patients or group participants can begin to understand and realize for themselves what is helpful and unhelpful. Ethics is the foundation for meditation because, for most people, acting unethically is destabilizing and not conducive to meditation. When we act ethically, our minds are more inclined to mental composure and thus more prepared to courageously cultivate mindful and concentrated attention, which is meditation.

Meditation

As mentioned earlier, in groups, after we have talked about wisdom and wise actions, I (MH) will often ask the question: How does one cultivate wisdom? Some participants say wisdom comes from reading or hearing wise words or logical reasoning. Most will say, however, that wisdom comes from life experience. From this point, I provide one rationale for mindfulness practice as being a tool to understand our life experience and cultivate wisdom.

In an effort to combine the contemporary with the traditional, Ven. Bodhi defined mindfulness as: 'to remember to pay attention to what is occurring in one's immediate experience with care and discernment' (12). The inclusion of the terms 'remembering', 'care', and 'discernment' indicate the context that mindfulness was designed to be embedded within: that of the eight-fold path. The Pali term for mindfulness is *sati*, which literally means memory. As a mental factor, *sati* is the act of remembering the present and keeping the present in mind. Its opposite is forgetfulness (13). The practice of mindfulness involves remembering to track, with attention, the changing aspects of body, mind, and life. According to Wallace and Hodel, (14) mindfulness (*sati*) involves retrospectively remembering things from the past, thus being able to cultivate wisdom, prospectively remembering to do something in the future, thus being mindful to act in accordance with wisdom, and present-centred recollection, in order to stay connected with current realities.

Right concentration refers to the gathering of attention and settling it into one place in a way that is not harmful. Right effort refers to the motivating energy behind right mindfulness and right concentration. Effort needs to be balanced as neither too much nor too little. Effort is often described as courageous (15) because, in the process of energetic mindfulness and concentration, we may uncover and face up to things about ourselves that may be painful and uncomfortable.

The calm and insight aspects of meditation

Theravada Buddhist meditation has two aspects: calm and insight. The calm aspect of meditation provides the focus and clarity to see psychological patterns, and the insight aspect provides understanding. The calm aspect of Buddhist meditation usually emphasizes concentration and absorption while the insight aspect emphasizes inquiry and analysis. According to the teachings, (6) the Buddha was like a physician who prescribes specific medication for specific ailments. He taught different types of meditation depending on the particular temperaments of his students and the context within which he encountered them. The varieties of meditation practices available can be classified within the categories of either calm or insight. Mindfulness of breath, for example, is a common calm meditation practice, and the practice of mindfulness in the context of the four foundations of mindfulness (see below) is regarded as an insight practice. Calm meditations are stabling and centring. They serve to relax the body, calm the mind, and bring peace to the heart. Insight meditations, on the other hand, serve to deconstruct problems that are created from misunderstanding and misperceiving. Insight helps us see and understand our lives, the world, and ourselves realistically.

As can be seen in Table 13.1, the two aspects of calm and insight work together in mutually supportive ways, and a lack of balance between them can be problematic. Insight without calm presence can be quite distressing because we may see what is happening in our lives but not have the psychological resources to cope. On the other hand, being calm and relaxed without any understanding may be directionless. The benefits of balancing insight and calm as practised in Buddhist meditation can be generalized to working skilfully with a range of clinical presentations. When working with those who are suffering the effects of trauma, for example, it is important that individuals have the opportunity to soothe and center themselves when their emotions become overwhelming. This process of balancing the stabilizing effects of calm meditation with the deconstructing aspects of insight meditation can be found, in our view, in the protocol of eye movement desensitization and reprocessing (EMDR) (16), which is often used with people suffering with the effects of a trauma. Before the process of desensitizing and reprocessing is initiated, patients establish skills in

Table 13.1 Functions and features of calm and insight

Calm	Insight
Integrates/stabilizes	Dismantles/deconstructs
Sustained attention and focus on a single object	Mindfulness and penetrative inquiry into characteristics of immediate experience
Stills the mind and absorbs into experience	Understands phenomena
Restores and rejuvenates	Develops understanding

being able to self-soothe by creating, psychologically, a 'safe place' (16). The safe place serves as a resource, and a calming respite and retreat, when the intensity of insight-based deconstruction of a trauma becomes overwhelming. As well as the safe place, EMDR uses a range of other calming, soothing, stabilizing, and centring strategies to ensure that a patient does not experience untoward and unhelpful reactions to the treatment.

With calm meditation, mindfulness serves to ensure that attention remains with a chosen object. With insight meditation, mindfulness becomes the key element and serves to help us understand experience. In groups and in individual therapy, I (MH) will usually explain that mindfulness has four foundations or domains. The four foundations of mindfulness are:

1. body, including posture, actions, physical sensations, and breath;
2. feeling, or the hedonic qualities of pleasantness, unpleasantness, or neither;
3. heart–mind, including moods, emotions, and states of mind in varying manifestations;
4. phenomena, including emotional, mental, and behavioural patterns analysed as either helpful or unhelpful (3).

When we track or monitor experience with mindfulness, we begin to understand it. The foundations of mindfulness are comparable to gears on a motor vehicle. We move back and forward between the foundations depending on the psychological terrain we travel on (3). The foundations are used and adapted dependent on temperament, issues, and context. Just like any approach to therapy where the intervention must be suitable for the presentation and 'a one size fits all' approach is risky, no one foundation is suitable for everything. As clinicians, we need to use clinical judgement in order to guide our patients with how and when to apply the different domains of mindfulness. For example, 'mindfulness of the breath' and 'body scan' are two common mindfulness of body practices taught in contemporary psychology. However, mindfulness of breath can often trigger panic attacks for those with panic disorder, while body scan can trigger abreactions for those who have been sexually violated (5). When we understand the breadth of meditation practices available, we can match particular practices with individual clinical presentations. More often than not, an individual needs to balance their insightful mindfulness practice with calming and soothing skills that include access to human connection and relationship qualities.

The four divine abodes

There is a set of calm meditation practices described by the Buddha as the 'four divine abodes'. They are aspirations for, and the cultivation of, loving-kindness, compassion, appreciative joy, and equanimity. Loving-kindness includes qualities of benevolence, warm friendliness, and universal goodwill. It involves the capacity to see the good in oneself and others, and it is based on nourishing happiness and warm relationships with oneself and others. Compassion includes sensitivity to suffering and the motivation to alleviate it (17). Appreciative joy arises in celebration and appreciation of the successes, virtues, good fortune, skills, and happiness of self or other. It also involves, in our opinion, gratitude. Equanimity is a grounded sense of being centred, stable, emotionally balanced, and unshaken in the midst of the inevitable highs and lows of life. It involves impartiality regarding attraction or aversion to beings, and treating all as equally worthy of kindness (14).

Emotions function within three interrelated systems: the avoid or threat system (fight, flight, and freeze); the approach, drive, or resource-seeking system (pursuing and wanting); and the attach, connection, and soothing system (bonding and safety) (18,19). The therapeutic power of the four divine abodes is evident in how compassion and other intentions of goodwill are considered as essential in balancing these emotional systems (20). Emotions are necessary for human survival, well-being and thriving, and are essential for communication and the welfare of our families and communities. In balance, emotions help us form relationships, motivate behaviour and save lives (21). The emotional systems can function in a healthy and balanced way, or be out of balance and therefore increase *dukkha*. Unwarranted stimulation of the threat system may reflect, for example, an anxiety disorder while an unbalanced drive system may reflect an addiction.

Strengthening the soothing and connection system with practices such as the four divine abodes are ways to regulate the threat system and balance the drive system. Cultivating the four divine abodes help us cope with life's difficulties. Warm compassionate connections with others have a powerful effect in soothing and helping us to bear that which is very difficult to bear. In addition, these four qualities form the basis of how one can relate to oneself. In synchrony with Carl Roger's (22) emphasis on the essentials of empathy, positive warm regard, and genuineness in an effective therapeutic relationship, a Buddhist therapist will most often endeavour to practise and model mindful presence and the four divine abodes in relationship with their patients, because they are embedded in the eight-fold path of wisdom, ethics, and meditation. In our opinion, training in the four divine abodes is an essential balance to mindfulness training in a clinical setting or a group programme format.

Summary of a Buddhist framework

The framework of Buddhism begins with the four truths. The fourth truth is the path of freedom that has eight factors grouped into three components: wisdom, ethics, and meditation. Meditation involves the cultivation of effort, mindfulness, and concentration and has two aspects: calm and insight. Meditation for calm emphasizes concentration while meditation for insight emphasizes mindfulness. One set of calm meditations consists of the cultivation of four relationship qualities called the 'divine abodes', which are helpful in meeting the ups and downs of meditation practice. Calm and insight balance and support each other. and promote wisdom.

The wisdom group of the path includes intentions based on letting go, goodwill, and harmlessness. These intentions lead to actions of body, speech, and mind that reflect our understanding and best intentions. The path is not only a way that leads to psychological freedom but is also a way of living this freedom. A graphical representation of this summary is provided in Fig. 13.1.

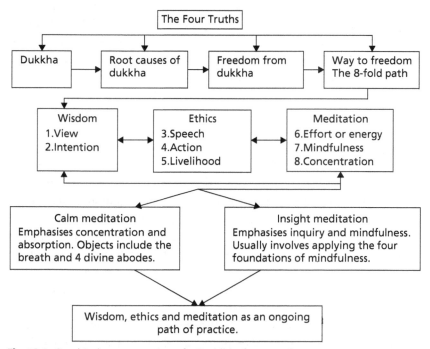

Fig. 13.1 Graphical representation of a Buddhist framework.

A brief history of mindfulness in health services

It was the work of Jon Kabat-Zinn beginning in 1979 that spurred interest in mindfulness in the contemporary psychology world. When Kabat-Zinn developed the mindfulness-based stress reduction (MBSR) (23) programme, he was strongly influenced by Buddhist practices (24). Nonetheless, he realized that in order for mindfulness as practised in MBSR to be accepted by both the public and the scientific community, it had to be presented in a contemporary scientific context and had to be detached from 'religion', which meant that it had to be distanced from Buddhism. His strategy was successful and, since the early 1980s, both lay and professional mental health interest and engagement in mindfulness have grown exponentially.

Marsha Linehan (25) was one of the first research practitioners to adapt mindfulness to the clinical setting with the development of dialectical behavior therapy (DBT). At the time DBT was developed, Linehan was a meditation practitioner and a teacher of Zen Buddhism. DBT incorporated mindfulness practices as skills to develop the ability to observe, describe, and participate in life, in a way that is effective, in the present moment and doing one thing at a time. In my view (LP), the dialectical principles that structure DBT can also be found in the middle (balanced with no extremes) path described in Buddhism. In addition, the wisdom component of the eight-fold path is reflected in the DBT concept of the wise mind, which is the balance between the rational mind and the emotional mind. DBT proved to be very helpful in reducing rates of deliberate self-harm and hospital admissions for individuals suffering with borderline personality disorder (25).

In the 1990s, Segal, Williams, and Teasdale (26) found that mindfulness-based cognitive therapy (MBCT) was effective in preventing the relapse of depression for individuals with a history of recurrent depression. Their research indicated vicious cycles between depressive affect and cognitions characteristic of depression (26). They proposed MBCT could break these vicious cycles via a distinctive way of relating to affect and thoughts, perceiving their emergence as mental events and promoting a disidentification with them. Studies have shown that for individuals with three or more depressive episodes, MBCT is as effective as pharmacotherapy in preventing recurrence of depression at a two-year follow-up (26).

Around the same time that MBCT was gaining scientific credibility, the seminal book on ACT (27) appeared on the bookshelves. Evolving separately from Buddhist traditions, ACT included mindfulness as one of its therapeutic factors. ACT has proved to be an innovative and effective treatment approach for a variety of clinical presentations (28).

A range of mindfulness-based approaches have continued to be developed in the twenty-first century and established as scientifically valid clinical strategies (29). With the advance of brain-scanning and biological-monitoring technology, research about the positive neurobiological correlations associated with meditation and mindfulness practices burgeoned. Just to mention a few discoveries, meditation and mindfulness have been correlated with positive changes in immune function (30), positive neuroplasticity, (31) and the ability to deactivate default mode networking when it is associated with depression and anxiety (32). In contrast to many positive health benefits, there is also a growing body of evidence that mindfulness training can have untoward negative side effects. It can, for example, exacerbate existing conditions as well as trigger anxiety, depression, and, in some cases, psychosis (33).

Differences between the contemporary and the traditional

In general, Buddhists have welcomed how mindfulness has become accessible to the contemporary world and had a positive impact on the reduction of human suffering. There has, nonetheless, been some discontent about the appropriation of mindfulness into contemporary psychology. Monteiro et al. (10) pointed out some of the differences between the contemporary and traditional approaches to mindfulness, and highlighted a few concerns expressed among Buddhist communities. These concerns included the following:

1. The practice of mindfulness has been de-contextualized from the eightfold path.
2. The scientific reductionist approach to defining mindfulness may have removed essential elements of what Buddhists call 'right mindfulness'.
3. Mindfulness as taught in contemporary settings is often devoid of any explicit reference to ethics.

Some of these concerns may be beginning to be addressed in the emergence of mindful compassion approaches, as demonstrated by compassion focused-therapy (20), breathworks, mindfulness, and compassion (34) and mindful self-compassion (35). These approaches emphasize compassionate motivation as equally important as mindfulness in the therapeutic endeavour. Compassionate motivations and actions are, in our view, cognate with ethics, and thus these later developments could be indications of a recognition that mindfulness is not just an isolated skill but an integral part of a system that includes wisdom, ethics, and meditation. The later mindful compassion approaches make explicit reference to the role of Buddhist psychology in their theories and practices (17).

Ven. Anālayo (36), in a paper comparing the Buddha's four foundations of mindfulness with contemporary mindfulness-based interventions (MBIs), acknowledges overlap with some practices such as mindfulness for pain and eating. However, he also highlights how the attitudes and rationales for mindfulness practice, in general, vary greatly. With Buddhist practice, the aim is clearly for the realization of complete psychological freedom. This entails practices that incline towards detachment from sensual pleasures and the reduction of what Buddhists see as the root causes of psychological suffering: greed, ignorance, and hatred. On the other hand, some practices with MBIs may incline to 'savouring' experience and increasing sensual desires rather than decreasing them. These differences point to how many of the theoretical frameworks that support mindfulness in contemporary psychology are different from the Buddhist approach.

Ven. Sujato, an Australian-born Buddhist monk, writes about the importance in meditation of theory and practice informing each other, and warns that: 'Theory without practice becomes a mere intellectual mind game; while practice without theory tends to drift without direction, or rather, directed by the personal delusions of the individual' (37).

Balancing theory with practice is also important in clinical psychology. Our theoretical frameworks provide the flexibility to adapt and fine-tune interventions to specific presentations. They enable a clinician to decide what to do in cases that lie outside what is catered for within a particular protocol, such as a manual. In addition, when things go wrong, such as when individuals experience negative side effects of a therapeutic strategy, frameworks help us find solutions and utilize effective alternatives. The foundation for the development of theoretical frameworks in contemporary psychology is the scientific method. This involves developing and testing hypotheses with empirical observation, quantification and measurement, objective inquiry, repeatability, and the capacity to share results for verification.

When Kabat-Zinn developed MBSR (23), he was light on theory and emphasized practice. In contrast, the approaches that emerged after MBSR created coherent, empirically supported frameworks to support their general technics and specific interventions. ACT, as one example, is based on relational frame theory (27). Like the Buddhist approach, ACT also utilizes mindfulness (contact with the present moment) as one factor within a context of other factors that are equally important.

There has been some discussion about the common ground between ACT and Buddhism (38). For example, both ACT and Buddhism are based on contextual frameworks. In our view, however, there are some significant differences. Buddhism elaborates and emphasizes the importance of focused attention or concentration, whereas with ACT the importance of meditative concentration seems not to be mentioned. In respect to ethics, clarifying valued directions are important in both ACT and Buddhism. However, the ACT framework does not distinguish between ethical and unethical values. In general, ACT therapists include compassion as a core principle in the ACT approach (38). However, this is not yet established as a guiding principle. When principles are only implied, it is easy to deviate from their gist.

According to Tirch et al. (38), Steven Hayes points out that ACT utilizes scientific methodologies to advance empirical knowledge and practical strategies while Buddhism does not. The sciences, including psychology and psychiatry, value objective quantifiable data that are third person and can be measured and compared. Buddhism, on the other hand, values subjective first-person experiences that may not be quantifiable and are therefore difficult to measure and objectively compare (11).

Reflections

Buddhism and the Buddhist approach to mindfulness, inclusive of its contextual connection to the four truths and the eight-fold path, add to the richness and range of clinical opportunities already available with mindfulness in mental health services. When a theoretical framework that supports mindfulness includes wisdom, it enables frank and curious exploration around this universally accepted value. When we have clarity about how wisdom includes understanding and wise intentions, this provides a rationale and the motivation to act in ways that are beneficial for self and other. Similarly, when the ethical nature of an individual's behaviours is considered as important on the path of psychological balance and healing, ethical actions can become the foundations of well-being and meaningful living. When we understand the balancing dynamics of calm and insight, it is possible to prescribe specific meditation practices for specific presentations and adjust the approach to what is needed. Furthermore, when intentions of goodwill and the cultivation of loving-kindness, compassion, appreciative joy, and equanimity are considered as essential aspects of human connection and therapy, it then opens the door to a large array of practices and strategies to help to sooth, support, and heal. Finally, when an approach to mindfulness has a framework that includes how the realization of suffering is also paradoxically linked to the realization of freedom, we may be more able to meet inevitably difficult experiences with acceptance, confidence, and skilfulness.

In summary, Buddhist mindfulness and the ancient theoretical framework of the Buddha's path have much to contribute to the advance and benefit of mental health care in Western cultures.

References

1. **de Silva P.** Buddhism and behaviour modification. *Behavioral Research and Therapy.* 1984;**22**:661–78.

2. **Bodhi B.** *The noble eightfold path: way to the end of suffering.* Onalaska, WA: BPS Pariyatti Editions; 2000.

3. **Huxter M.** Mindfulness and the Buddha's Noble Eight-Fold Path. In: *Buddhist Foundations of Mindfulness*, Mindfulness in Behavioral Health Series. Heidelberg: Springer International Publishing; 2015.

4. **Huxter M.** *Healing the heart and mind with mindfulness: ancient path, present moment.* Oxon, UK: Routledge; 2016.

5. **Huxter M.** Mindfulness as therapy from a Buddhist perspective. In: *Innovations and advances in cognitive behaviour therapy.* Bowen Hills, Qld: Australian Academic Press; 2007. p. 43–56.

6. **Bodhi B.** *In the Buddha's words: an anthology of discourses from the Pali Canon.* Boston, MA: Wisdom Publications; 2005.

7. **American Psychiatric Association (APA).** *Diagnostic and statistical manual of mental disorders.* Fifth edition. Washington, DC: APA; 2013.

8. **Andrews G, Creamer M, Crino R, Hunt C, Lampe L, Page A.** *The treatment of anxiety disorders: clinician guides and patient manuals.* Cambridge, UK: Cambridge University Press; 1995.

9. **Forsyth JP, Eifert GH.** *The mindfulness and acceptance workbook for anxiety: a guide to breaking free from anxiety, phobias, and worry using acceptance and commitment therapy.* Oakland, CA: New Harbinger Publications; 2008.

10. **Monteiro L, Musten F, Compson J.** Traditional and contemporary mindfulness: finding the middle path in the tangle of concerns. *Mindfulness.* 1 Feb 2014;**6**:1–13.

11. **Huxter M.** Buddhist mindfulness practices in contemporary psychology: a paradox of incompatibility and harmony. *Psychotherapy in Australia.* 2012;**18**(2):26–31.

12. **Shapiro SL.** The integration of mindfulness and psychology. *Journal of Clinical Psychology.* 2009;**65**(6):555–60, p. 556.

13. **Hwang Y-S, Kearney P.** *A mindfulness intervention for children with autism spectrum disorders: new directions in research and practice.* Heidelberg: Springer International Publishing; 2015.

14. **Wallace BA, Hodel B.** *Embracing mind: the common ground of science and spirituality.* Boston, MA: Shambhala; 2008.

15. **Pandita SU.** *In this very life: the liberation teachings of the Buddha.* Boston: Wisdom Publications; 1992.

16. **Shapiro F.** *Eye movement desensitization and reprocessing: basic principles, protocols, and procedures.* New York: Guilford Press; 2001.

17. **Gilbert P, Choden.** *Mindful compassion: using the power of mindfulness and compassion to transform our lives.* London: Constable & Robinson; 2013.

18. **Gilbert P.** *The compassionate mind: a new approach to life's challenges.* oakland, ca: New Harbinger Publications; 2010.

19. **Hanson R.** *Hardwiring happiness: the practical science of reshaping your brain and your life.* London: Rider; 2013.

20. **Gilbert P.** *Compassion focused therapy: distinctive features.* Hove, East Sussex: Routledge; 2010.

21. **Ekman P.** *Emotions revealed: recognizing faces and feelings to improve communication and emotional life.* New York: Times Books; 2003.

22. **Rogers C.** *On becoming a person: a therapist's view of psychotherapy.* Second edition. New York: Mariner Books; 1995.

23. **Kabat-Zinn J.** *Full catastrophe living: using the wisdom of your body and mind to face stress, pain, and illness.* New York: Guilford Press; 1990.

24. **Kabat-Zinn J.** Some reflections on the origins of MBSR, skillful means, and the trouble with maps. *Contemporary Buddhism.* 1May 2011;**12**(1):281–306.

25. **Linehan M.** *Cognitive-behavioral treatment of borderline personality Disorder.* New York: Guilford Press; 1993.

26. **Segal ZV, Williams JMG, Teasdale JD.** *Mindfulness-based cognitive therapy for depression: a new approach to preventing relapse.* New York: Guilford Press; 2002.

27. **Hayes SC, Strosahl KD, Wilson KG.** *Acceptance and commitment therapy: an experiential approach to behavior change.* New York: Guilford Press; 1999.

28. **Hayes SC, Follette VM, Linehan MM.** *Mindfulness and acceptance: expanding the cognitive-behavioral tradition.* New York: Guilford Press; 2011.

29. **Didonna F.** (ed.). *Clinical handbook of mindfulness.* New York: Springer-Verlag; 2009.

30. **Davidson RJ, Kabat-Zinn J, Schumacher J, Rosenkranz M, Muller D, Santorelli SF,** et al. Alterations in brain and immune function produced by mindfulness meditation. *Psychosomatic Medicine.* 2003 Aug;**65**(4):564–70.

31. **Treadway MT, Lazar SW.** The neurobiology of mindfulness. In: **Didonna F** (ed.), *Clinical handbook of mindfulness.* New York: Springer; 2009, pp. 45–57.

32. **Brewer JA, Worhunsky PD, Gray JR, Tang Y-Y, Weber J, Kober H.** Meditation experience is associated with differences in default mode network activity and connectivity. *Proceedings of the National Academy of Sciences of the USA.* 13 Dec 2011;**108**(50):20254–9.

33. **Farias M, Wikholm C.** *The Buddha pill: can meditation change you?* London: Watkins Publishing; 2015.

34. **Cusens B, Duggan GB, Thorne K, Burch V.** Evaluation of the breathworks mindfulness-based pain management programme: effects on well-being and multiple measures of mindfulness. *Clinical Psychology & Psychotherapy.* Feb 2010;**17**(1):63–78.

35. **Germer CK, Neff KD.** Self-compassion in clinical practice. *Journal of Clinical Psychology.* 2013 Aug;**69**(8):856–67.

36. **Anālayo B.** Mindfulness-based interventions and the four satipaṭṭhānas. *Mindfulness.* 1 Apr 2019;**10**(4):611–5.

37. **Sujato B.** *A history of mindfulness.* Taiwan: The Corporate Body of the Buddha Education Foundation; 2005. Available from: http://santifm.org/santipada/wp-content/uploads/2012/08/A_History_of_Mindfulness_Bhikkhu_Sujato.pdf

38. **Tirch D, Schoendorff B, Silberstein LR, Gilbert P, Hayes SC.** *The ACT practitioner's guide to the science of compassion: tools for fostering psychological flexibility.* Oakland, CA: New Harbinger Publications; 2014.

Chapter 14

Judaism

Haim Belmaker, Rael Strous, and
Pesach Lichtenberg

History

The Jewish religion originated in the land of Israel in the period beginning 1000
BCE but did not reach a systematized theology and practice in writing until the
early period of the modern era 100–200 CE. In the period around 1000 BCE,
the biblical narrative relates that the Hebrew people had arrived after a long
period of slavery in Egypt and made their way into the land of Canaan after a
period of 40 years of wandering in the desert (1, 2). To modern scholars, the
Hebrew religion developed in the land of Israel in the period of 1000–500 BCE
as an indigenous development from the cultures that had existed there previously (3). Indeed, considerable evidence suggests that Hebrew is closely related,
if not identical to, the languages of Moab, Ammon, Edom, and Phoenician,
the neighbouring peoples. None of them in the many existing written or cultic
archeological relics show any evidence of having believed in one god, monotheism. Each people had its own local deity whom it worshipped and whom it
expected would provide for its prosperity, victory in wars, and rain in the appropriate agricultural seasons. The Hebrew God was known as 'YHWH', sometimes pronounced as Yahweh and sometimes as Jehovah. The earliest biblical
text suggests that he was seen as a local god of the Hebrew people who could
become angry if his citizens were not loyal, could reward his citizens on some
occasions with victory in battle, and could often perform arbitrary acts that
some may state would not meet our modern standards of justice, such as calling
for the destruction of the Amalekites or the sacrifice of Abraham's son as a ges-
ture of obedience. The concept of Yahweh as one God, and the only God whose
providence extended worldwide, seems to have been developed after about 750
BCE by the prophets of the two Hebrew-speaking kingdoms, Israel in the north
and Judah in the south, and whose writings from this period until 500 BCE are
preserved in the books of Isaiah, Jeremiah, and other prophetic books of the
Hebrew Bible (4, 5).

This period of about 750–500 BCE, when religious writings were assembled and sanctified, is generally parallel to the chronology of the development of the sacred writings of Buddhism and Hinduism in India, Confucianism in China, and Zoroastrianism in Persia (1). There is no evidence of cross-influence between the religious developments in the early Middle East and religious developments in the Indus Valley or the Yellow River Valley. These religious developments seem to have been independent, although approximately simultaneous. Their body of religious thought constitutes the basis for much religious thought around the world today. This seminal period of religious and philosophical foment has been referred to as the 'Axial Age' by the psychiatrist and philosopher Karl Jaspers (quoted in (6)). Of course, around the same period, philosophy was extensively developed in Greece but did not become attached to a series of rules and rituals for daily life that constituted a religion in the same sense. Social laws existed long before this time, are evident in codes such as the laws of Hammurabi in Mesopotamia, and included clear moral injunctions to aid the orphan and widow, to be just in commerce, to avoid murder and thievery, etc. However, in Mesopotamia, these rules were not ascribed to the will of the multiple deities who were less involved in a moral sense in the lives of mortals (3, 4).

The early prophetic religion that developed in Israel 750–500 BCE ascribed the power of the moral code to the will of the deity with the role of the Bible being central to Jewish belief and practice. While orthodox Jews believe that all five books of the Torah (Pentateuch) are written by God and are therefore immutable, many in the reform and conservative sects of Judaism believe that some or all of these five books of the Torah were written by man. This has had profound consequences, leading to different levels of religious practice among the various streams of Judaism. Therefore, if the Torah is divine, then the same God that instructs the individual to refrain from murder or stealing, told the individual as well to refrain from eating milk and meat together, keeping the Sabbath as well as respecting his parents. The majority of Jews today are completely secular and view the Bible text more like old family stories than received truth (7). Most modern scholars (3, 4) consider the earliest written version of the Bible to be the book of Deuteronomy which, according to this theory, was apparently written by the temple priests and presented to King Josiah in 622 BCE. The Deuteronomic group of authors may also have authored the books of Joshua, Judges, Samuel, and Kings, and some of the other writings that were later codified as the Hebrew Bible according to this approach. The Deuteronomic authors had a harsh sense of justice and saw God's will in all of history. Therefore, if a people were exiled, if a drought occurred, if earthquakes caused mass devastation, all of these were the will of the omnipotent deity (Yahweh) and a punishment for misdeeds. These misdeeds could be social misdeeds, such as lack of welfare for the orphan and widow, or stealing from the poor; but more often these misdeeds were worship of deities other than God and particularly worship of any sculpture or idol of a deity (3, 4). Archeological evidence from this period shows that many homes in the Hebrew-speaking kingdoms of Israel in the north and Judah in the south had small idols to multiple gods including the Canaanite gods of Baal or Ashteret and others (2). Thus, the official religion of Yahweh worship was not universally accepted or observed. It was therefore not difficult for the theologians of the Yahweh school of the time to justify the fall of the northern kingdom of Israel, its total destruction in 722 BCE by the Assyrians, and subsequent exile; or the fall of Jerusalem and the kingdom of Judea in 586 BCE and the exile of its people to Babylonia. The YHWH theologians explained the disasters as punishment by God for worship of other gods and idols. Archeological evidence of the Hebrew-speaking exiles in Babylonia has been found, as well as archeological and other evidence of their return to Israel in about 500 BCE when the more liberal Persian empire conquered Babylon and allowed the Jews to return and construct the Second Temple. In Babylonia, these Judean exiles had faced the task of adapting their religion outside the land of Israel, outside their usual agricultural livelihood and without the temple sacrifices, which constituted the major organized focus of worship during the First Temple (5) and resumed its centrality in the Second Temple, after 500 BCE and until its destruction in 70 CE. Animal sacrifice ended in 70 CE but its memory is preserved in the daily prayers of Jewish people to this day (5).

In the Babylonian exile, much of the Jewish biblical scripture was codified and organized. Evidence for this includes the use of Persian words and concepts in those biblical books. The Jewish religion became a universalist one in the sense that God was seen as being all-powerful and exclusive. However, it remained a religion of a specific people in the sense that only the Jews maintained a particular relationship with God as his chosen people (3–5).

After the return from Babylon in 500 BCE, the Judean state existed as a province within the Persian empire and later the Hellenistic empire after Alexander the Great conquered Judea and Jerusalem in 333 BCE. Hellenistic influences affected Jewish culture, as can be seen in numerous Greek words and concepts in the later books of the Hebrew Bible. Tension existed between the Greek Hellenistic culture and the Hebrew culture. Judaism, as it developed during this Second Temple period, developed a powerful emphasis on following the detailed rules that Jews felt originated in divine order in the ancient scriptures.

These rules included universal social rules against murder, theft, adultery, as well as specific rules such as the prohibition of leavened bread during the spring festival of Passover; the commandment to build and live in small temporary structures (*sukot*) during the fall harvest festival; the prohibition against eating pig meat; or the commandment to put a small parchment with biblical verse on the entrance to the door of every home. Many commentators have noted that the Jewish religious concepts seem to give equal weight to commandments such as thievery and pork eating, which all derive in Judaism from the same biblical laws. During the late Second Temple time, the concept of punishments from God via destruction or drought in this life was modified to include belief in an afterlife where God would reward or punish those who had kept or broken his commandments. This theological advance was of course much more concurrent with the reality that is clear to most observers of human life to the effect that good people often have difficult lives and vice versa. However, not all the Jewish groups in the Second Temple period accepted these changes in the same way. Historical sources, such as Josephus (8), describe a political religious party called the 'Sadducees', which emphasized a religion based on the temple sacrifices and the early biblical religion, ignoring any concept of the afterlife, and focusing on the pure and an exclusive and uninterpreted literal meaning of the written law arising from the five books of Moses (the Pentateuch or Torah). The Pharisees, on the other hand, while accepting the temple sacrifices, emphasized personal piety in the home, study in learned academies called 'yeshivas' by the masses of the people, and the acceptance of new rabbinical explanations that was open to interpretation and discussion of the biblical law. There was a third group whose detailed writings and remains we may have found at Qumran: these are called the 'Dead Sea Scrolls' and are also discussed in contemporary historical documents such as Josephus (8) that emphasized aestheticism, celibacy, and belief in an imminent messianic advent. This group's ideas reflect partly the ferment in Judea and Jerusalem after the Roman Empire took over the Hellenistic empire and began to enforce restrictive legislation on Jewish culture and autonomy. The Jewish groups had conflicting ideologies but were a fertile ground for the development of new religions such as Christianity, which developed at that time and accepted the Hebrew Bible as its Old Testament and the sayings, parables, and prophesies of a particular Jewish rabbi named Jesus as its New Testament. Semitic peoples in Arabia had always had contact with the Hebrew Semites of the land of Israel and the religious leader Mohammed in the seventh century CE clearly from his writings had much contact with Jews in the Arabian Peninsula. His teachings and prophecies, transmitted in the Koran, which forms the basis of the new religion Islam, included many stories from the Hebrew Bible as well the concept of one God.

Judaism over the past 2000 years has been shaped by three factors: 1) The destruction of Jewish independence and the Second Temple by Roman forces in 70 CE in a bloody crushing of the Jewish revolt; 2) the rejection of Judaism by the two daughter religions, Christianity and Islam, which persecuted Judaism both in Christian Europe and in Muslim North Africa and the Middle East; and 3) the persistence of the Jewish refugees from the land of Israel as a religious minority spread throughout Europe, Muslim North Africa, and the Middle East without political independence but with incredible devotion to their religious texts, both the Hebrew Bible and the commentaries on it that form the Talmud, and the consequent obedience to the numerous religious laws described in those commentaries. Jews continued throughout a 2000-year exile to speak Hebrew not as a daily language but as an international communication with other Jews and in the study of the Bible; to observe the biblical rules and customs as interpreted by the rabbis in the Second Temple period (and after); and to hope for return to their ancient homeland at the first available opportunity.

The relationship of Judaism to psychiatric illness and to the psychology of the human soul has of course varied over the three millennia of Judaism's development and change. The biblical emphasis on punishment, destruction, and catastrophe is painful to the modern ear but may have been a reflection of the day-to-day life of peoples in the ancient Middle East, and perhaps the prophesies of hope for the future were more unique to their religious understanding. The role of literacy and studying the biblical texts that became a requirement for Judaism in the Second Temple period has had a tremendous effect on Jewish personality and the attitude of Jews toward learning, up and to including the modern era. Jews today are split strongly between those who accept the ancient system of rabbinic rules called the 'Halacha' and those who do not. Most do not. What is important to note is that, although theology and belief in a deity is one of the core principles of faith and thus of the religion, Judaism per se is actually a religion based more on 'doing' than 'believing'. Thus it is less critical what one believes that what one does—both in terms of action between man and God and between man and man.

While there is no evidence that there is a higher incidence of obsessive compulsive disorder (OCD) among those who do accept the elaborate system of rules and regulations, from personal observation it appears that when OCD is present, the intensity and expression of OCD may be more profound). The messianic ideals and beliefs of a future period of peace and glory that is not mentioned in the Bible, but has become a central core of Jewish belief since Second Temple times, can often be involved in manic states in bipolar disorder in Jewish people. Both these matters will be discussed below.

Cultural sensitivity and mental illness in the Jewish community

In recent years, the importance of cultural sensitivity and the adjustment of mental health services to the diversity of religious and ethnic populations has been increasing. Cultural competence describes the ability of services to meet the cultural, social, and linguistic needs of people from different cultures and religions. What at times complicates and makes the process interesting is the variety of religious practice within religions and various ethnicities. The introduction of The Diagnostic and Statistical Manual of Mental Disorders-5 emphasizes the importance of understanding the culture of the patient when determining the diagnosis (9). Within Judaism, there are several varied expressions of formal religion ranging in levels of commitment and practice to Jewish ritual and religious behaviour. The principal major divisions of these denominations within Judaism range from the least vigorous ritual behaviour laden 'Reform', to the 'Conservative', 'Modern Orthodox', and 'Ultra-Orthodox' (haredi) expressions of Judaism. In general, orthodox Jews may be differentiated from non-orthodox Jews in their level of stringent adherence to religious law (Halacha) based on the literacy of their belief that the Torah is divine (the 'word of God') and thus one cannot choose what to practise or not—it is a 'package deal'.

Arguably, the largest growing and, at the same time most insular of these subgroups, is that of the haredi Jewish camp. Though this group emerged as a nineteenth-century reaction to the encroachments of modern European society, they see themselves as the principal expression of 'authentic Judaism'. While they often confine themselves to their own detached communities, thus protecting themselves from outside 'negative' influences, complete detachment from majority culture can never be attained. Changes may be noted as well in the awareness of mental health, psychiatric illnesses, and the importance of psychiatric care, which is increasing among the haredi population around the world. Frameworks and services tailored and adapted to the haredi sector are developing in both the treatment and the rehabilitation systems. These include, most notably, attention to sexual abuse, eating disorders, and trauma. Therapists in these settings, as well as therapists in other systems that service the haredi sector, meet and discuss issues related to the connection between psychiatry and the religious and spiritual world, and define the unique needs and characteristics of care in this area. It is incumbent upon the therapist who works and treats patients in this population to understand the world of the haredi patient, including his outlook on the concept of mental illness, in order to promote the sensitivity of cultural competence by mental health caregivers with these patients.

Jews and mental health

While specific issues of mental illness may be noted in various subcategories of religious and cultural Jewish observance among Jews, various generalities have been described indicating associations between religious practice and mental health in Jews. For example, Rosmarin et al., (10) have noted less anxiety and depression in those with higher levels of faith in God. In addition, in another study by members of their team (10), it has been found that 'positive strategies' of religious coping can be correlated with improved mental health consequences in those faced with stressors or crises in their lives. Thus, while religious coping in general is common among Jews and often a positive bearing on the Jewish individual (10), at times this may have a negative effect. As described by Rosmarin et al. (10), 'spiritual struggles' as defined by emotionally inappropriate beliefs and approaches based on religious grounds, can lead at times to poorer physical and mental health for Jews. However, among Orthodox Jews, it appears that spiritual struggles lead to better mental (and physical) outcomes—possibly related to resilience or growth in the face of adversity as a result of strong religious faith (10).

With regard to Jewish religious ritual, it has been shown that such daily observance of Jewish commandments of biblical and rabbinic origin is associated with less anxiety and depression (10, 11). It may be suggested that an important aspect of this manifestation is the fact that prayer, which may mitigate anxiety (12), constitutes such an important part of daily practice of religious observant Jews, having to pray three times a day, most ideally in the context of at least a 10-man quorum in a synagogue or other improvised prayer venue (reviewed in (13)). In addition, Korbman et al. (13) in a review of the subject, have described how trust and mistrust in God, as one of the core fundamental foundations of Judaism, are associated with anxiety and depression among Jews. More specifically, they indicate how trust in God leads to less anxiety and depression with mistrust associated with more depression (14, 15). They also discuss the benefits of gratitude, how gratitude features prominently in Jewish values and ritual practice, and how gratitude in turn is associated with more robust mental health in individuals, especially when faced with adversity. These mechanisms of coping among Jews and their association with better mental health outcomes may be noted in the specific scale, termed the 'JCOPE', which was established by Rosmarin et al. (10) and which shows, for example, the critical role of positive or negative religious coping in Jews and its relationship to depression. This religious coping occurs not only at the level of the individual but, based on the central and pivotal role that the Jewish community as a whole plays in the life of the religiously affiliated Jew, the individual can rely on the community for support and assistance. This also appears to mitigate the presence or expression of mental illness among Jews.

Psychiatry and the religious Jew

In many patients with mental ill health diagnoses or problems, religion and faith help patients find meaning in their illness and in coping with the difficulties they must face. Among the subpopulation who are stringent in their Jewish religious faith, most indicate that religion and faith give hope, purpose, and meaning to their lives and illness. Furthermore, in the recovery process, religion influences their adaptation within society. However, the downside of this practice may be noted in a subset of religious observant individuals who may exhibit increased distress and anxiety (10) as a result of strict standards that they may apply to themselves, and which may become overwhelming in various contexts when demands for scrupulosity are higher, such as around Jewish festivals (Passover most notably) and nuances of Jewish ritual.

With regards to extreme stress and depressive states, religion can also be very significant in a person's choice of suicide: in most who are strong believers, strict faith lowers the chance of suicide (prohibition and fear of punishment). However, in rare cases, stringent religion in the ultra-orthodox may increase the risk of suicide with the hope of reaching heaven and being close to God (16). The positive effect of religion on reducing addictions should also be considered. In Orthodox Jewish practice, it is considered sinful to damage one's own body in any way (including the practice of tattooing). Thus, religion mitigates the risk of addictions. Unfortunately, few ultra-orthodox patients share their beliefs about religion with their therapist and doctor in treatment. This is due to the large element of distrust that exists if the patients feel that their mental health caregiver does not, or cannot, understand their world of ultra-orthodox Jewish religious practice (18, 19). Thus, any disparity of faith and religious affiliation between patients and caregivers may become a stumbling block in communication between the two. Since, in the United States for example, studies have indicated that psychiatrists are less religious than other physicians, and definitely less religious than the general population (18), a significant gap may arise in patient and caregivers' world views, and psychiatrists do not always refer to religion in the patient's world. The second reason orthodox and ultra-orthodox Jewish patients do not trust their secular or modern-orthodox style mental health caregiver is more historical. Several psychological theories have referred to religion as primitive, and to miracles and supernatural experiences as a cause of mental health disorders. In the field of science and medicine, research advances have helped to find biological and psychosocial explanations for many psychiatric disorders. Thus, a disparity exists in weltanschauung between the world views. Overall, observations and studies point to the importance of considering beliefs and religions in treatment, and especially in rehabilitation of religious patients suffering from psychiatric disorders (19). This is not only ethical and professional, but also improves and encourages accessibility and collaboration in clinical care.

Psychiatry in a haredi (ultra-Orthodox) population

More recently, within the Jewish population in Israel and in the Jewish diaspora, there has been a significant demographic increase in the haredi sector. According to forecasts, the proportion of the ultra-Orthodox population in Israel, for example, is expected to increase from 11% in 2015 to 20% in 2040 and 32% in 2065 (20). Therefore, special issues need to be addressed in the religious orthodox and haredi worlds. Religious haredi and the professional raise many issues related to the patient's religion and socio-cultural affinity. Being familiar with concepts of Jewish religion and developing cultural sensitivity to these issues, which are of utmost importance to individuals in this community, can promote treatment compliance offered to haredi individuals.

1. Religious literature—discussions in Jewish law and religious sources regarding patient and mental health

    Beyond religious belief, Jewish religion is present in deeds, behaviour, thoughts, and throughout life. Therefore, many references to human psychology can be found in Judaic and Sages' writings, and reference to a variety of complex mental health and treatment situations. The Talmud and Halachic literature refer to some patients with psychiatric disorders with the concept of 'shoteh'. In the Babylonian Talmud, Tractate Chagigah (page 3B), a shoteh, most closely described in modern-day terminology as the psychotic individual, is not defined by his speech or his thoughts, but by his behaviour: 'who goes out at night alone', 'who sleeps in the cemetery', 'who rips his clothes', and also 'who loses everything they give him'. The Talmud adds that the shoteh is behaving in this manner in an illogical, disorganized way. The Talmud is aware that the severity and progression of the disease can vary between people (21). It should be noted that the term 'shoteh' is not a medical or psychiatric concept but a legal one. The Talmud also refers to 'shoteh' in order to circumscribe his capabilities and responsibilities. The complexity of this view is the paradox created in which, on the one hand, there is compassion for the patient who is expressed as being exempt from religious and civil responsibility, and on the other hand defines responsibilities of the community, including the court to protect the shoteh while simultaneously safeguarding society when necessary (22).

A. Psychiatric patient and observance: Halachic rulers addressed questions related to the 'shoteh' status of mental health. A 'shoteh' who goes through periods of psychotic state and periods of remission must maintain religious obligations during remission; however, he is exempt when in a psychotic state.

B. Forced treatment: The Bible actually may refer to forced incarceration of people appearing insane: 'for every man that is mad, and maketh himself a prophet, that thou shouldest put him in the stocks and in the collar' (Jeremiah 29:26; Jewish Publication Society translation). The Talmud in Tractate Baba Kama (p. 20) states that locking a person inside a room causes harm and should be compensated. According to this, coercion in psychiatric treatment is allowed only in a situation where there is a potential danger to humanity. However, when there is no danger to life, every person has the right to decide for themselves whether they want treatment or not, even in a psychotic state. These concepts are not intended to influence the therapist's decision to the extent that the law requires a framework of forced treatment, but it is important to understand how the religious Jewish world addresses these issues.

C. Pregnancy and psychiatry: when continued pregnancy presents a clear danger to the mother, such as a serious exacerbation of a psychotic condition, including suicidal behaviour or violent outbreak, rabbis can authorize abortion, like other life-threatening medical conditions. On the subject of contraception, most rabbis permit the practice when a further pregnancy would be presumed to cause a psychotic crisis and pose a significant health risk to a woman (23).

D. Approach to Sabbath observance: the question of life-saving religious law exemptions for the Sabbath (permitting to desecrate certain laws of the Torah for the sake of saving human life) on the Sabbath is also relevant in the field of mental health—both for the physician and the community. For example, in schizophrenia, the prevalence of suicidal behaviour throughout life is about 10% and, in an acute psychotic state, the likelihood of self-harm or other violence is even more common. The doctor should treat the 'shoteh' on a Sabbath as well, because in a psychotic state he is considered 'a patient in danger'. Mental disorder is no less dangerous than a physical illness in terms of life-threatening risk and the life of those with psychiatric disorders must also be saved.

E. Privacy: there is a well-known rule of Jewish law among the Orthodox Jewish population that stipulates that a man and woman who are not married are not allowed to be alone together in a closed place. This obviously has repercussions for the Orthodox therapist and patient—from either side. However, for the purposes of psychotherapy and psychiatric treatment, the Halacha (Jewish law) would state for the orthodox individual that no third person in the room is required if certain rules are followed, such as making sure that other people are in the clinic and can enter. It should be noted that, on this subject, there is a parallel in the secular world that one may request the presence of another person during a medical examination. However, medical institutions with expertise in gender, employ men who treat women and women who treat men in a way that is based on understanding and sensitivity to the issue.

2. Expressions of unique psychiatric disorder manifestations in the haredi patient

Culture influences the expression of psychiatric disorders (24). This is no less important in orthodox Jewish religious circles wherein the mental health caregiver needs to be aware and informed of the different groups in the range of religious expression in order to differentiate between normative thoughts, behaviour, and speech or psychopathology in these areas. In this context, it would be important for the mental health caregiver to ascertain the importance of belief and religious practice in the individual's life and how this affects their mental health status.

A. Psychosis: in the ultra-Orthodox sector, content of psychosis can be different. Several specific themes are often evident. These include thoughts related to the Messiah, special connection with a deceased religious leader, or persecutory thoughts that include prophets or angels. The importance and centrality of the community in the ultra-Orthodox population, and especially in Hasidic communities, can also influence psychotic content. Persecutory thoughts about 'publishing about me in a community newspaper', 'talking about me in the synagogue', etc. are common. Since the question of 'piety or pathology' may be unclear, often looking at general function outside the thoughts and salience of the ideological preoccupation may assist in the differentiation between pathology and extreme religious but non-psychotic behaviour.

B. Obsessive compulsive disorder (OCD): there has been a perception in the past that the prevalence of bothersome obsessive thoughts and compulsive behaviour is higher among the religious population. However, several studies have shown that the prevalence of OCD is relatively stable across different cultures (25). Nevertheless, what appears to be clear is that the expression of the illness may be enhanced and more severe as a result of strict Halacha (religious Jewish law), which encourages more intense and pious practice of religious practice and ritual. In the ultra-Orthodox sector, overly strict observance of laws, becoming obsessive and compulsive in nature, with respect to ritual purity, 'clean thoughts' and prayer (26) are often clearly manifest. This would be in cases where scrupulosity is clearly extreme and affects function in various areas including social, occupational, ritual practice, and emotional stability. Examples include hand washing beyond the halachic requirements, excessive number of immersions in the mikvah (ritual bath), repeating the same prayer many times until the correct intention is achieved, time spent in the bathroom and shower, etc. (27). This is most usually over and above the halachic requirement according to rabbinic opinions. What assists in the evaluation or monitoring of any perceived unusual behaviour is understanding whether the behaviour is according to the norms of the particular religious sect, whether such considered obsessive behaviour results in impaired functioning in other areas, whether the behaviour bothers the individual, and whether it leads to significant discomfort or even suffering on the part of the patient ('ego dystonic') (28). Thus, while cooperation and consultation with a competent rabbinic authority when questions of religious practice affect mental health are always important, when it comes to the assessment and management of OCD, it is particularly critical.

C. Eating disorders: There are indications of an increase in the prevalence of eating disorders in Jewish women in general, and in orthodox and haredi women and men (29). No matter how ultra-orthodox parents believe their children are protected and guarded from outside influences, opinions about thinness and striving for perfection still exist and persist even in this subpopulation. Many ultra-Orthodox families do not tend to recognize the disorder and seek help only when the girl is on the verge of hospitalization or death. This is reinforced by the fear that haredi girls who are undergoing treatment in non-orthodox mental health treatment facilities may abandon the haredi world of religious belief and practice. The hesitancy regarding recognizing the existence of an eating disorder is influenced by the stigma that exists in the haredi world regarding mental illness and the importance of thinness in order to obtain a better 'arranged marriage partner'. Some believe that haredi Jewish girls may turn to an eating disorder to gain control and perfection as they see it, and in trying to cope with various traumas. What is clear is that eating disorders are not less common in such Jewish communities (30–32). The community has become aware that eating disorders are a serious problem that can pose a risk of death, and that the most effective treatment will come from people with cultural sensitivity to this subpopulation of patients (32).

3. Issues related to the Orthodox and ultra-Orthodox society and the community to which the patient belongs

   A. Stigma, confidentiality, and access to care

   The social stigma in haredi communities toward psychiatric illness, along with the centrality of the community in human life, affects family communication with others in the community setting and their ability to share illness-related issues with people outside the immediate family (33). Exposing such information could harm the potential of family and community matchmaking for marriage (26, 34). Due to the stigma of mental illness and the potential for affecting marriage matchmaking for the individual involved as well as for direct family members, mental illness is often not disclosed and often remains untreated as a result. This is in order that people in the community do not hear about or see the individual in treatment institutions. Thus, the effort to keep the psychiatric illness a secret can keep the individual and family unit from getting the help they need. The issue of secrecy and privacy of mental illness is important in all cultures and communities, but in the haredi community there is great sensitivity to this issue, both because of the possible consequences of the stigma and because it is a relatively closed and connected community where many people know each other or the family. The stigma and importance of secrecy, as well as other factors that will be described later, often result in avoidance of treatment in the haredi population, or rejection of the initiation of treatment. Today, major efforts are being invested in order to educate the community about mental illness and encourage early intervention, thus providing access to psychiatric care to reduce delay in treatment delivery and improve prognosis.

   B. Addressing unprofessional factors involved in treatment

   The place of the religious leader or Rabbi in the haredi community is profound. In this community, it is commonplace for the patient to seek to consult their rabbi in making all important decisions. Thus, Rabbis who are familiar with the field of mental health can have a positive impact on the person's cooperation with evaluation and treatment. On the other hand, some may oppose treatment and result in resistance to particular treatment or hospitalization. With the consent of the patient and after signing a confidentiality waiver, it is sometimes important and necessary to have direct communication between the physician or therapist and the rabbi, all in the best interests of the patient.

C. Unique accommodations in psychiatric outpatient and rehabilitation settings

In the haredi society, there is a tendency to refrain from utilizing mental health services, partly due to the lack of trust in non-haredi professionals, as well as the perceived conflict between 'modern' and 'traditional' treatment methods, or to general opposition to the laws and the secular establishment (35). Some haredi patients reject treatment and refuse to be admitted to public hospitals because of their fear, or that of their family, that they will not be able to maintain religious observance or will lose religious identity. Thus, in order to encourage psychiatric treatment and hospitalization in this subpopulation, religious sensitivities must be addressed, and patients and their families reassured (35). These accommodations include a variety of aspects: (a) enabling active observance and participation in unique religious activities while hospitalized (for example, prayer services, Torah learning, etc.), (b) avoiding activities and exposure that violate the lifestyle of haredi people (for example, TV with open channels, open internet, structured separation between men and women, etc.).

Mental health rehabilitation and recovery have now become a major goal in psychiatric care. Rehabilitation is strongly influenced by cultural aspects. Environmental expectations, gender roles, and priorities are influenced by the community in which people live. In the haredi sector, for example, Torah study is a major preoccupation, and daily routine is full of activities and functions around religious observance and activity (tefillin, prayer, etc.). In the rehabilitative treatment process, emphasis is placed on the person's return to significant premorbid activities and pastimes, and their role in society. In view of this, religious study time should be given therapeutic significance, just as any other therapeutic or occupational therapy group in a psychiatric ward. Participation in learning for the haredi individual provides a sense of value and belonging, a connection to community and life outside the hospital, and an opportunity to practise cognitive and social skills. Paying attention to the community rehabilitation system is also of great importance to the sensitivity and adaptation of the needs of the haredi population (36).

Thus, there is a close and extensive relationship between religion and belief and mental health and psychiatry. This association is reflected in the influence of the religious and spiritual world of people with psychiatric illnesses on the manifestations and expression of their illness and their implications for functioning, as well as their coping and recovery processes (37). Accordingly, this relationship should be reflected in the adaptation of unique psychiatric care services to the *haredi* population, in order to support recovery and rehabilitation processes, and to provide appropriate psychiatric care.

Messianism and mania

While most of the behaviours accompanying individuals in manic states do not require separate consideration in this text, we do wish to devote the next section to a discussion of the messianic ideas that can be a central part of manic episodes. The term 'messiah' is a rough transliteration for the Biblical word meaning 'the anointed one', referring to the ritual of rubbing with sacred oil the heads of the king and high priest in ancient Israel. The Pentateuch does not refer to a historic figure who will redeem the world, though the prophets do make vague references to such a possibility, particularly in Isaiah. The indeterminacy of the descriptions has provided fertile ground for Jewish–Christian polemics throughout the centuries.

The messianic idea is firmly embedded in Judaism (38). Jews have thought about messiahs, and occasionally been messiahs, for at least 2000 years. While Jesus is unquestionably the most prominent in a long line of messiahs (39), countless others have tried to assume the mantel of saviour.

Psychiatric legend has it that (40), though Christians in the throes of a manic psychosis may believe that they are God, based on what many believers consider to be the precedent at the basis of their religion, the unequivocally unitarian Jew can only aspire to be the Messiah. Our clinical experience with divine Jews, as well as larger contemporary phenomena in the Jewish religious world, have blurred this dichotomy.

Messianism can have different non-mutually exclusive versions, and these can be reflected in psychopathology:

1. Messianism may be *restorative*, in the sense of restoring the rule of King David's dynasty and the ritual at the site of the destroyed Temple Mount. Some people believe themselves to be the messiah and await their coronation upon the restored Davidic throne. Past history provides many precedents, not necessarily pathological, for these beliefs. Rabbi Haim Vital (1542–1620) from Safed, a respected kabbalist in the circles of the pathbreaking mystic,

Rabbi Isaac Luria, wrote a riveting autobiography, *The Book of Visions* (Sefer haHizayon), where the author brings multiple demonstrations of his messianic identity, which seemed to have little effect upon his outward behaviour. A contemporary psychiatrist might unfairly diagnose him with a psychotic disorder. Undoubtedly, the most interesting Jewish messiah after Jesus was Shabbetai Tzvi (1626–1676), an often troubled, intermittently charismatic figure who in 1666 briefly convinced most of the Jewish world that he was indeed the long-awaited redeemer (41). He has been retrospectively diagnosed with bipolar disorder, which would explain many of his excesses. The Ottoman ruler's demand that Tzvi convert to Islam on pain of decapitation had immediate anti-manic effects, and Tzvi outwardly left Judaism, but reverberations of his manic episodes resound to the present day.

A contemporary psychiatrist working with Jewish populations will almost inevitably meet a person believing himself (or, more rarely, herself) to be cast in a messianic role. His patient may be ecstatic about the impending redemption or driven to suicide by the weight of the responsibility; may nurture his secret in private or set out to trumpet the news everywhere; may secretly immerse himself in mystical contemplations or seek to gather an army of adherents. The patient may cooperate with the psychiatrist, or react to any enquiries with paranoid suspicion.

2. Messianism may be *apocalyptic*, a harbinger of a catastrophically upended world brought about by God's fury. The Armageddon legend, based on the prophecy appearing in the book of Daniel, is merely the best known of these scenarios. For many patients, messianism may be the delusional interpretation afforded to an inchoate fear of existential destruction. The terror animating the person is projected onto a grand stage of universal cataclysm. This individual will often prefer to be released from any messianic anticipation.

   Jewish lore tells a tale of two messiahs (Babylonian Talmud, Sukkah, 52a). The first to appear, Messiah son of Joseph, will bring news of redemption and will lead the Jewish people to war, in which the messiah will perish. His violent demise will pave the way for the coming of the final redeemer, Messiah son of David. A psychiatrist would do well to inquire whether the messiah whom he is examining is of the stock of Joseph or of David. If the response is the former, it behoves the psychiatrist to conduct a particularly detailed assessment of suicidality.

3. Messianism may also be *utopian*, wherein the laws of nature, or human nature itself, are altered, and the creation attains a state of perfection not known since Eden. A popular idea in Jewish spirituality is that people are God's partner in repairing the world's imperfections, and the Messiah is seen

as leading the way. Some who see themselves cast in this role may quietly bide their time, collecting the signs of the Messiah's arrival and awaiting the inevitable salvation of the world, but others will meet the psychiatrist in a state of euphoria or manic agitation, which can become aggressive if the psychiatrist is perceived as colluding to thwart the desired End of Days.

As always, cultural currents affect the content of psychopathological thought. Contemporary Judaism is astir with messianic ideas, promulgated by spiritual and political leaders of varying stripes. Certain Hassidic groups—such as Habad and Breslav (40)—maintain a high tension of messianic expectation among their members. These ideas disperse though the community by the usual personal and virtual channels, and seemingly secularized Jews may also access messianic ideas in times of psychotic distress or elation. Though it is difficult to compare with past eras, it is possible that these ideas are more rampant today, and the psychiatrist is likely to meet the permutations and reverberations of these fantasies.

In treating patients beset with messianic excitement, the psychiatrist will as ever be wise not to rely exclusively on psychopharmacological interventions. The patient may be expressing a personal striving for a better world, which should be respected. Acting in this way, the psychiatrist will be cementing the therapeutic alliance, empowering his or her patient, and advancing the goals of recovery.

> A 23-year-old man has been immersed in mystical literature in recent months. He begins to have visions of people's souls, and believes that he has identified the Messiah. He goes to the Western Wall of the destroyed Temple, Judaism's holiest site, undertakes intense prayer, and utters a sacred vow not to eat, drink, or communicate till he coerces the Messiah to appear. The next morning, he is brought into the department for a coerced hospitalization, bearing a diagnosis of catatonia. The treating psychiatrist, familiar with the tradition of sacred vows, performs a religious ritual for annulling the force of the sacred vow. The patient is sent home within several hours. Years later, he gains a degree in clinical psychology and partners with the psychiatrist in establishing alternatives to psychiatric inpatient departments (41).

A useful metaphor when treating manic or psychotic individuals with religious Jewish backgrounds is that of the Shattering of the Vessels. This is a venerable idea central to the creation myths of the Kabballah that describe how, in the drama of creation, God's light was so overwhelming that parts of creation ('vessels') meant to contain the light were shattered, dispersing the sacred light throughout the unredeemed world. This creation crisis became the source of evil, but also the basis for redemption.

A patient in the throes of a manic episode can relate to this tale. They may feel overwhelmed with energy, with a divine light. The psychiatrist can sensitively speak of this creation story, discuss the dangers of a catastrophic break, and refer to therapy, or medication, as a method for strengthening the vessels so they do not shatter.

Jerusalem syndrome

The Jerusalem syndrome refers to individuals with redemptive delusions centring upon the city of Jerusalem and featuring the imminent appearance there of the Messiah (42). Cases dating back to the fourteenth century have been reliably described (43). Like other geographically linked psychiatric syndrome (e.g. Stendhal Syndrome for visitors to the aesthetic charms of Florence and Italy, or Paris Syndrome for Japanese tourists arriving in Paris), Jerusalem Syndrome is not recognized by the standard nosological manuals, which would presumably assign to individuals showing the relevant symptoms a diagnosis within the rubric of schizophrenia spectrum and other psychotic disorders in the DSM-V (9), or a form of schizophrenia or 'acute and transient psychotic disorder', depending on duration, according to the ICD-10 (44).

According to the definition suggested above for Jerusalem Syndrome, it can appear regardless of religion, and Jerusalem psychiatrists will report many Jews drawn to local messianic fantasies. However, the cases that receive the most public attention are those of pilgrims, typically evangelical Christians, arriving in Jerusalem, who, once here, overcome by the spiritual energies of the city and inspired by the many holy sites, ascend into a religious ecstasy anticipating the imminent appearance of the Saviour, or perhaps descend into a paranoid maelstrom of fear of the anti-Christ. Possibly apocryphal lore tells of tourists previously enjoying sound mental health who lose their sanity on the via Dolorosa or at sites similarly pregnant with history and meaning, but are brought back to health by continuing on the next leg of their tour of the Eastern Mediterranean, away from the Holy Land. But while brief, isolated psychotic episodes can occur, in or out of Jerusalem, undoubtedly the vast majority of these episodes will occur for people with past backgrounds of psychosis. Indeed, the recurrence or exacerbation of a pre-existing psychosis may be what made the tourist choose the destination in the first place:

> A 35-year-old woman, with two psychiatric hospitalizations in her twenties, recently joined a Pentecostal congregation in Texas, USA. While on a trip in a Western African nation, she became anxious about devils she perceived to be pursuing her. Opening the Bible for reassurance, she chanced upon the word 'Jerusalem', and grasped that she was being summoned there to bring news of Jesus's return to save the world. She quickly flew to Israel, but within three days her strange and disruptive behaviour at the hostel in the Old City of Jerusalem caused her to be hospitalized. Her family was notified, and through the embassy she was returned to her community to continue her hospitalization.

Conclusions

The historical and textual analysis of the Bible into multiple sources, some of which are corroborated by archaeology and some of which are contradicted by archaeology, has led to a new scientific understanding of the development of Biblical Israelite religion and its gradual development into rabbinic Judaism. The psychiatrist, as a scientific physician, is therefore able to understand the Judaism of his Jewish patients, not as an absolute faith that must be accepted or rejected, but as a human phenomenon that has developed over time and has multiple functions and purposes in the lives of individual patients. These can be utilized for therapeutic purposes and handled with cultural sensitivity once understood by the psychiatric clinician. The special needs of the minority haredi, or ultra-orthodox stream within modern Judaism presents special issues and challenges that should be studied by psychiatrists who work with this patient population. The role of ritual in the Jewish tradition must be understood in order to distinguish religious rituals from OCD; similarly, the importance of messianic beliefs in Jewish history and religion should be evaluated carefully in patients with Jewish backgrounds who may have psychoses with messianic grandiosity.

Dedication

This chapter is dedicated to the memory of Helen Belmaker Barkai.

References

1. **Harari Y.** *Sapiens: A brief history of humankind.* New York: Harper; 2015.
2. **Finkelstein I, Silberman N.** *The Bible unearthed: archaeology's new vision of ancient Israel and the origin of its sacred texts.* New York: Touchstone; 2002.
3. **Hayes C.** *Introduction to the Bible.* New Haven: Yale University Press; 2012.
4. **Kugel J.** *How to read the Bible: a guide to scripture, then and now.* New York: Free Press; 2008.
5. **Schama S.** *The story of the Jews: finding the words 1000 BC—1492 AD.* New York: Ecco; 2014.
6. **Armstrong K.** *The great transformation: the beginning of our religious traditions. first.* New York: Knopf; 2006.
7. **Updike J.** *Roger's version: a novel.* New York: Random House (Kindle version); 2012.
8. **Flavius J.** *The Jewish war.* Reissued edition. London: Penguin Classics; 1984.
9. *Diagnostic and statistical manual of mental disorders.* DSM–5. Washington DC: American Psychiatric Association; 2013.
10. **Rosmarin DH, Pargament KI, Krumrei EJ, Flannelly KJ.** Religious coping among jews: development and initial validation of the JCOPE. Journal of Clinical Psychology 2009;**65**:670–83. Available from: https://doi.org/10.1002/jclp.20574

11. **Krumrei EJ, Pirutinsky S, Rosmarin DH.** Jewish spirituality, depression, and health: an empirical test of a conceptual framework. International Journal of Behavioral Medicine 2013;**20**:327–36. Available from: https://doi.org/10.1007/s12529-012-9248-z

12. **Ellison CG, Bradshaw M, Flannelly KJ, Galek KC.** Prayer, attachment to god, and symptoms of anxiety-related Disorders among U.S. Adults. Sociology of Religion: A Quarterly Review 2014;**75**:208–33. Available from: https://doi.org/10.1093/socrel/srt079

13. **Korbman M, Appel M, Rosmarin D.** Judaism and health. In: **von Dras D**, (ed.), *Better health through spiritual practices: a guide to religious behaviors and perspectives that benefit mind and body*, Santa Barbara, California: Praeger; 2017.

14. **Pirutinsky S, Rosmarin DH, Pargament K, Midlarsky E.** Does negative religious coping accompany, precede, or follow depression among orthodox jews? *Journal Of Affective Disorders*. 2011;**132**:401–4.

15. **Rosmarin DH, Pirutinsky S, Greer D, Korbman M.** Maintaining a grateful disposition in the face of distress: the role of religious coping. *Psychology of Religion and Spirituality*. 2016;**8**:134–40. https://doi.org/10.1037/rel0000021

16. **Huguelet P, Mohr S, Jung V, Gillieron C, Brandt PY, Borras L.** Effect of religion on suicide attempts in outpatients with schizophrenia or schizo-affective disorders compared with inpatients with non-psychotic disorders. *European Psychiatry*. 2007;**22**:188–94. https://doi.org/10.1016/j.eurpsy.2006.08.001.

17. **Borras L, Mohr S, Gillieron C, Brandt PY, Rieben I, Leclerc C,** et al. Religion and spirituality: how clinicians in Quebec and Geneva cope with the issue when faced with patients suffering from chronic psychosis. *Community Mental Health Journal*. 2010;**46**:77–86. https://doi.org/10.1007/s10597-009-9247-y.

18. **Curlin F, Odell S, Lawrence R, Chin M, Lantos J, Meador K,** et al. The relationship between psychiatry and religion among U.S. physicians. *Psychiatric Services*. 2007;**58**(9):1193–8.

19. **Mohr S, Pierre-Yves Brandt M, Borras L, Gilliéron C, Huguelet P.** Article toward an integration of spirituality and religiousness into the psychosocial dimension of schizophrenia. *American Journal of Psychiatry* 2006;**163**(11).

20. **Malach G, Choshen M, Cahaner L.** Statistical report on ultra-orthodox society in Israel. Center for Religion, Nation and State. 2016.

21. **Strous R.** The shoteh and psychosis in Halacha with contemporary clinical application. *Torah U'Madah*. 2004;**12**:158–78.

22. **Marx T.** *Halaka and handicap: Jewish law and ethics on disability*. 1993.

23. **Iggerot M.** Even ha-Ezer n.d.;1.

24. **Krzystanek M, Krysta K, Klasik, Aczyk I,** Krupka-Matusz. Religious content of hallucinations in paranoid schizophrenia. *Psychiatr Danub*. 2012 Suppl 1:S65–9.

25. **Huppert JD, Siev J, Kushner ES.** When religion and obsessive-compulsive disorder collide: treating scrupulosity in ultra-orthodox jews. *Journal of Clinical Psychology*. 2007;**63**:925–41. https://doi.org/10.1002/jclp.20404

26. **Vinker M, Jaworowski S, Mergui J.** Obsessive compulsive disorder (OCD) in the ultra-orthodox community--cultural aspects of diagnosis and treatment. *Harefuah*. 2014;**153**:463–6.

27. **Bonchek A, Greenberg D.** Compulsive prayer and its management. *Journal of Clinical Psychology*. 2009;**65**:396–405.

28. **Greenberg D, Witztum E.** *Sanity and sanctity: mental health work among the ultra-orthodox in Jerusalem.* New Haven: Yale University Press; 2001.

29. **Latzer Y, Stein D,** Witztum E. Treating ultra-orthodox adolescents with eating disorders in Israel: culturally-sensitive interventions, difficulties, and dilemmas. *J Clin Psychol.* 2019 Aug;75(8):1455–68.

30. **Feinson M, Meir A.** Disordered eating and cultural distinctions: exploring prevalence and predictors among women in Israel. *Israel Journal of Psychiatry and Related Sciences.* 2014;**51**:145–53.

31. **Feinson M, Meir A.** Disordered eating and religious observance: a focus on ultra-orthodox jews in an adult community study. *International Journal of Eating Disorders.* 2012;**45**:101–8.

32. **Pinhas L,** Heinmaa M;, Bryden P, **Bradley S, Toner B.** *Disordered Eating in Jewish Adolescent Girls.* 2008;**53(9):601–8.**

33. **Paradis C, Cukor D, Friedman S.** *Cognitive-behavioral therapy with orthodox Jews.* Washington DC: American Psychological Association; 2006.

34. **Greenberg D, Buchbinder J, Witztum E.** Arranged matches and mental illness. *Psychiatry.* 2012;75:342–54.

35. **Bilu Y, Witztum E.** Between sacred and medical realities: culturally sensitive therapy with jewish ultra-orthodox patients. *Science in Context.* 1995;8:159–73. https://doi.org/10.1017/S0269889700001939

36. **Greenberg D, Kalian M, Witztum E.** Value-sensitive psychiatric rehabilitation. *Transcult Psychiatry.* 2010;47:629–46.

37. **Spero MH.** *Handbook of psychotherapy and Jewish ethics: Halakhic perspectives on professional values and techniques.* New York: Feldheim; 1986.

38. **Scholem G.** *The Messianic idea in Judaism.* New York: Schocken Books.

39. **Flusser D.** *Jesus.* Jerusalem: Magnes Press and Hebrew University; 1998.

40. **Perez, L.** The messianic psychotic patient. *Israel Annals of Psychiatry and Related Disciplines.* 1980;**15**:364–74.

41. **Scholem G.** *Sabbatai Sevi: the mystical Messiah.* Princeton, NJ: Princeton University Press; 1973.

42. **Bilu Y, Mark Z.** Between Tsaddiq and Messiah: A comparative analysis of Chabad and Breslav Hassidic groups. In: **Garb Y, Wexler P** (eds), *After spirituality: studies in mystical traditions.* New York: Peter Lang; 2012, pp. 47–78.

43. **Lichtenberg P.** From the closed ward to Soteria: a professional and personal journey. *Psychosis* 2017;9:369–75. Available from: https://doi.org/10.1080/17522439.2017.1373842

44. **Bar-el Y, Durst R, Katz G, Zislin J, Stauss Z, Knobler H.** Jerusalem syndrome. *British Journal of Psychiatry* 2000;176:86–90.

45. **Kalian M, Witztum E.** Jerusalem syndrome as reflected in the pilgrimage and biographies of four extraordinary women from the 14th century to the end of the second millennium. *Mental Health, Religion & Culture.* 2002;5:1–16. https://doi.org/10.1080/13674670110068505

46. **World Health Organization (WHO).** *The ICD-10 classification of mental and behavioural disorders: clinical descriptions and diagnostic guidelines.* Geneva: WHO; 1992.

Chapter 15

Non-religion, atheism, and mental health

Miguel Farias and Thomas J. Coleman III

Introduction

Given the established link between religiosity and positive mental health, does it mean that being an atheist or agnostic presents a health risk? Or, on the contrary, is it possible that the non-religious might endorse a belief system and engage in activities which fulfil a similar role in promoting health—as religious beliefs and practices do for religious individuals? This chapter provides a tentative answer to these questions. Because this subject is deeply embedded in a cultural view that perceives religious people as 'better' than the non-religious, a view which has shaped the work of psychological and medical researchers, we will begin the chapter by deconstructing some of the key misconceptions about non-religious individuals. After this, we will review the evidence comparing mental health outcomes for the non-religious with those of religious individuals.

Atheists do not believe in anything

Scientists have studied the relationship between religiosity and health for over a century (1), starting with Galton's (2) pioneering study of whether the royal family lived longer because they had millions of people praying for them—they didn't. In contrast, it is only in the past decade that researchers have begun to explore the potential health consequences of non-religiosity (3). Given that psychologists have been studying religion for over a hundred years, it has clearly taken a very long time to ask what these individuals might believe in, and whether these beliefs might have similar psychological functions to religious ones. There is now a corpus of research showing that atheists and agnostics endorse a variety of ontological, epistemological, and ethical beliefs about reality (4, 5). Experimental psychological research has uncovered that beliefs in science or in progress are strengthened when non-religious individuals are exposed to high levels of uncertainty, existential anxiety, or stress (6,

7), suggesting that these are meaningful beliefs than non-religious individuals cling to in times of need (8). If this suggestion is correct, it radically changes our understanding of beliefs and their functional role: the benefits of beliefs are probably not driven by their supernatural content but by the process of believing, which causally and meaningfully gives structure to the world and events in everyday life.

Belief in science or progress naturally does not exhaust the varieties of beliefs non-religious individuals might espouse. Humanism, positivism, existentialism, Marxism, and transhumanism are other well-known examples of non-religious belief systems within Western culture. How any of these beliefs interact with health is unknown. We have clearly come a long way from when atheists were classified by personality psychologists as adherents of 'extremes of social, political, and religious outlook' like fundamentalists and communists (9). However, as we now describe, the stereotypes about the lack of moral qualities in atheists are very much alive.

Atheists are a-moral and rationalist

It is a well-documented phenomenon that the perception of prejudice and discrimination is associated with negative mental health consequences (10). Expressed atheism and other religious dissent is often met with scorn, ridicule, and even violence (11, 12); further to this, perceived discrimination among self-identified atheists is associated with lower levels of psychological wellbeing (13–15). Research suggests that prejudice against atheists stems from their lack of belief in God (16). More specifically, the popular perception that belief in God is necessary to maintain one's moral character seems to be the root of prejudice toward atheists. As a consequence, across a variety of religious and cultural backgrounds, research indicates that atheists are viewed as untrustworthy and immoral (17); in the USA, atheists are less accepted than any other ethnic, religious, or minority group (18, 19). Stereotypes targeting atheists are not limited solely to issues of morality, though, and studies (20, 21) demonstrate that it is not uncommon for them to be viewed as angry, unhappy, cynical, joyless, and incapable of experiencing moments of profundity and awe.

The idea that non-religious individuals are less moral has recently been contradicted in a large cross-cultural study of atheists and agnostics across Western and Eastern countries (China, Japan, England, USA, Brazil, and Denmark). Participants were asked to rank, out of a list of 50 values, the five that made their lives most meaningful. This list included values such as science, nature, love, infinity, family, sex, etc. Surprisingly, there was remarkably high agreement between non-religious individuals and the general population of these countries. When it comes to 'finding meaning in the world and your own life', the values that ranked highest for all were 'family' and 'freedom' (22).

These results not only contradict the stereotype of atheists and agnostics as less moral, but it shows that they share moral world views that are similar to those of the general population.

Concerning rationality, starting in 2012, various psychological experiments conducted in the USA and then Canada apparently showed that non-religious individuals had a more rational–analytical thinking style, which contrasted with the more intuitive style of religious people (23–25). Neuroimaging evidence corroborated this by claiming that the non-religious were more able to inhibit supernatural thoughts, which was correlated with a higher activation of the right inferior frontal gyrus (26). However, in the past few years, new evidence from cross-cultural and neural stimulation data emerged that contradicted the older studies. It was found that, with some exceptions, such as in the USA, atheists and agnostics are overall not higher on rational thinking than religious individuals (27) (although see a recent study by Stagnaro and colleauges (28)); another set of studies was also not able to find any differences in cognitive styles between these populations and showed that the stimulation of the right inferior frontal gyrus was not associated with a decrease of religious beliefs or attributions (29).

There are a number of other misconceptions about the non-religious, such as that they don't engage in self-transcendence or don't have rituals similar to those of religious individuals. That atheists are able to experience awe, self-transcendence, and even delight in mysticism is clear from the literature. We can refer to work by Coleman (4, 30, 31) and colleagues (90) on profound experiences among atheists. Additionally, empirical research from Silver and colleagues (32) identified six types of atheists, such as the 'ritual atheist/agnostic' type, who appreciate and participate in ritual activities, and a recent book by John Gray (33) also discusses various types of atheism, in which the last two chapters are dedicated to mystical atheists. Finally, there is also emerging fieldwork depicting how atheists engaging with mindfulness meditation report an array of self-transcendent experiences (34).

Less well known is that some non-religious, and admittedly a minority, have created ritual ceremonies. The most recent example is that of the Sunday Assemblies in the UK and the USA, which mimic Christian Evangelical services where religious songs are replaced by upbeat pop tunes and the sermon can focus on topics such as science, literature, or feminism (35). This ritual creation from the non-religious is something that stretches back much further. August Comte, the well-known father of sociology and of the theory of positivism created a 'positive religion' intently focused on humanist values of compassion, love, and self-knowledge (36) (see also the account by Comte's friend, John Stuart Mill (37)). There were several of these churches in France, the UK, and even in Brazil, where they held services, processions, and rituals of baptism,

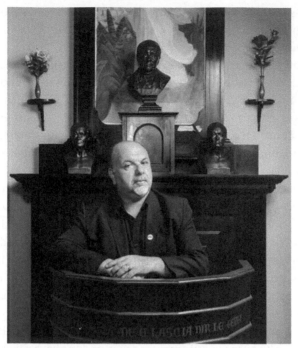

Fig. 15.1 The priest of the last active church of Positivism sitting by the altar of the Positivist Church in Porto Alegre, Brazil.
Photograph reproduced courtesy of Aubrey Wade, aubreywade.com.

wedding, as well as funerals. As far as we know, only one Positivist church in the world remains active—in the south of Brazil where its leader is attempting to grow its membership (see Fig. 15.1).[1]

To summarize: non-religious individuals hold various types of beliefs that are meaningful to them and may help them cope with adverse events in life, and they don't seem to differ from religious individuals concerning moral priorities or in cognitive style. Lastly, although rare, they can also create and engage with rituals that closely mirror that of Western religions.

Methodological problems

It is unfortunate that psychologists and medical researchers invested in the study of religion and its health correlates have for almost a hundred years

---

[1] For a video that shows parts of their services, see the short documentary 'Understanding unbelief in Brazil' by Ariane Porto: https://www.youtube.com/watch?v=9pDKyVDgJvA

neglected the study of the non-religious. The prejudices against this population is methodologically transparent when the non-religious are treated in the negative—simply as people who lack belief in God. There are several reasons such a 'negative approach' to conceptualizing non-religion has endured in social scientific research on mental health. First, the varieties of non-religious experience and identification do not enjoy the same deep historical structure and elucidation as their religious compatriots. Although in no way absent across history (38), deviations from the culturally prevailing religion have historically been met with ridicule, scorn, and even death (39). As a result, the different ways in which an individual might be non-religious have not been articulated to the degree that religious variety has been (e.g. Catholics, Sufi, Protestant, etc.). Second, and relatedly, although the large, national, and multinational surveys, used to cull mental health and other data from, usually include a variety of religious self-identifications to select, ways in which a non-religious individual might self-identify in positive terms, such as humanist or naturalist, are not included. Third, when studies do measure religiosity or belief as a continuous variable, atheists and non-religious individuals are often conceptualized as occupying the low end of these continuums (40). Two consequences of this are: 1) it confuses a zero or low score on a religiosity scale with the absence of theistic belief (5); and 2) it creates a biased comparison, whereby the mental health of atheists and the non-religious is predicted by constructs they reject and/or do not value, while the mental health of theists and the religious is predicted by constructs that are believed in and valued (41). To use an analogy, this would be the same as using the low end of an omnivore scale to draw inferences about the psychology of vegans, or measuring the mental health of devout Muslims based on their rejection of Christianity or Hinduism, for example. Defining atheism and non-religion by what is lacking does not provide a solid footing from which to explore mental health in the non-religious.

In spite of its methodological shortcomings, the existing research on non-religion and mental health is still informative, because it points to a puzzle that can be solved in part, we argue, by enriching our conceptualizing of non-religion and atheism. What is this puzzle? It is the interesting observation, first identified by Galen and Kloet (42–44) that strongly non-religious and atheistic individuals appear to experience similar salutary effects to those well-documented to be experienced by strongly religious individuals. In the next sections, we provide a necessarily selective review of the existing research.

Non-religion, atheism, and mental health: a review

The enduring relationship between religiosity and health is well documented (1), but, as is often the case, the proverbial devil is in the details. For lacking religion, does the 'non-religious man assume a tragic existence', as once proclaimed by historian of religion Mircea Eliade (p. 203)? (45) According to Schumaker (46), being non-religious contributes to maladaptive psychological outcomes by depriving the individual of the health benefits bequeathed by religion. Such sentiments are echoed by some researchers who view religion as a sui generis source of meaning and psychological health that cannot be fulfilled in secular ways (47–49). Given the putative benefits associated with religiosity, which cover a variety of domains related to psychological and physical well-being (see the other chapters in this volume for a review), this position would be understandable if the non-religious had been a very unusual, minority sample; admittedly they are in some countries but that is not the case in most Western countries, and some Eastern ones, particularly Japan and China, where there are significant proportions of non-religious individuals (50). We will now focus on the evidence available on the non-religious and mental health starting with meaning in life.

Meaning in life

The perception of meaning in life is an important component of mental health. One reason non-religiosity is viewed as a health liability is due to the assumption that the non-religious either struggle with or are deprived of life meaning. There is considerable evidence that religion is an important aspect of meaning in life for religious individuals (51). However, it is only recently that researchers have sought to compare theists and atheists, and this has challenged the assumption that atheists have deficits in perceived meaning in life and related constructs.

In one study, Schnell and Keenan (52) compared a German sample of self-identified atheists recruited from an online forum with a representative German sample of religious 'nones' with 'Religionists'. They found that the nones, followed by the atheists, reported an overall lower degree of life meaningfulness compared with the religious individuals. However, it is possible that the content of some of the meaningfulness scale items exacerbated any real difference, because they could be interpreted as having theistic undertones (e.g. 'I think my life has a *deeper* meaning', our emphasis), something that might have placed atheists at an a priori disadvantage. Overall, though, there was no difference in the degree of experienced crises of meaning between atheists and the religious group.

Schnell was able to identify three different sub-types of atheists based on their commitment to different sources of meaning, two of which valued several sources of meaning (e.g. knowledge, individualism, community) more strongly than religious individuals. In a more recent study using an American sample,

Nelson and colleagues (53) asked atheists and theists to list sources of personal meaning in life. They found that, compared with theists, atheists were more likely to report statements that the researchers coded as having 'no meaning' in life. However, one of the two examples the authors give for this code ('I don't find my life meaningful in any objective sense') appears to be a non-answer to the researchers' central question asking for *personal* sources of meaning in life, which would exclude exactly the type of response they included in their analysis. More interestingly, atheists were more likely to report sources of life meaning that did not fit the researchers' coded scheme. In addition, compared with theists, atheists reported less presence of meaning in life *but* theists also reported a greater need for meaning.

In a sample of atheists affiliated with various secular organizations in America, Caldwell-Harris and colleagues (15) found that atheists were just as likely as theists to respond affirmatively to statements about finding meaning in life experiences and having a sense of purpose. In a different study with American undergraduate students and a general sample, Sedlar and colleagues (54) found that atheists were just as likely as theists to experience struggles with ultimate meaning and purpose. Furthermore, in a nationally representative American sample, Speed, Coleman, and Langston (55) compared two proxies for lack of meaning in life: the presence of nihilistic (perceived lack of purpose) and fatalistic attitudes (nothing one can do to change one's life), and found no differences between atheists, non-religious individuals, or theists, nor any difference based on whether individuals were raised in (non)religious households. They did, however, find that atheists and the non-religious were more likely than theists to agree that meaning in life is endogenous (i.e. self-generated). Finally, a large cross-cultural study of atheists and agnostics across Western and Eastern countries found that when it comes to 'finding meaning in the world and your own life' the values that ranked highest for both non-religious individuals and the general population were 'family' and 'freedom' (22).

In this large cross-cultural survey of six countries, they found that both atheists/agnostics and religious individuals valued family and freedom above other potential sources of meaning, such as God, love, or science. But there is mixed evidence for this similarity of sources of meaning. For example, a study of a highly secularized country, Denmark, found that religious individuals were more attached to vertical transcendent sources of meaning (spirituality and religiosity) than atheists, who preferred self-actualization values (e.g. achievement, freedom, individualism) (91). Similar results have been reported for the UK (92), though this study also found that spiritual 'New Age' individuals scored as high as atheists in values of self-actualization. To make things more complicated, the Danish study (91) indicated that some of the worldview differences between religion and non-religious individuals disappeared when controlling for age and gender, which led them to conclude that most sources of meaning are common human values, regardless of one being religious or not. But this rings counter-intuitive. We would expect that holding a religious worldview implies the availability and frequent use of religious explanations in everyday life. Early models of attribution theory applied to religion predicted exactly that (93), but these have been robustly disconfirmed by various studies showing that even very religious individuals tend to make more naturalistic than religious explanations in their everyday lives, and to see God as a distal rather than a proximal cause (94, 95); the exception to this seems to be when religious individuals are faced with life-threatening events (96).

These findings need to be understood in the light of culture and history. It is likely that when religious worldviews are used by most people and life is embedded in a rich tapestry of religious rites, individuals will more often resort to religious worlviews. But, as historians have highlighted, the rise of Protestantism in the West brought with it a tsunami of changes—from the erosion of religious ideas and rites to the advent of modern science (97)—that secularized much of our way of finding religious causation in our lives. The similarities found between unbelievers and religious individuals when it comes to explaining life events are thus unsurprising

In sum, these studies add nuance to our understanding of the relationship between meaning in life and non-religion in two ways. First, they suggest that whether or not atheists and theists perceive equal levels of meaning in life depends in part on how open-response data is coded and how measures of meaningfulness are worded. Second, they suggest that there may be no negative consequences if and when atheists do report lower levels of meaningfulness, although further research is needed to understand this, especially outside the USA and Europe. The perception that meaning in life is something particularly difficult for atheists to achieve, or that religion is the sine qua non of meaning in life, is not supported by the current data. In other words, the absence of religion does not appear to leave behind what Yaden and colleagues (57) and Crescioni and Baumesiter (58) have argued as some kind of meaning gap. In fact, Heintzelman and King (59) reviewed 195 studies using two common measures of meaning in life and found fewer than five studies with sample mean scores below the scale mid-point. In other words, meaning in life appears to be a common component of human life regardless of (non)-religiosity. Finally, we also found that atheists and religious individuals espouse similar naturalistic explanations in their daily lives.

Non-religion and general well-being

It is generally well known that religious people have high levels of well-being. A review of the literature found that, out of 72 studies, 56 found a positive relationship between religiosity and well-being, and only one reported a negative relationship (1). If non-religiosity carries a penalty, we might expect the least religious countries to be associated with lower levels of well-being. However, at the societal level, countries that are the least theistic often fair better than countries with high numbers of religious individuals. For example, they have higher overall socioeconomic development (60), and report higher levels of happiness (61), lower rates of homicide and sexually transmitted diseases (62), better quality of life, and better governmental services (63). Moreover, across 33 countries, participation in a non-religious organization correlated with equal or higher levels of self-rated health than participation in a religious organization (64). Although a country's level of secularization is not always and everywhere correlated with an increase in well-being (65), greater numbers of non-religious individuals in a country generally correlate with a wide range of positive health outcomes (66).

Let us look closer at sub-samples from various countries where the published data reveal either a pattern of null results when comparing theists/atheists and religious/non-religious or find that the non-religious report experiencing equivalent levels of psychological well-being. For example, in a 2011 field study that included 360 participants from 29 countries who were walking the Camino de Santiago in Spain, Farias, Coleman, and colleagues (67) found no differences between positive/negative affect and self-reported mental health problems between atheists and theists. Similarly, samples of Italian (68) and American (69) participants have not found differences between atheists and theists on life satisfaction and subjective well-being. Looking only at self-identified religious compared with non-religious individuals in a systematic random sample from Kyoto, Roemer (70) found no differences in levels of psychological distress.

Even in samples of American children and teenagers, DeCamp and Smith (71) found that, when controlling for known protective factors, such as the quality of one's parental relationship, there is no difference in the amount of antisocial behaviour (e.g. alcohol use and vandalism) exhibited based on (non) religiosity.

When researchers do find statistically significant differences between samples, the effect size is often small, and whether the differences are of practical significance is difficult to establish. For example, a study with 821 theists and atheists in Puerto Rico found that theists reported higher life satisfaction;

however, atheists experienced higher psychological flourishing, and both differences were very small in effect size (72).

One consistent finding across various studies has been that of a U-shape curve, where the most strongly religious and non-religious show better health outcomes than the moderately religious and less strongly non-religious. This finding has been been identified in the USA (66, 73, 74), including in the US prison population context (75) and among South Asian migrants in the USA (76), Turkey (77), Israel (78), and East Germany (79).

We may ask: if the non-religious are able to reproduce the positive functions of beliefs, do they also experience the potential negative consequences of adhering strongly to a worldview, as happens with religious individuals when they experience desecration or sacred loss (46)? The answer is yes. New research on atheist members of a death metal worldview show that they experience higher positive effect and pro-social attitudes when listening to their preferred music; on the other hand, they are able to experience sacred loss and desecration of their death metal objects, as if these were religious, and feel particularly angry and depressed when this happens (80).

What of experimental studies that contrast religious with non-religious individuals? These are rare and often biased. To give one specific example, that of pain tolerance and alleviation and the role of belief. Waccholtz and Pargament (81) reported that a spiritual affirmation meditation (e.g. God is love) led to greater pain tolerance than a secular affirmation condition (e.g. I am good). Along similar lines, in a functional resonance magnetic stimulation experiment, Wiech, Farias, and colleagues (82) compared pain alleviation in practising Catholics versus non-religious individuals while they were contemplating either a religious or a secular portrait. They found stronger pain alleviation in the religious group as well as a stronger activation of the ventrolateral prefrontal cortex, a region known to drive top-down inhibitory circuits. Both these studies suffer from the same methodological constraint: they were unable to provide the non-religious group with a condition (affirmation or image) that might have had the same strength of meaning as the religious condition had for the other group. A more recent experiment compared non-religious with religious postgraduate students on various psychophysiological measures while exposing them to acute stress. Here they used a more balanced priming method, where both types of participants either wrote about a very important event in their lives where religion or science had been particularly meaningful, or, in the control condition, they wrote about their favourite season (83). The results showed no difference in outcomes for either group and no differences between the experimental and control groups, suggesting that neither religious nor secular beliefs were particularly useful in helpful participants cope with acute stress.

The literature on atheism and well-being is still in its infancy and the findings reported above are often crude. As we reported in the previous paragraph, there are studies suggesting that religious individuals may accrue special benefits but, overall, this research has a much more developed and extensive battery for assessing the varieties of religious experiences and beliefs than of non-religion. By contrast, atheists are usually clumped together as a single type of individuals, and we are often left with a simplistic, inaccurate portrayal, or—even worse—a caricature. For this literature to develop, there needs to be a more sophisticated understanding of the varieties of atheist world views, including of beliefs, value priorities, and life goals.

Conclusion: rethinking the study of religion, non-religion, and health

There is a world of research to undertake in order to understand who the non-religious are, the variety of their beliefs and worldviews, as well as practices, and how these might interact with mental health. There is no doubt that the literature is limited and contentious. It is important to note that there is a slow trickle of recent literature that represents, in some ways, a backlash at the findings we have presented here. For example, some survey work suggests that atheists and agnostics may sometimes experience higher levels of physical health but not of psychological health or well-being like religious individuals (84). Another example from social psychological research highlights that the non-religious can be dogmatic and prejudiced towards their outgroups (e.g. non-liberal or religious groups), and show a lack of flexibility in taking a different perspective (85–87). None of this is particularly unexpected or surprising and it has certainly not been our intention here to present the non-religious as superior—morally or otherwise—to religious individuals. What we have attempted here was, on the one hand, to point out the historical neglect, and the conceptual and methodological biases on this topic. On the other hand, we reported the variety of non-religious beliefs and how these non-religious individuals may experience health benefits that mirror the findings from the literature on religion and health. The reasons for this are unclear but may be associated with their beliefs, meaning systems, but also their social networks and secular rituals (including meditation).

There is one final reason why this work is important and will have repercussions beyond the understanding of the non-religious per se: it may well be that the salutary effects of religion have little to do with the supernatural contents of beliefs and rituals, but with the strength of beliefs and the actions enacted in rituals. If that is the case, then we will have to entirely review the literature on mental health and religion, as well as many suppositions in the psychology of religion.

Acknowledgements

This work was supported by the John Templeton Foundation as part of the 'Understanding Unbelief' project (grant ID: 60624).

Bibliographical References

1. **Koenig H.** Religion, spirituality, and health: the research and clinical implications. *ISRN Psychiatry.* 2012;1–33. doi: 10.5402/2012/278730

2. **Galton F.** Statistical inquiries into the efficacy of prayer. *International Journal of Epidemiology.* 1872/2012;**41**(4):923–8. doi: 10.1093/ije/dys109

3. **Hwang K, Hammer J, Cragun R.** Extending religion-health research to secular minorities: issues and concerns. *Journal of Religion and Health,* 2009;**50**(3):608–22. doi: 10.1007/s10943-009-9296-0

4. **Coleman III T, Silver C, Holcombe, J.** Focusing on horizontal transcendence: much more than a 'non-belief'. *Essays in The Philosophy of Humanism.* 2013;**21**(2):1–18. doi: 10.1558/eph.v21i2.1

5. **Farias M.** The psychology of atheism. In: **S Bullivant** and **M Ruse,** (eds), *The Oxford handbook of atheism.* Second edition. Oxford: Oxford University Press; 2013, pp. 468–482

6. **Farias M, Newheiser A, Kahane G, de Toledo, Z.** Scientific faith: belief in science increases in the face of stress and existential anxiety. *Journal of Experimental Social Psychology.* 2013;**49**(6):1210–3. doi: 10.1016/j.jesp.2013.05.008

7. **Rutjens B, van Harreveld F, van der Pligt, J.** Step by step: finding compensatory order in science. *Current Directions in Psychological Science.* 2013;**22**(3):250–5. doi: 10.1177/0963721412469810

8. **Coleman III T, Sevinç K, Hood R, Jong, J.** An atheist perspective on self-esteem and meaning making while under death awareness. *Secular Studies.* 2019;**1**(2):204–28. doi: 10.1163/25892525-00102002

9. **Vetter G, Green, M.** Personality and group factors in the making of atheists. *Journal of Abnormal and Social Psychology.* 1932;**27**(2):179–94. https://doi.org/10.1037/h0075273

10. **Major B, O'Brien L.** The social psychology of stigma. *Annual Review of Psychology.* 2005;**56**(1):393–421. doi: 10.1146/annurev.psych.56.091103.070137

11. **Cragun R, Kosmin B, Keysar A, Hammer J, Nielsen, M.** On the receiving end: discrimination toward the non-religious in the United States. *Journal of Contemporary Religion.* 2012;**27**(1):105–27. doi: 10.1080/13537903.2012.642741

12. **Hammer J, Cragun R, Hwang K, Smith, J.** Forms, frequency, and correlates of perceived anti-atheist discrimination. *Secularism and Nonreligion.* 2012;**1**:43. doi: 10.5334/snr.ad

13. **Brewster M, Hammer J, Sawyer J, Eklund A, Palamar, J.** Perceived experiences of atheist discrimination: instrument development and evaluation. *Journal of Counseling Psychology.* 2016;**63**(5):557–70. doi: 10.1037/cou0000156

14. **Cheng Z, Pagano L, Shariff, A.** The development and validation of the Microaggressions Against Non-religious Individuals Scale (MANRIS). *Psychology of Religion and Spirituality.* 2018;**10**(3):254–62. doi: 10.1037/rel0000203

15. **Doane M, Elliott M.** Perceptions of discrimination among atheists: consequences for atheist identification, psychological and physical well-being. *Psychology of Religion and Spirituality.* 2015;**7**(2):130–41. doi: 10.1037/rel0000015

16. **Swan L, Heesacker, M.** Anti-atheist bias in the United States: testing two critical assumptions. *Secularism and Nonreligion.* 2012;**1**:32–42.

17. **Gervais W, Xygalatas D, McKay R.** et al. Global evidence of extreme intuitive moral prejudice against atheists. *Nature Human Behaviour.* 2017;**1**(8). doi: 10.1038/s41562-017-0151

18. **Edgell P, Gerteis J, Hartmann, D.** Atheists as 'other': moral boundaries and cultural membership in American society. *American Sociological Review.* 2006;**71**(2):211–34. doi: 10.1177/000312240607100203

19. **Edgell P, Hartmann D, Stewart E, Gerteis, J.** Atheists and other cultural outsiders: moral boundaries and the non-religious in the United States. *Social Forces.* 2016;**95**(2):607–38. doi:10.1093/sf/sow063

20. **Caldwell-Harris C, Wilson A, LoTempio E, Beit-Hallahmi, B.** Exploring the atheist personality: well-being, awe, and magical thinking in atheists, Buddhists, and Christians. *Mental Health, Religion & Culture.* 2011;**14**(7):659–72. doi: 10.1080/13674676.2010.509847

21. **Meier B, Fetterman A, Robinson M, Lappas C.** The myth of the angry atheist. *Journal of Psychology.* 2015;**149**(3):219–38. doi: 10.1080/00223980.2013.866929

22. **Bullivant S. Farias M, Lanman J, Lee, L.** *Atheists and agnostics around the world: interim findings from 2019 research in Brazil, China, Denmark, Japan, the United Kingdom and the United States.* London: St. Mary's University; 2019, pp. 1–24.

23. **Gervais W, Norenzayan A.** Analytic thinking promotes religious disbelief. *Science.* 2012;**336**(6080):493–6. doi: 10.1126/science.1215647

24. **Pennycook G, Cheyne J, Seli P, Koehler D, Fugelsang, J.** Analytic cognitive style predicts religious and paranormal belief. *Cognition,* 2012;**123**(3):335–46. doi: 10.1016/j.cognition.2012.03.003

25. **Shenhav A, Rand D, Greene, J.** Divine intuition: cognitive style influences belief in God. *Journal of Experimental Psychology: General.* 2012;**141**(3):423–8. doi: 10.1037/a0025391

26. **Lindeman M, Svedholm A, Riekki T, Raij T, Hari, R.** Is it just a brick wall or a sign from the universe? An fMRI study of supernatural believers and skeptics. *Social Cognitive and Affective Neuroscience.* 2012;**8**(8):943–9. doi: 10.1093/scan/nss096

27. **Gervais WM, van Elk M, Xygalatas, D.** et al. Analytic atheism: a cross-culturally weak and fickle phenomenon? *Judgment and Decision Making.* 2018;**13**(3):268–74.

28. **Stagnaro M, Ross R, Pennycook G, Rand, D.** Cross-cultural support for a link between analytic thinking and disbelief in God: evidence from India and the United Kingdom. *Judgement and Decision Making.* 2019;**14**(2):179–86.

29. **Farias M, van Mulukom V, Kahane G.** et al. Supernatural belief is not modulated by intuitive thinking style or cognitive inhibition. *Scientific Reports*. 2017;7(1). doi: 10.1038/s41598-017-14090-9

30. **Coleman III TJ, Silver CF, Hood Jr, RW.** ' … if the universe is beautiful, we're part of that beauty.'—A 'neither religious nor spiritual' biography as horizontal transcendence. In: **H Streib** and **R Hood** Jr, (eds), *Semantics and psychology of spirituality*. Dordrecht, NL: Springer; 2016, pp. 355–72.

31. **Coleman III TJ, Swhajor-Biesemann A, Giamundo D, Vance C, Hood Jr, RW, Silver CF.** 'Experimenting with ideologies … '—A 'more spiritual than religious' Zen Buddhist. In: **H Streib** and **R Hood Jr**, *Semantics and psychology of spirituality*. Dordrecht, NL: Springer; 2016, pp. 339–53.

32. **Silver CF, Coleman III TJ, Hood Jr, RW, Holcombe J.** The six types of nonbelief: a qualitative and quantitative study of type and narrative. *Mental Health, Religion & Culture*. 2014;17(10):990–1001. doi: 10.1080/13674676.2014.987743

33. **Gray, J.** *Seven types of atheism*. London: MacMillan Publishers; 2018.

34. **Rahmani M.** Understanding unbelief in the mindfulness subculture. In: **L Lee, S Bullivant, M Farias** and **J Lanman**, (eds), *Cultures of unbelief*. Oxford University Press. Forthcoming.

35. **Price ME, Launay J.** Increased wellbeing from social interaction in a secular congregation. *Secularism and Nonreligion*. 2018;7(1):6. doi: 10.5334/snr.102

36. **Comte A.** *The catechism of positive religion: or summary exposition of the universal religion in thirteen systematic conversations between a woman and a priest of humanity*. Cambridge, MA: Cambridge University Press; 1852.

37. **Mill JS.** *August Comte and positivism*. Cambridge, UK: Cambridge University Press; 2015, orig. 1866.

38. **Coleman III TJ, Messick K, van Mulukom V.** New cognitive and cultural evolutionary approaches to atheism. In: **J Lane** and **Y Lior**, (eds), *The Routledge handbook of evolutionary approaches to religion*. Routledge; Forthcoming.

39. **Bremmer J.** Atheism in antiquity. In: **M Martin**, (ed.), *The Cambridge companion to atheism*. Cambridge, UK: Cambridge University Press; 2007;11–26.

40. **Coleman III TJ, Jong J.** Counting the nonreligious: a critical survey of new measures. In: **A Ai, P Wink, RF Paloutzian** and **K. Harris**, (eds), *Assessing spirituality and religion in a diversified world: beyond mainstream perspective*. Cham, Switzerland: Springer International Publishing; 2020;87–116.

41. **Coleman III TJ, Hood Jr R, Streib H.** An introduction to atheism, agnosticism, and nonreligious worldviews. *Psychology of Religion and Spirituality*. 2018;10(3):203–6. doi: 10.1037/rel0000213

42. **Galen L, Kloet J.** Mental well-being in the religious and the non-religious: evidence for a curvilinear relationship. *Mental Health, Religion & Culture*. 2011;14(7):673–89. doi: 10.1080/13674676.2010.510829

43. **Galen L.** Atheism, wellbeing, and the wager: why not believing in God (with others) is good for you. *Science, Religion and Culture*. 2015;2(3):54–69. doi: 10.17582/journal.src/2015/2.3.54.69

44. **Galen, L.** Focusing on the nonreligious reveals secular mechanisms underlying well-being and prosociality. *Psychology of Religion and Spirituality*. 2018;10(3):296–306. doi: 10.1037/rel0000202

45. **Eliade, M.** *The sacred and the profane.* San Diego: Harcourt, Brace; 1987, orig. 1957.

46. **Schumaker J.** Mental health consequences of irreligion. In: **J Schumaker**, (ed.), *religion and mental health.* First edition. New York: Oxford University Press; 1992, pp. 54–69.

47. **Hood R, Hill P, Spilka B.** *The psychology of religion: an empirical approach.* Fifth edition. New York: Guilford Press; 2018.

48. **Pargament, K.** *The psychology of religion and coping: theory, research, practice.* First edition. New York: Guilford; 1997.

49. **Park C, McNamara P.** Religion, meaning, and the brain. In: **P McNamara**, (ed), *Where God and science meet: how brain and evolutionary studies alter our understanding of religion.* First edition. Westport: Praeger; 2006, pp. 67–89.

50. **Keysar A.** Religious/non-religious demography and religion v. science: a global perspective. In: **P Zuckerman** and **J Shook**, (eds), *The Oxford handbook of secularism.* Oxford: Oxford University Press; 2017:553–86.

51. **Park C.** Religion and meaning. In: **R Paloutzian** and **C Park**, (eds), *Handbook of the psychology of religion and spirituality.* Second edition. New York: Guilford; 2013, pp. 357–79.

52. **Schnell T, Keenan W**. Meaning-making in an atheist world. *Archive for the Psychology of Religion.* 2011;**33**(1):55–78. doi: 10.1163/157361211x564611

53. **Nelson T, Abeyta A, Routledge C.** What makes life meaningful for theists and atheists? *Psychology of Religion and Spirituality.* 2019;13(1):111–8. doi: 10.1037/rel0000282

54. **Sedlar A, Stauner N, Pargament K, Exline J, Grubbs J, Bradley D.** Spiritual struggles among atheists: links to psychological distress and well-being. *Religions.* 2018;9(8):242. doi: 10.3390/rel9080242

55. **Speed D, Coleman III TJ, Langston J.** What do you mean, 'What does it all mean?' *Atheism, Nonreligion, and Life Meaning.* SAGE Open. 2018;8(1):215824401775423. doi: 10.1177/2158244017754238

56. **Bullivant S, Farias M, Lanman J, Lee L.** *Atheists and agnostics around the world: interim findings from 2019 research in Brazil, China, Denmark, Japan, the United Kingdom and the United States.* London: St. Mary's University: 2019, (pp. 1–24).

57. **Yaden D, Iwry J, Smith E, Pawelski J.** Secularism and the science of well-being. In: **P Zuckerman** and **J Shook**, (eds), *The Oxford handbook of secularism.* Oxford: Oxford University Press; 2017, pp. 554–570.

58. **Crescioni A, Baumesiter R.** The four needs for meaning, the value gap, and how (and whether) society can fill the void. In: **J Hicks** and **C Routledge**, (eds), *The experience of meaning in life: classical perspectives, emerging themes, and controversies.* First edition. Dordrecht: Springer; 2013, pp. 3–15.

59. **Heintzelman S, King L.** Life is pretty meaningful. *American Psychologist.* 2014;**69**(6):61–74. doi: 10.1037/a0035049

60. **Barber N.** Country religiosity declines as material security increases. *Cross-Cultural Research.* 2012;**47**(1):42–50. doi: 10.1177/1069397112463328

61. **Rees, T.** The happiness smile [Blog]. 2009. Available from: https://www.patheos.com/blogs/epiphenom/2009/08/happiness-smile.html

62. **Paul G.** The chronic dependence of popular religiosity upon dysfunctional psychosociological conditions. *Evolutionary Psychology.* 2009;7(3): 147470490900700. doi: 10.1177/147470490900700305

63. **Zuckerman M, Li C., Diener E.** Religion as an exchange system: the interchangeability of God and government in a provider role. *Personality and Social Psychology Bulletin.* 2018;**44**(8):1201–13. doi: 10.1177/0146167218764656

64. **Upenieks L, Foy S, Miles, A.** Beyond America: cross-national context and the impact of religious versus secular organizational membership on self-rated health. *Socius: Sociological Research for a Dynamic World.* 2018;**4**: 237802311879595. doi: 10.1177/2378023118795954

65. **Yu C, Trier H, Slama M.** A data mining and data visualization approach to examine the interrelationships between life satisfaction, secularization and religiosity. *Journal of Religion and Health.* 2018;**58**(1):271–88. doi: 10.1007/s10943-018-0737-5

66. **Zuckerman P.** Atheism and societal health. In: **S Bullivant** and **M Ruse,** (eds), *The Oxford handbook of atheism.* Oxford: Oxford University Press: 2013:468–82.

67. **Farias M, Coleman III TJ, Bartlett, J.** et al. Atheists on the Santiago Way: examining motivations to go on pilgrimage. *Sociology of Religion.* 2019;**80**(1):28–44. doi: 10.1093/socrel/sry019

68. **Villani D, Sorgente A, Iannello P, Antonietti A.** The role of spirituality and religiosity in subjective well-being of individuals with different religious status. *Frontiers in Psychology.* 2019;**10**. doi: 10.3389/fpsyg.2019.01525

69. **Moore J, Leach M.** Dogmatism and mental health: a comparison of the religious and secular. *Psychology of Religion and Spirituality.* 2016;**8**(1):54–64. doi: 10.1037/rel0000027

70. **Roemer M.** Religion and psychological distress in Japan. *Social Forces.* 2010;**89**(2):559–83. doi: 10.1353/sof.2010.0049

71. **DeCamp W, Smith J.** Religion, nonreligion, and deviance: comparing faith's and family's relative strength in promoting social conformity. *Journal of Religion and Health.* 2019;**58**(1):206–20. doi: 10.1007/s10943-018-0630-2

72. **González-Rivera J, Rosario-Rodríguez A., Rodríguez-Ramos E, Hernández-Gato I, Torres-Báez L.** ¿Realmente son los creyentes más felices que los ateos? Medidas de Bienestar en una Muestra de Ateos y Creyentes en Puerto Rico. *Interacciones. Revista De Avances En Psicología.* 2019;**5**(1):51. doi: 10.24016/2019.v5n1.160

73. **Coleman III TJ, Jong J.** Counting the nonreligious: a critical survey of new measures. In: **A Ai, P Wink RF Paloutzian** and **K. Harris.** (eds), *Assessing spirituality and religion in a diversified world: beyond mainstream perspective.* Cham, Switzerland: Springer International Publishing; 2020:87–116.

74. **Weber S, Pargament K, Kunik M, Lomax J, Stanley M.** Psychological distress among religious nonbelievers: a systematic review. *Journal of Religion and Health.* 2011;**51**(1):72–86. doi: 10.1007/s10943-011-9541-1

75. **Drakeford, L.** Mental health and the role of religious context among inmates in state and federal prisons: results from a multilevel analysis. *Society and Mental Health.* 2019;**9**(1):51–73. doi: 10.1177/2156869318763248

76. **Stroope S, Kent B, Zhang Y, Kandula N, Kanaya A, Shields A.** Self-rated religiosity/spirituality and four health outcomes among US South Asians. *Journal of Nervous and Mental Disease.* 2020;**208**(2):165–8. doi: 10.1097/nmd.0000000000001128

77. **Yeniaras V, Akarsu T.** Religiosity and life satisfaction: a multi-dimensional approach. *Journal of Happiness Studies.* 2016;**18**(6):1815–40. doi: 10.1007/s10902-016-9803-4

78. **Brammli-Greenberg S, Glazer J, Shapiro, E.** The inverse u-shaped religion—health connection among Israeli jews. *Journal of Religion and Health.* 2018;**57**(2):738–50. doi: 10.1007/s10943-018-0577-3

79. **Hanel P, Demmrich S, Wolfradt U.** Centrality of religiosity, schizotypy, and human values: the impact of religious affiliation. *Religions.* 2019;**10**(5):297. doi: 10.3390/rel10050297

80. **Messick K.** *A psychological study of the sacred in metal music culture* (PhD thesis). Coventry: Coventry University; 2019.

81. **Wachholtz A, Pargament K.** Is spirituality a critical ingredient of meditation? Comparing the effects of spiritual meditation, secular meditation, and relaxation on spiritual, psychological, cardiac, and pain outcomes. *Journal of Behavioral Medicine.* 2005;**28**(4):369–84. doi: 10.1007/s10865-005-9008-5

82. **Wiech K, Farias M, Kahane G, Shackel N, Tiede W, Tracey I.** An fMRI study measuring analgesia enhanced by religion as a belief system. *Pain.* 2008;**139**(2):467–76. doi: 10.1016/j.pain.2008.07.030

83. **Farias M, Newheiser A.** The effects of belief in God and science on acute stress. Psychology of consciousness: *Theory, Research, and Practice.* 2019;**6**(2):214–23. doi: 10.1037/cns0000185

84. **Hayward R, Krause N, Ironson G, Hill P, Emmons R.** Health and well-being among the non-religious: atheists, agnostics, and no preference compared with religious group members. *Journal of Religion and Health.* 2016;**55**(3):1024–37. doi: 10.1007/s10943-015-0179-2

85. **Uzarevic F, Saroglou V.** Understanding nonbelievers' prejudice toward ideological opponents: the role of self-expression values and other-oriented dispositions. *International Journal for the Psychology of Religion.* 2019; 30(3): 1–17. doi:10.1080/10508619.2019.1696498

86. **Uzarevic F, Saroglou V, Clobert, M.** Are atheists undogmatic? *Personality and Individual Differences.* 2017;**116**:164–70. https://doi.org/10.1016/j.paid.2017.04.046

87. **Uzarevic F, Saroglou V, Muñoz-García A.** Are atheists unprejudiced? Forms of nonbelief and prejudice toward antiliberal and mainstream religious groups. *Psychology of Religion and Spirituality.* 2019;13(1):81–93. doi: 10.1037/rel0000247

88. **Uzarevic F, Coleman III TJ.** The psychology of nonbelievers. *Current Opinion in Psychology.* 2021;**40**:131–8. doi: 10.1016/j.copsyc.2020.08.026

89. **Coleman III TJ, Messick K.** Keeping the secular deck intact. *Implicit Religion.* 2019;**22**(1):58–65. doi: 10.1558/imre.40119

90. **Preston J, Shin F.** Spiritual experiences evoke awe through the small self in both religious and non-religious individuals. *Journal of Experimental Social Psychology.* 2017;**70**:212–21. doi: 10.1016/j.jesp.2016.11.006

91. **Pedersen H, Birkeland M, Jensen J, Schnell T, Hvidt N, Sørensen T, La Cour P.** What brings meaning to life in a highly secular society? A study on sources of meaning among Danes. *Scandinavian Journal of Psychology.* 2018;**59**(6):678–90. doi: 10.1111/sjop.12495

92. **Farias M, Lalljee M.** Holistic individualism in the age of Aquarius: measuring individualism/collectivism in new age, catholic, and atheist/agnostic groups. *Journal for the Scientific Study of Religion.* 2008;**47**(2):277–89. doi: 10.1111/j.1468-5906.2008.00407.x

93. **Spilka B, Shaver P, Kirkpatrick L.** A general attribution theory for the psychology of religion. *Journal for the Scientific Study of Religion*. 1985;24(1):1. doi: 10.2307/1386272

94. **Lupfer M, Brock K, DePaola S.** The use of secular and religious attributions to explain everyday behavior. *Journal for the Scientific Study of Religion*. 1992;31(4):486. doi: 10.2307/1386858

95. **Lupfer M, Layman E.** Invoking naturalistic and religious attributions: a case of applying the availability heuristic? The representativeness heuristic? *Social Cognition*. 1996;14(1):55–76. doi: 10.1521/soco.1996.14.1.55

96. **Loewenthal K, Cornwall N.** Religiosity and perceived control of life events. *International Journal for the Psychology of Religion*. 1993;3(1):39–45. doi: 10.1207/s15327582ijpr0301_6

97. **Brooke J.** *Science and religion*. New York: Cambridge University Press; 1991.

Chapter 16

African religions, spirituality, and mental health healing practices

Olatunde Ayinde, Akin Ojagbemi,
Victor Makanjuola, and Oye Gureje

Introduction

It is a universal human experience to seek meaning and purpose in life. This is often achieved through partaking in activities that give value to one's life and help in the experience of connectedness to self, to the community and to a higher being, which may in turn lead to a feeling of wholeness, harmony, and of hope (1–4). In many cultures around the world, the vehicle for this uniquely human quest is 'spirituality', defined in this chapter as a search for meaning and purpose and for a relationship with the transcendent (5).

While 'spirituality' may or may not be associated with, or originate from, a religion (6, 7) in many contexts globally, religion is the most common vehicle for connectedness to a higher being in many settings including the African setting. Religion as used here connotes an organized system of belief, practices, symbolic objects, places, and officials that facilitate closeness to a sacred reality (6, 7). In Africa, 'spirituality' and religion are often used interchangeably and the epistemological distinction between them is almost non-existent.

The origin of religions on the African continent, as elsewhere, is a subject of considerable debate. However, there seems to be some evidence to suggest that religion arose as a by-product of psychological mechanisms that evolved in humans for reasons such as survival and social interaction (8). Some cognitive psychologists (8) believe that the psychological foundations of religion include the cognitive tendency to find causal explanation for natural events and the ability to recognize that other people have intentions and desires. These mechanisms are responsible for our ability to imagine purposeful agents behind naturally occurring events and phenomena. African religions may also trace their origin to the experiences and deep reflections of the ancestors of African peoples in response to the yearnings of the human spirit to find meaning within the context of Africa's diverse cultural heritage (9).

Whatever the origin, the reality is that religion has been part of African peoples from the dawn of history and continues to serve as the glue that holds together entire communities of peoples that are not related by birth. A Gallup survey of adults in 114 countries found that between 85% and 100% of respondents in Africa admitted that religion was important in their daily lives (10). In a more recent nationwide panel study in South Africa (11), between 89.6% and 91.8% identified themselves as religiously affiliated, while 88.0%–90.3% perceived religion to be important in their lives. These findings are only rivalled by those reported from South-East Asian countries (10).

From birth to death, every event in the life of an African is infused with religious rituals and meanings—daily life events and family life, important thresholds in life, kinship, occupation, leadership, social structure, and interactions. Gyekye captures the ubiquitous presence of religion in African societies in these words: 'to be born into African society is to be born into a culture that is intensely and pervasively religious and that means, and requires, participating in the religious beliefs and rituals of the community' (12). Mbiti (13) expressed a similar sentiment: 'to be is to be religious in a religious universe. These ideas drive the philosophical understanding of African myths, customs, traditions, beliefs, morals, actions and social relationships.' To Africans, religion is not an aspect of life; it is ' . . . the glorification of everyday life, imagined and enacted through customs and ritual performance, in folk tales and proverbs, creation myths, prayer and invocation, music and dance' (14).

African conception of religion and African religions

In African thought systems, it is almost an impossible task to isolate religion and give it a concrete or precise definition. However, in an attempt to bring an African understanding to the description of religion, Beyers defines religion as 'the continual participation in traditions (myths and rituals) passed on from one generation to the next' (15). For an African, religion is inextricably woven into the entire fabric of life, of being and existence. It dominates language, thought patterns, social relationships, attitudes, ethics and, philosophical dispositions. Religion in the African context goes beyond beliefs, worship, and ceremonies. It is the final source of reference in terms of morals and ethics, tradition, culture, and custom, a guide for daily living and social relationships, and the place of the individual in the overall socio-political scheme of society.

Perhaps, the most important function of religion among Africans is that of personal and ethnic identity, as well as a framework for kinship with members of one's family, alive or dead (13). According to Mbiti, to exist at all as a human being in a traditional African community is to be completely immersed in its beliefs, traditions, ceremonies, and festivals. In other words, for Africans, religion is intimately linked to tribal and communal identity as well as kinship. Therefore, in practice, there is no unitary African religion. Thus, Africa has a multiplicity of ethnic groups, each with their own unique culture, language, norms, and religion (16, 17). It is for this reason, for example, that one can refer to a 'Yoruba religion' in that ethnic group in Nigeria or an 'Akan religion' in Ghana.

African religions are almost entirely focused on a celebration of life in the here and now, a continuing, dynamic, communal relationship among entities both physical and supernatural, in time and space, 'a concern for community and the expression of common humanity' popularly known as 'Ubuntu' in Bantu languages (14). Related to this is the African affirmation of differences and diversity in religious persuasion, a striking capacity to accommodate religions different from theirs. Africans approach religion with an attitude that 'the road to the market cannot be a single one; there are several roads to the market' (Yoruba proverb). Perhaps the reason why Africans are able to be very tolerant of other religions is the very nature of their belief system. The pantheon of often indeterminate number of deities, spirits, and ancestors co-exist quite harmoniously in the African's mind, each deity with his own niche. The organizational structure of the pantheon is quite flexible. There is a chief god who is not too concerned about the day-to-day running of affairs and has delegated most functions to lesser gods, deities, and spirits. A person is therefore at liberty to pour libations to or offer sacrifices to countless other spiritual entities without necessarily violating any oath of allegiance to his own family god, if this is what the medicine man has prescribed. Unlike the God of Islam or of Christianity, neither the chief god nor his lesser companions in African traditional religions are jealous or demand absolute loyalty; the adherents of one deity are quite free to join adherents of another deity to worship, celebrate, and provide solidarity during festivals. Fundamentalism is therefore unheard of in African traditional religion.

African religious cosmology

Despite the plurality of religions and the diverse ways of religious expression on the continent, African religions share many essential features, such that some scholars of religion have concluded that the same philosophy underlies all of them. According to Turaki (18), some of these common features include the belief in a Supreme Being, belief in spirits and divinities, the cult of ancestors, and the use of magic, charms, and spiritual forces. Indeed, other scholars have suggested that it is possible to recognize some core traits of nearly all African religions to enable scholars to speak of a traditional African religion (ATR), in the singular generic sense (19).

In African religious cosmology, the transcendent is imagined as both a dynamic, impersonal power that permeates the entire universe, and also as a personal, immanent reality that has influence over all human activities (15). The universe is envisioned as a living, dynamic entity, with two parallel spheres. The physical realm is the abode of man, animals, plants, and the rest of animate beings, as well as phenomena and inanimate objects. The spiritual sphere is the abode of God, deities (or gods), and spirits. Yet, there are also a few African cultures that hold strong beliefs about gods that live close to the earth and spirits that roam the earth (20). Man is the centre of this religious ontology; one form of ontological existence presupposes the other and all forms exist in complete unity and harmonious balance (13).

Apart from these ontological categories of existence, there also exists a power, a life force or energy that permeates the entire universe. The ultimate source and controller of this power is a Supreme Deity, who has granted access to some of its power to lesser deities or gods and spirits. In African traditional religion, it is believed that a special category of humans exits: witches, wizards, priests, and medicine men who have the ability and knowledge to access, manipulate, and use this mystical power for either good or evil in the community. The African religious world view is holistic, with little distinction between the physical and the spiritual world: men become spirits and return to their place of origin in the spiritual realm when they die, living men can be inhabited by spirits, and so can inanimate objects and phenomena: 'everything and everyone is connected to everything and everyone else' (15).

The idea of God in the Christian or Islamic fashion, or a Supreme Deity in African religions, poses a bit of controversy. Some scholars of African religions opine that the idea of God is a Eurocentric concept that missionaries brought to Africa in a bid to find a deity close to their God in the African pantheons in order to ease their missionary work, and that the idea of a deity is more polytheistic than monotheistic among African cultures. Other scholars maintain that the notion that Africans do not subscribe to the idea of a supreme God is incorrect.

What appears to be more correct, however, is that the organization of spiritual personages in African religions is often patterned after the social-political structures and realities of the culture in question, with a Supreme

Being at the apex of the hierarchy (13). Although this Being is perceived personally, contact with him is only possible through mediators and councillors: gods, spirits, and ancestors. The worship and veneration of these mediators do not detract from the Supreme Being and is an indication of the worship of God (19). This is a fundamental difference between African religions and the Abrahamic religions, in which God is portrayed as being fiercely jealous and demanding in absolute loyalty and worship. Mbiti notes that there is hardly any African culture without the notion of a Supreme Deity, albeit known by different names in different cultures (13). God is perceived as being all-powerful and all-knowing, with no beginning and no end. God is both transcendent and immanent, and is involved in the daily affairs of men. In many cultures, he is considered to be the king, ruler, and master of the universe. Creation and sustenance of life is attributed to him. God is also considered to be the origin of human traditions, consisting of moral code and rules for ethical living. Morality flows from God to humans through the ancestors. In some cases, God can also afflict individual humans or entire communities with calamities, diseases, or mental illness as a form of punishment when they commit certain offences or contravene certain rituals (13). In African religions, the worship of God is not primarily for redemption or for paradise but for continued sustenance in the here and now.

African religions are also characterized by the worship and/or veneration of a huge number of spiritual beings, spirits, and the 'living dead' (13). Gods, deities, or divinities are manifestations of God, his associates, or his children in the spiritual abode. In some cases, they are deified humans or national heroes. Their number and attributes vary from culture to culture. There are divinities of death, thunder, war, iron, fertility, as well as river and mountain divinities. Each is a messenger of God and acts as an intermediary between God and man. Each deity has its own specialty and it is not uncommon for the worshipper of a river deity to approach the priest of the fertility god to solve a fertility problem without causing any rancour between the gods. Spirits are lower in hierarchy to gods but superior to men, and were either created ab initio, or are the end point of humans when they die. Spirits are invisible and are believed to be ubiquitous. They can be benevolent or malicious, can sometimes be employed by witches and medicine men to cause harm or illness, and are commonly believed to be involved in the causation of mental illness and epilepsy. Spirits are also believed to possess persons to cause illness or to act through them as mediums. They can be approached through mediums, traditional healers, and diviners to convey important information, such as the cause of a mental illness, from the spiritual world to men. Spirits can reside in men, animals, plants, rivers, mountains, inanimate objects, and phenomena. They are generally feared but can be appeased through sacrifices and prayers.

Ancestors are deceased members of the family or community who have attained an elevated status in the spiritual realm. They function essentially to mediate between their descendants and God and deities. They are the conduits through which traditions and moral behaviour flow from God to man, and they are often consulted for personal, family, and communal problems and decisions. A close relationship with them is supposed to bring spiritual harmony and good fortune, while neglecting them is considered to be dangerous and can lead to misfortune. Ancestors also act as guardians of family affairs and daily activities, traditions, and moral behaviour. Ancestors are believed to accompany and act as guides to their earthly descendants through their cyclical journey through birth, childhood, adolescent, adulthood, death, and sometimes rebirth, and are an essential part of the initiation rites and rites of passage at each of the crossroads of life, having navigated these dangerous journeys themselves successfully in their own time. Political and moral authority as well as the family and social structures of society are often claimed to flow directly from the ancestors who act as the custodians of society's morals and social structure. Persons who have died through suicide or who did not procreate while alive are commonly believed to be denied elevation to the status of ancestors.

Worship in African religions can take the form of private communion or communal expressions of worship manifested in prayers, invocations, appeasement, salutations, sacrifice, and offerings. These are often accompanied by rich symbolism, rites and ritual, colourful visual and oral arts forms as well as music, dance, and general outpouring of emotion. Community elders, kings, and other traditional leaders, as well as herbalists and traditional healers are believed to have both political and sacred powers, and therefore feature prominently in communal worship.

Laws, customs, norms, rules, observances, and taboos often have sacred values and contravening them can bring about personal and/or communal calamity and illness as judgement and punishment from the spiritual world. Respect and obedience to parents and authority figures may assume a religious significance. Interpersonal difficulties often take on religious significance such that quarrels and misunderstandings may become occasions for accusation of witchcraft, sorcery, and magic. In almost all African religions, the spirit of men never die; children are born, grow old, die, and return to the spirit world where they either become ancestors or are reborn, in a cyclical fashion. With very few exceptions, African religions have no notion of heaven or hell.

Aspects of African religions and spirituality relevant to mental health theory and practice

Mental wellbeing, resilience, and risk factors for mental illness

As it is in practically all religions, there are elements of African religions that promote mental well-being and confer some measure of resilience. Some of the hypothesized mediators of the salutary effects of religion on mental well-being include social support, security in personal and communal identity, coping, positive emotions such as a sense of purpose, meaning, self-confidence, hope and acceptance engendered by religious beliefs, as well as other unknown psychological mechanisms (21). However, two proposed mechanisms need to be particularly emphasized. There is an intense focus of African religions on communal existence and relationship. The advantages this may confer on mental well-being include social support and solidarity in times of stress and adversity. As African cultures are largely socio-centric or collectivist, it is important to understand that in religion, as in therapies, families, kinship, tribes, or clans can play an important role. The pervasive influence of religion in everyday life may be a veritable source of daily comfort, meaning, and security. However, this may also become counterproductive, as mundane relationship failures and adversity may take on serious spiritual connotations. For example, a quarrel with a parent leading to the parent withdrawing 'parental blessing' is a serious situation with possible psychological impacts. Similarly, adversity may also become more significant as a risk factor for mental illness. For example, infertility and suicide have profound religious and spiritual dimensions in the African religious context, such that these conditions impose additional burdens of risk. That is, the fact of being infertile or of having a family member who died by suicide may be interpreted as indicative of more profound spiritual meaning for self and for one's family. Perhaps a deity has been offended or an ancestor is visiting retribution for some infraction. There may also be additional concerns that a person who dies by suicide would be denied the elevation to ancestorhood and its perks, or that the spirit of someone who dies childless would lose the chance of communicating with the physical world after death. It is therefore of benefit to enquire in clinical settings whether otherwise understandable adversity and loss has some religious significance to warrant special spiritual support in addition to bio-psycho-social management.

Traditional healers commonly double as religious leaders and advisers in all aspects of life (13). The counsel they offer for psychosocial difficulties that do not rise to the level of psychopathology, as well as the mediation between their clients and their ancestors for advice on day-to-day decisions and problems, may be a source of psychological resilience (22). It is common for traditional healers to offer supplications and sacrifices to ward off evil spirits, illness, and adversity. These rituals and sacrifices have been hypothesized to have psychotherapeutic effects (23, 24). Some of these practices and the beliefs underlying them have often been taken along to their new religions by converts to Islam and Christianity (25). It is therefore important that mental health practitioners enquire and explore about such beliefs and to what degree they influence patients' world view, even when such patients do not profess African religions.

Causal attribution of mental illness and religious interpretation of psychopathology

Elements of African traditional religion are relevant to causal attribution of illness, including mental illness. Even though biological and psychosocial factors are believed to play a role in the aetiology of mental disorders, there are often additional supernatural causes (26–28). Many Africans express beliefs that mental illnesses result from curses, witchcraft, demon possession, and punishment for sin committed at various times either by the patient, their family, or community. In addition, beliefs that mental illnesses are contagious through body fluids are often expressed (29). The most commonly expressed biological causes of mental illnesses include head trauma (especially in childhood), fevers, and psychoactive substance abuse (30). Others include stress and hereditary factors. When beliefs in bio-psych-social causation of mental illnesses are expressed, such illnesses are thought to have initially started as a 'spiritual attack' (31). In other instances, witches can take advantage of diseases with primary biomedical causation to make them more severe or run a chronic unremitting course.

Supernatural causal attribution, in addition to other health system factors, have been shown to influence help-seeking behaviour, stigma, and delay in accessing effective conventional mental health care (32–35). For example, beliefs that mental illnesses may be contagious, and are the result of punishment for wrongdoing may result in, negative attitudes and stigmatization of patients and families by members of their community (36). Traditional remedies for wrongdoing may include ritual cleansing that restores social balance and reintegration into community life (37).

Healing and African religions

Traditional healing in the African context is faith healing according to African religions. Healing in traditional medicine is a much broader concept than the provision of care for health problems. Traditional African healing may also comprise consultation for clairvoyance (38) as well as for solutions to a wide range of social and economic challenges, including prowess in career, dating, fertility, and finances (39). The major categories of African traditional healers include herbalists, diviners, shrine priests, and witchcraft practitioners (38). However, many combinations, such as herbalist and Christian or herbalist and Islam have also been identified. In general, an eclectic approach to healing is not uncommon with a healer drawing from experience in herbalism, divination, and use of rituals. A majority of African traditional healers provide both physical and mental health services (38). Their practice is often a reflection of the absence of a strict mind–body dichotomy in the African conceptualization of health and ill health. In general, healers have received training through many years of apprenticeship and rely on signs and symptoms to make a diagnosis (38).

The management of patients by African traditional healers involves history taking (during which they inquire about presenting complaints, duration of illness, circumstances surrounding the onset of illness), a 'physical examination' and investigation (often by consulting some oracles). Diagnosis may be commonly made through divination and/or analyses of the presenting signs and symptoms. Treatment options include the use of herbs, rituals, sacrifices, and sorcery. For mental health conditions, approaches such as scarification and flogging (40) are also not uncommon. These practices often reflect a belief about a need to drain bad blood or to drive away demons possessing the patients. The common currency of interaction between the healer and the people they serve is the belief system. Hence, the healer is in a way a custodian of the beliefs related to causation and treatment of mental illness. He has the power and skills to invoke good spirits and gods for healing, appease angry ancestors, cast out malevolent spirits, and communicate with the spiritual world to find the cause of illness and the indicated treatment. These beliefs help form explanatory models of causes and treatment as well as the course of various mental illnesses. Traditional healers also use animal and plant materials, some of which have been known to have active pharmacological properties. However, some of these agents have more symbolic or sacramental functions, with some simply having names that rhyme with their functions, and are used symbolically in therapeutic chants and incantations (41).

African religions, help-seeking behaviour, and global mental health

Healing practices based on African traditional religions are the de facto mental health care in most of Africa (38). Healers are more in number than mental health professionals and are more readily accessible to the community. In a survey of patients with schizophrenia in Xhosa-speaking South Africa, 84%

had consulted traditional healers for their symptoms (42). Conservative estimates from other African countries—for example, Nigeria—suggest that approximately 60% of patients using traditional healing as the first point of contact for a variety of health conditions do so because of a mental illness (43). An important reason for the popularity of traditional healing in Africa is that users find the underlying tenets of traditional healing practices to be congruent with their own beliefs, values, and norms (32). African traditional healing is also generally perceived to have efficacy for prevention, treatment, and rehabilitation of mental health conditions. A study in Ethiopia, which explored the possible contributions of traditional healing to the healthcare delivery system, found that 57.2% of the population endorsed the efficacy of traditional healing for the treatment of mental illnesses (44). Several other African studies have demonstrated perceived efficacy of traditional healing practices for mental disorders by the community (45, 46).

Traditional healing practices substantially tap into the psychological, social, and spiritual basis of health and ill health. Healers explore these three dimensions in arriving at the cause of illness and in proffering treatment options. For this reason, they are particularly effective in mental health conditions for which psychological, social, and spiritual explanations and treatments are efficacious. A recent systematic review (47) assessed the effectiveness of treatment of traditional healers in low- and middle-income countries, including countries in Africa, and found evidence of effectiveness for common mental disorders such as anxiety and depression, as well as psychosocial concerns that do not reach a diagnostic threshold. These are conditions known to be more commonly amenable to psychosocial interventions. Among the common elements of psychological treatment recognized in traditional healing include catharsis and cognitive restructuring, as well as elements of hope and faith (23). The traditional healer has also been described as a social organizer who incorporates into their treatment efforts at restoring social and spiritual harmony and balance, renewal of family structures, restoration of community identity, and social cohesion (23).

A continent in transition: interactions of African religions with Islam, Christianity, globalization, and modern politics

African religions have gone through three partly overlapping phases in the history of the continent. Precolonial African religions enjoyed a monopoly of influence on the total way of life of African peoples. The second phase corresponds with a period of gentle evangelization of African peoples and, if there was any clash at all with African traditional religions, it was subtle and African people found ways of making Abrahamic religions coexist with traditional religions with minimal conflict. This was accomplished by either simultaneously holding two different religious world views, or by merging those views into a somewhat coherent whole, or by the partial acceptance and rejection of concepts.

One of the results of these processes is the rise of the independent Christian churches where Africans have managed to practise a syncretic form of Christianity that gives Africans freedom to design their own Christian liturgy that is rich in songs, dance, rituals, and active emotional displays (48). They are able to express their traditional religious ethos and solidarity, which may include fortification against evil spirits and enemies, as well as regular prayers for healing, sustenance, and prosperity. Emerging from this second phase and overlapping with it is a third phase in which there is a clear growth of Christian and Islamic fundamentalism on the continent. In this phase, more extreme views about the supremacy of one religion over the other, and jostling for dominance among them, are producing friction and even violence.

The rise of Christian and Islamic fundamentalism is taking place against the backdrop of globalization and the pervasive influence of Western cultures. So, while there is tension between the two Abrahamic religions seeking prominence, both are in apparent agreement in regard to the place and status of African traditional religions: they are now cast as backward, fetishistic, and evil. Their adherents are regarded as relics of an embarrassing past. On the other hand, Islam and Christianity are viewed as modern, progressive, salvific religions associated with economic prosperity and status. The adherents of African religions in most of post-colonial Africa are now becoming the minority because most traditional communities have been overtaken by Islam and Christianity. Furthermore, it would seem that African religions no longer enjoy the monopoly of influence they once had on the religious life and social cognition of Africans.

Even so, several scholars of religion have suggested that religious conversion for Africans is often never complete (49). An indication of this is that elements of African religious beliefs and practices continue to survive as part and parcel of the liturgy of African independent churches, such as the Aladura Church Movement in Nigeria (48), in the music and healing rituals of the Gnawa cults in Morocco, and Candomblé in Afro-Caribbean countries (14). Across Africa, different demographic segments of the society professing one or other Abrahamic religion have reason to consult traditional healers. Hence, elements of African religions continue to exert a powerful influence on thoughts, emotions, and behaviour of Africans at the subconscious level, and deserve a generous attention in mental health service provision on the continent.

Practical considerations and competence for mental health practitioners working on the continent

Psychiatrists working on the continent need to recognize and admit their own religious world view, which may likely be one of Islam or Christianity, while working with persons who profess African religions. The temptation to view the belief systems in African traditional religions with disdain is ever present and should be overcome in clinical settings. Not only should practitioners be open-minded by using beneficial elements of the belief systems for therapeutic purposes while discouraging the harmful ones with respect and dignity, they should also be aware of psychosocial stressors that may be related to religious beliefs, and address them appropriately. There is room for collaborative care models incorporating useful elements of African religions into conventional care, and reducing potentially harmful beliefs and practices. Future research would need to tease out which elements of, and to which extent, African religious views continue to influence attitudes and behaviours that promote mental well-being and resilience, as well as the harmful elements to de-emphasize in mental health care.

References

1. **Hassed CS.** Depression: dispirited or spiritually deprived? *Medical Journal of Australia.* 2000;**173**:545–7.
2. **Humphreys J.** Spirituality and distress in sheltered battered women. *Journal of Nursing Scholarship.* 2000;**32**:273–8.
3. **McSherry W.** Education issues surrounding the teaching of spirituality. *Nursing Standard.* 2000;**14**:40–3.
4. **Puchalski CM, Vitillo R, Hull SK,** et al. Improving the spiritual dimension of whole person care: reaching national and international consensus. *Journal of Palliative Medicine.* 2014;**17**:642–56.
5. **Swinton J.** Healthcare spirituality: a question of knowledge. In: **R Cobb, C Puchalsk, B Rumbold** (eds), *Oxford textbook of spirituality in healthcare.* New York: Oxford University Press; 2012:99–104.
6. **Koenig HG, McCullough ME, Larson DB.** *Handbook of religion and health.* New York: Oxford University Press; 2001.
7. **Mbiti JS.** *Introduction to African religion.* London: Heinemann; 1975.
8. **Atran S, Norenzayan A.** Religion's evolutionary landscape: counterintuition, commitment, compassion, communion. *Behavioral and Brain Sciences.* 2004;**27**:713–30.
9. **Opoku KA.** African traditional religion: an enduring heritage. In: **Olupona J, Nyang S** (eds), *Religious Plurality in Africa: Essays in Honour of John S Mbiti.* Berlin: Mouton de Gruyter; 1993:67–82.

10. **Gallup Inc.** Religiosity highest in world's poorest nations. *Gallup.com.* 2010.

11. **Tomita A, Ramlall S.** A nationwide panel study on religious involvement and depression in South Africa: evidence from the South African national income dynamics study. *Journal of Religion and Health.* 2018;**57**:2279–89.

12. **Gyekye K.** *African cultural values: an introduction.* Accra: Sankofa Publishing Company; 1996.

13. **Mbiti JS.** *African religions and philosophy.* Portsmouth, NH: Heinemann; 1976.

14. **Ward K.** African Traditional Religion. In: **Palmer M** (ed.), *World religions: a comrehensive guide to the religions of the world.* London: Times Books; 2004:86–93.

15. **Beyers J.** What is religion? An African understanding. *HTS Teologiese Studies/ Theological Studies.* 2010;**66(1):341.**

16. **Heine B, Nurse D.** *African languages: an introduction.* Cambridge, UK: Cambridge University Press; 2000.

17. **Kpanake L.** Cultural concepts of the person and mental health in Africa. *Transcult Psychiatry.* 2018;**55**:198–218.

18. **Turaki Y.** *Christianity and African gods: a method in theology.* Potchefstroomse Universiteit vir Christelike Hoër Onderwys; 1999.

19. **Krüger JS, Lubbe G, Steyn HC.** *The human search for meaning: a multireligious introduction to the religions of humankind.* Pretoria, SA: Van Schaik; 2009.

20. **Sundermeier T.** *Was ist religion? Religionswissenschaft im theologischen kontext; ein studienbuch.* Kaiser Gütersloher Verlagshaus, Gütersloh; 1999.

21. **Moreira-Almeida A, Lotufo Neto F, Koenig HG.** Religiousness and mental health: a review. *Revista Brasileira de Psiquiatria.* 2006;**28**:242–50.

22. **White P.** The concept of diseases and health care in African traditional religion in Ghana. *HTS Teologiese Studies/Theological Studies.* 2015;**71**:7.

23. **Cheetham RW, Griffiths JA.** The traditional healer/diviner as psychotherapist. *South African Medical Journal.* 1982;**62**:957–8.

24. **Awanbor D.** The healing process in African psychotherapy. *American Journal of Psychotherapy.* 1982;**36**:206–13.

25. **Aina OF.** 'Psychotherapy by environmental manipulation' and the observed symbolic rites on prayer mountains in Nigeria. *Mental Health, Religion & Culture.* 2006;**9**:1–13.

26. **Cohen JC, Montoya JC.** *Using technology to fight corruption in pharmaceutical purchasing: lessons learned from the Chilean experience.* Washington, DC: World Bank Institute; February 2001.

27. **Gureje O, Lasebikan VO, Ephraim-Oluwanuga O,** et al. Community study of knowledge of and attitude to mental illness in Nigeria. *British Journal of Psychiatry.* 2005;**186**:436–41.

28. **Makanjuola R.** Yoruba traditional healers in psychiatry. I. Healers' concepts of the nature and aetiology of mental disorders. *African Journal of Medicine and Medical Sciences.* 1987;**16**:53–9.

29. **Ojagbemi A, Gureje O.** The importance of faith-based mental healthcare in African urbanized sites. *Current Opinion in Psychiatry.* 2020;**33**:271–7.

30. **Iheanacho T, Stefanovics E, Ezeanolue EE.** Clergy's beliefs about mental illness and their perception of its treatability: experience from a church-based prevention of

mother-to-child HIV transmission (PMTCT) trial in Nigeria. *Journal of Religion and Health*. 2018;**57**:1483–96.

31. **Kpobi L, Swartz L, Keikelame MJ.** Ghanaian traditional and faith healers' explanatory models for epilepsy. *Epilepsy & Behaviour*. 2018;**84**:88–92.

32. **Gureje O, Nortje G, Makanjuola V**, et al. The role of global traditional and complementary systems of medicine in the treatment of mental health disorders. *Lancet Psychiatry*. 2015;**2**:168–77.

33. **Ae-Ngibise K, Cooper S, Adiibokah E**, et al. 'Whether you like it or not people with mental problems are going to go to them': a qualitative exploration into the widespread use of traditional and faith healers in the provision of mental health care in Ghana. *International Review of Psychiatry*. 2010;**22**:558–67.

34. **Sorsdahl K, Stein DJ, Grimsrud A**, et al. Traditional healers in the treatment of common mental disorders in South Africa: *Journal of Nervous and Mental Disease*. 2009;**197**:434–41.

35. **Burns JK, Tomita A.** Traditional and religious healers in the pathway to care for people with mental disorders in Africa: a systematic review and meta-analysis. *Social Psychiatry and Psychiatric Epidemiology*. 2015;**50**:867–77.

36. **Henok A, Lamaro T.** Knowledge about and attitude towards epilepsy among Menit community, Southwest Ethiopia. *Ethiopian Journal of Health Sciences*. 2017;**27**:47–58.

37. **Adjei P, Akpalu A, Laryea R**, et al. Beliefs on epilepsy in Northern Ghana. *Epilepsy & Behaviour*. 2013;**29**:316–21.

38. **Esan O, Appiah-Poku J, Othieno C**, et al. A survey of traditional and faith healers providing mental health care in three sub-Saharan African countries. *Social Psychiatry and Psychiatric Epidemiology*. 2019;**54**:395–403.

39. **Peltzer K.** Utilization and practice of traditional/complementary/alternative medicine (TM/CAM) in South Africa. *African Journal of Traditional, Complementary and Alternative Medicines*. 2009;**6**:175–85.

40. **Keikelame MJ, Swartz L.** 'By working together and caring for one another we can win this fight': A qualitative exploration of a traditional healer's perspectives of care of people with epilepsy in a South African urban township in Cape Town. *Epilepsy & Behaviour*. 2018;**79**:230–3.

41. **Makanjuola R, Jaiyeola A.** Yoruba traditional healers in psychiatry. II. Management of psychiatric disorders. *African Journal of Medicine and Medical Sciences*. 1987;**16**:61–73.

42. **Babb DA, Pemba L, Seatlanyane P**, et al. Use of traditional medicine by HIV-infected individuals in South Africa in the era of antiretroviral therapy. *Psychology, Health & Medicine*. 2007;**12**:314–20.

43. **Odinka PC, Oche M, Ndukuba AC**, et al. The socio-demographic characteristics and patterns of help-seeking among patients with schizophrenia in south-east Nigeria. *Journal of Health Care for the Poor and Underserved*. 2014;**25**:180–91.

44. **Birhan W, Giday M, Teklehaymanot T.** The contribution of traditional healers' clinics to public health care system in Addis Ababa, Ethiopia: a cross-sectional study. *Journal of Ethnobiology and Ethnomedicine*. 2011;**7**:39.

45. **Abbo C.** Profiles and outcome of traditional healing practices for severe mental illnesses in two districts of Eastern Uganda. *Global Health Action*. 2011;**4**:7117.

46. **Sorketti EA, Zainal NZ, Habil MH.** The treatment outcome of psychotic disorders by traditional healers in central Sudan. *International Journal of Social Psychiatry.* 2013;59:365–76.

47. **Nortje G, Oladeji B, Gureje O**, et al. Effectiveness of traditional healers in treating mental disorders: a systematic review. *Lancet Psychiatry.* 2016;3:154–70.

48. **Dada AO.** Old wine in new bottle. *Black Theology.* 2014;12:19–32.

49. **Nadel SF.** *Nupe religion.* Abingdon, Oxon: Routledge; 1954.

Chapter 17

Spiritual but not religious

Bruno Paz Mosqueiro

Introduction

Past few decades have been marked by an increased interest in the subject of spirituality and mental health outcomes as evidenced by a growing number of scientific publications about the impact of religiosity/spirituality (R/S). Most people worldwide report that R/S constitutes a very significant part of their lives and consistent evidence demonstrates the benefits of R/S beliefs and practices to mental health and well-being. Moreover, many people, regardless of religious affiliation, seem to search for more profound experiences of meaning, purpose, and transcendence, especially those facing adversities, loss, illness, and suffering, but also individuals experiencing feelings of emptiness or unhappiness despite access to a satisfactory and comfortable life, relationships, resources, pleasures, and professional achievements. Spirituality and religiosity, then, emerge as significant sources of meaning, hope, and awakening in face of the challenging circumstances of life.

In such a scenario, recent surveys reveal a significant number of people, especially among Western countries, describing themselves as 'spiritual but not religious' (SBNR), trying to differentiate their beliefs and faiths from those usually purposed by religious institutions and from those people without religious beliefs, such as atheists or agnostics [1].

According to the Pew Research Center Global Religion Landscape, around 16.3% of the global population (1.1 billion people) are not affiliated to any religious institutions, but, still, many of them do hold religious or spiritual beliefs [2]. Furthermore, different studies report that 27% of people in the United States describe themselves as SBNR [3], 19% in England [4] and 13.5% in a sample of depressed patients in Brazil [5].

What are the implications to mental health practice of this new way of people expressing their R/S? What are the concerns and most relevant questions about SBNR people in mental health research? How should those spiritual and personal beliefs be addressed in clinical practice? Asking those questions, this chapter presents an overview of the evidence about R/S and mental health of

SBNR individuals, and discusses the clinical implications and potential ways to address R/S in light of different mental health approaches.

Spirituality: a search for understanding

Spirituality is indeed a very recent concept in mental health. The idea of spirituality, independent of religious backgrounds, appears to be a recent phenomenon in human history. Until the twentieth century, religion and spirituality were viewed as being the same (6).

Actually, spirituality can be a quite difficult concept to define. Different definitions of spirituality have been proposed and used, but none is completely accepted (also see Chapters 1 and 2 of this volume). For some authors, it would be very difficult to differentiate spirituality from religiosity, and the combined term 'religiosity/spirituality' is usually seen in scientific literature related to both terms in a more broader concept. The limitation tin defining spirituality is reflected in the difficulties to access and measure spirituality in quantitative assessments. Not uncommonly, positive mental health constructs, such as hope, peace, purpose, and well-being are included in the measures of spirituality (7).

Interestingly, William James anticipated some concepts about spirituality that would expand over the next few decades, studying an individual subjective, inner, religious attitude of the soul, beyond religious organizations (8). According to William James

> Were one asked to characterize the life of religion in the broadest and most general terms possible, one might say that it consists of the belief that there is an unseen order, and that our supreme good lies in harmoniously adjusting ourselves thereto. This belief and this adjustment are the religious attitude in the soul (9).

James Fowler, otherwise, proposes a distinction but also a degree of interdependence between religion and faith (10). Religion could be understood as the cumulative tradition of 'various expressions of the faith of people in the past', constituted by 'texts of scripture or law, narratives, myths, prophecies, revelations, symbols, oral traditions, music, arts, ethical teachings, theologies, creeds, rites, liturgies, architecture and other elements'.

> Faith at once deeper and more personal than religion is the person's or group's way of responding to transcendent value and power as perceived and grasped through the forms of cumulative tradition. Faith and religion, in this view, are reciprocal. Each is dynamic, each grows or is renewed thought its interaction with the other. (10, p. 9)

The definition of religion seem to be clear and much more readily in comparison with the broadened definitions of spirituality in literature. This is reflected in research where most validated instruments are designed to measure the perceived degree of religiosity and its different dimensions. Therefore, one commonly used definition, especially relevant for research, distinguishes religion as an organized system of symbols, rituals, and practices designed to facilitate closeness to the sacred and transcendent. Spirituality, otherwise, has been defined as the personal quest for understanding questions about life, meaning, purpose, connected to the sacred and transcendent, which could lead or arise from religious affiliations or communities (11).

Spirituality as a personal experience

Recently, the term 'spiritual but not religious' has started appearing in the media, representing people that identify themselves in a new position of spiritual beliefs, not identified with 'atheists' and 'agnostics' on one side or 'religious traditional organizations' on the other (12–14).

In fact, SBNR people are probably not a clearly defined group of individuals, encompassing different R/S beliefs and practices. Furthermore, the very definitions of spirituality provided by people vary and this is probably another key issue within this kind of research (15). To some authors, the heterogeneity of SBNR beliefs across different populations will create a concern about its validity as a distinct concept with a defined group of believers. However, the consistency of reports across different geographical places reinforces the idea that the concept of SBNR requires genuine consideration and further research. Different authors provide terms and expressions that refer to those individuals and these include 'non-affiliated believers', 'believing without belonging', 'religious nonaffiliated theists', 'spiritual seekers', 'unchurched believers', 'religious privatism' and, of course, 'spiritual but not religious' (16).

Roof (17) distinguished an increasing number of people in the United States who were leaving traditional religious groups since 1960 and found that these followed emergence of 'new religions'. The author called 'highly active seekers' a group of educated individuals searching for spiritual development and growth, on individualized journeys, independent of religious traditions and worship (17). SBNR people would also belong to alternative spiritual movements, including holistic groups, alternative medicine practices, Yoga classes, Reiki, and spiritualist organizations. It seems that the identification of a person as SBNR really goes beyond a simple affiliation to religious groups and sometimes might not be a stable condition along life, encompassing experiences from diverse religious traditions and spiritual settings along time (16). In common, some of them share views about the *science and material reality not as the only way to undercover responses about life and truth, a questioning about secular worldviews and an objection toward conservatism in religions (13).*

A few possible reasons can be hypothesized in order to explain the expressive rise in SBNR and unaffiliated people in the United States: 1) the delay in marriage and parenthood, that traditionally bring people back to religious institutions; 2) a contemporary view of religious identification with right-wing politics, making social liberal people more prone to political detachment from religious organizations; 3) the views and policies regarding religion and secularization in Western cultures; and 4) more individualistic patterns of interpersonal relationships in postmodern society, with younger people being less engaged with organized institutions (16).

One reason for the increasing number of SBNR individuals may also be due to some culturally disseminated views of religion among more secular cultures. Religious groups are sometimes criticized as rigid, strict, and authoritarian. Moreover, some religious institutions might be viewed as distant or indifferent to ordinary people's claims, needs, and experiences. Hence, religious organizations sometimes appear to be obstacles to more individual spiritual journeys. According to Bartunek (2019), a Catholic priest in the United States, referring to close people in his life:

> I met people who (…) had grown up in religious households, but their religion had never felt spiritual. In fact, for many of them, the trappings of religion seemed to be an obstacle to real spiritual experience. They found spirituality outside of religion and spite of religion. These friends sometimes described themselves as spiritual but not religious. (18)

Spirituality and secularization

Wallach, in a comprehensive integrative perspective, states that the scientific progress and advances would be integrated with religious ideas and human experiences into a coherent world view by a 'non-dogmatic, secular spirituality a natural, even necessary, consequence for our culture and its rationality'. By spirituality, the author 'means the experiential core of any religion, as opposed to its doctrinal-dogmatic clothing', not necessarily detached from religious institutions, but certainly from any kind of dogmatisms or fundamentalisms (19).

The growing number of SBNR people in this perspective would reflect a renewal of religious and spiritual beliefs in Western societies, despite the wave of secularization especially in European countries observed after the end of World War II (20, 21). Indeed, religious and spiritual beliefs actually represent significant sources of meaning and purpose in life even in more secular societies (22).

In that regard, contrary to predictions made in the early twentieth century, reasoning and scientific advances do not overcome religiosity and spirituality. In a historical perspective, for instance, religious content has largely disappeared from science since the XIX century, 'but this does not mean that religious beliefs were no longer to be found among scientists (…) scientists with religious convictions have often found confirmation of their faith in the beauty and elegance of the mechanisms their research uncovers' (23). According to this point of view, the same would be true in society, where advances in science and technology have brought new insights, undercovering new motivations and needs, and that could represent a source of flourishing of diverse spiritual or religious ideas, not necessarily a suppression of them (also see Chapters 2 and 3 in this volume).

Spiritual but not religious: a global epidemiological perspective

According to the Pew Research Center (2), including surveys from 230 countries worldwide, 83,7% of people in the world are religious affiliated and 16.3% report no affiliation to any religious group. The religious unaffiliated include atheists, agnostics, and people who were not identified with a religious denomination in surveys. Considering the overwhelming majority of religious believers in the world, including the unconventional faiths and unchurched believers, Stark stands that 'the World is more religious than it has ever been' (20).

The religious unaffiliated are differentially distributed in the world and reflect distinct cultural and regional backgrounds (2). Most religious unaffiliated are concentrated in Asia and the Pacific (76%), specifically in China (62.2%); an additional number reside in Europe (12%), North America (5%), Latin America and the Caribbean (4%), and less frequently in Africa (2%) and the Middle East (1%). The countries with the largest absolute number of unaffiliated are China (62.2% of world unaffiliated), Japan (6.2%), the United States (4.5%), Vietnam (2.3%), Russia (2.1%), South Korea (2.0%), Germany (2.0%), France (2.0%), North Korea (1.5%), and Brazil (1.4%),whereas the countries with the largest percentages of unaffiliated (compared with their own population) are the Czech Republic (76%), North Korea (71%), Estonia (60%), Japan (57%), Hong Kong (56%), and China (52%). Interestingly, some of the countries with more religious unaffiliated historically imposed laws and policies with restrictions to religious expression (20, 24). It's not clear how many of those would identify themselves as SBNR, but, many of unaffiliated people do hold religious or spiritual beliefs (24).

In the United States, the Pew Research Center reported an increasing number of individuals who see themselves as religious unaffiliated in the past decade (2). But that does not reflect a necessary decrease in R/S beliefs in American society. The religious 'nones' (16.4% of the American population) comprise mainly people describing themselves as 'nothing in particular' (12%–17%) and to a lesser extent atheists (2%–4%) and agnostics (3%–5%). Furthermore, 7 million people in the United States (3% of the American population) report as identified with 'other faith' including 'personal religious beliefs and people who describe themselves as spiritual', a group that would be close to the definition of SBNR.

A survey in the United States using different methodological approaches reveals that an increasing number of people identify themselves as SBNR, reaching up to 27% of American population in 2017 (3). According to the research, from 2012 to 2017, there was an increase of 8% in the people describing themselves as SBNR. The questionnaire did not specifically ask if individuals were SBNR, but the results were based on the combination of two questions ('Do you think of yourself as a religious person, or not?' and 'Do you think of yourself as a spiritual person, or not?'). SBNR individuals were thus identified as those who responded 'no' to the first question and 'yes' to the second. Interestingly, 37% of SBNR individuals were not affiliated to religious groups, but 35% were Protestants, 14% Catholics and 11% members of other faiths, including Islam, Judaism, Buddhism, or Hinduism. These reports highlight the complexity of spiritual beliefs transcending the barriers of religions, but also reflect the challenges to the definition and assessment of SBNR.

Interestingly, some people who eventually describe themselves as SBNR, considering that they are not directly bounded to a specific religious tradition, would be better described as 'spiritual and multi-religious', considering their multiple search for experiences and attendance to different religious groups and traditions (25). A recent Brazilian survey (n = 1,169), for instance, identified that around one-third of Brazilians have switched religions over time, 26.3% changing their religion to another religion, and 10.4% becoming non-religious (25). Furthermore, 10.4% of adults and 8.8% of adolescents in Brazil report attendance to more than one religious group (26).

Mental health research

Importantly, a few methodological concerns must be presented in order to evaluate the studies about the SBNR population. The first is that there are still very few studies in literature regarding this population and most of them were not directly designed to study SBNR individuals. Most studies were performed in order to address religious beliefs and practices of major religious groups, and little research has been inclusive of religious minorities, atheists, agnostics, or SBNR groups (27). Second, most validated instruments to measure religious beliefs and practices are designed to evaluate R/S characteristics of predominant religious groups or, eventually, non-religious. Third, the very different

presentations, sets of beliefs, and cultural backgrounds might be another potential bias to mental health research and to generalizing those findings to SBNR
individuals worldwide. For instance, a young adult with spiritual beliefs and
practices living in a large European city and secularized Western culture might
be different from the same young adult in a small community and traditional
culture in Asia or from an eclectic spiritual background in Latin America. The
setting where the study is conducted is additionally very relevant, and this context must be well recognized. For instance, the protective effects of religiosity
over depressive symptoms seem to be higher in clinical samples compared with
general population studies (28). And finally, the prospective follow-up of individuals, controlling for other relevant psychosocial characteristics, such as social support, educational levels, and income, are certainly very important issues
to consider before further conclusions can be drawn from studies.

Clearly, consistent findings in scientific publications report the benefits of
those individuals who regularly attend religious activities and institutions (29,
30). Religious attendance, for instance, has been demonstrated to be a consistent protective factor to depression and suicide, and correlated to positive
mental health and human flourishing (29, 31, 32).

Limited research has investigated the mental health outcomes among SBNR
individuals. The third *National Psychiatric Morbidity Survey* in England, a
community-based survey with a large sample size of 7,403 respondents, included for the first time variables on religious and spiritual beliefs to evaluate
their association with mental health and psychiatric treatments (4). Participants
could state whether they had a religious or spiritual understanding of life or neither. Over 35% of respondents had a religious understanding of life, 19% had a
spiritual understanding without religious participation, and 46% were not religious or spiritual. Individuals with a spiritual understanding of life without
religious participation, after adjustments, were more likely to use psychiatric
medications, use recreational drugs, or have generalized anxiety disorder,
phobia, or eating disorder. No differences were found in psychotic disorders,
alcohol-drinking patterns, perceived happiness, and social support between
groups. The authors concluded, 'there is increasing evidence that people who
profess spiritual beliefs in the absence of a religious framework are more vulnerable to mental disorders'. Certainly, the cross-sectional association between
variables would be a limitation to further causal inferences. Nevertheless, it is
entirely possible that religious groups and practices really provide a supportive
environment to spiritual growth and development, with higher resources
leading to more healthy mental outcomes.

Another study (1) compared SBNR with religious affiliated and non-religious
individuals in 1,013 internet-recruited participants from the United States.

Contrary to other reported surveys, SBNR in this sample was represented by older women and with higher income. SBNR people scored higher in schizotypy measures (the Schizotypal Personality Disorder Scale). They also had higher scores on mystical experiences and connectedness (measured by the Mystical Experiences Scale), and were more likely to report paranormal beliefs (the Paranormal Belief Scale). The higher income, notably, in the SBNR group, may suggest that those experiences seem to be very adaptive in this sample or that higher income might provide material conditions and security to explore spirituality more deeply, compared with other groups. It is also possible that people with higher incomes were more likely to have access to the internet and hence more likely to respond to the survey, thereby making generalizability of these findings problematic.

The Landmark Spirituality and Health Survey (LSHS) examined 3,010 individuals representative of the US population, comparing religious affiliated (n = 2401), atheists (n = 83), agnostics (n = 189), and people with no religion preference (N = 329). A notable strength of this study was the more reliable assessment with in-person interviews and absolutely reduced percentage of non-responders. Religious individuals did have worse health on some individual measures including body mass index, number of chronic conditions, and physical limitations compared with atheists and agnostics, who otherwise had worse positive psychological functioning characteristics, social support relationships, and health behaviours. Religious affiliated individuals, compared to all groups, reported higher optimism, gratitude, compassion, forgiveness, and the highest levels of meaning in life, giving and receiving more social support. One interesting finding of this study was that religious non-affiliated individuals were more similar to religious affiliated in all measures, compared with atheists and agnostics (33).

Another study compared atheists, agnostics, religious affiliated, and people with religious beliefs but not affiliated (non-affiliated theists), in a representative sample of 1,714 individuals in the United States contacted by phone. Although with a reduced response rate (24.5%), physical and mental health were significantly worse for non-affiliated theists compared with other seculars and religious affiliates on most outcomes (34).

Along with reported findings, a recent Brazilian survey in a cross-sectional analysis distinctly evaluated the perceived levels of religiosity and spirituality of 1,046 Brazilian adults. The study revealed that, having higher levels of both spirituality and religiousness were more correlated to better outcomes (quality of life, optimism, happiness) than having just higher spirituality or none. (35).

Overall, religious affiliated individuals report better mental health outcomes compared with spiritual believers without religious participation. Nevertheless, considering the limited number of studies, there is no doubt that further research is necessary to understand the reported higher mental health symptomatology in SBNR individuals. A few points to be clarified in the future might include: (1) methodological improvements in definition and measurement of beliefs and practices among SBNR people; (2) a more comprehensive perspective including studies from different countries and cultural backgrounds, and diverse clinical settings and communities; and (3) prospective high-quality studies to allow clearer causal inferences about SBNR beliefs and mental health.

Clinical practice

The assessment of spiritual beliefs and mental health care of SBNR individuals should be guided by a person-centred approach, fostering therapeutic alliance, based on empathy, mutual respect, and shared goals (36). The World Psychiatric Association position statement on religion, spirituality and psychiatry specifies that spiritual assessments should be open, respectful, compassionate, and culturally sensitive to R/S beliefs and practices (37). This means that clinicians and mental health professionals should be open to listening and understanding the unique array of beliefs and practices reported by patients.

Religious communities often provide support and guidance to many patients. For those with strong spiritual beliefs who do not belong to organized faith communities, the health professionals' support might be very helpful in face of suffering and failing health. Alternative or complementary medicine practices might provide a context and tools to address R/S issues with some of those SBNR patients (38).

The clinical assessment of spiritual beliefs and practices of SBNR individuals should follow established guidelines for spiritual assessments to health care (see also Chapters 18 and 19) (39). Spiritual struggles and conflicts over religious or spiritual questions represent a source of suffering and distress, leading many patients to leave their religious communities, and these should therefore also be assessed and addressed in the mental health care of SBNR patients (40). In different circumstances, spiritual struggles are windows of opportunity and pathways to self-examination, wisdom, and spiritual growth (40, 41). Some SBNR patients might previously have been religious affiliated and facing religious struggles and conflicts, and they might eventually benefit from reconnecting to their R/S tradition or searching for a different R/S affiliation or group (see also Chapter 23). Furthermore, positive R/S coping strategies in a patient-centred approach could be identified and reinforced in clinical care as significant sources of well-being and resilience for many patients regardless of their religious affiliation (39).

James Fowler's stages of faith (10) constitute one framework to understanding spiritual growth journeys from different religious or spiritual perspectives. It is worth noting that more mature faith stages contemplate the capacity to accept diverse R/S views and will require an integration of personal beliefs, self-awareness, and flexibility. That does not necessarily mean that SBNR people are more mature compared with religious affiliated in contemplating pluralistic and comprehensive perspectives of reality. Indeed, SBNR individuals probably represent a very heterogeneous group, encompassing not only those with a deep spiritual reflection and commitment to their beliefs, philosophical principles, and trajectories, but also individuals with self-centred spiritual perspectives and immature personality, searching for different R/S experiences without serious commitment but with a more deep reflection and self-transformation.

According to research, different spiritual domains are potentially related to spiritual beliefs that could be measured and integrated to healthcare settings. The World Health Organization's cross-cultural initiative (WHOQOL project), for instance, aiming to understand what aspects of spirituality contribute to quality of life, developed a multidimensional measure of spirituality and quality of life, validated across 18 countries, appropriated to different religious, spiritual, or personal beliefs from different cultural backgrounds, including assessments of domains connection, awe, faith, hope, purpose, strength, wholeness, and purpose (42).

Diverse psychotherapeutic approaches are additionally helpful in addressing patients' R/S needs in clinical practice. In that regard, spiritually integrated psychotherapy (SIP) is increasingly common, addressing spiritual or religious contents in a context of psychological framework (43). A growing number of patients, religious affiliated or not, search for spiritual understanding and growth within psychotherapy (44). Sometimes, in a first encounter, patients may well be reluctant to discuss those experiences with therapists, concerned about how it would be interpreted, especially with patients and professionals from completely different cultural backgrounds: the same way that therapists might be reluctant to address those experiences directly with patients because of worries regarding ethical issues or lack of training and theoretical background about SIP (39).

An open, respectful, and interested consideration of patients' beliefs might be a first step to a deeper understanding of patients' R/S. Experiences of 'sacred or spiritual experiences' in psychotherapy, for instance, usually represent profound life-changing events, able to provide meaning, purpose, coherence, and healing, not uncommonly experienced beyond the barriers of religious denominations (45). They are described as experiences with God, a higher power or spiritual realm, defined by characteristics of transcendence, boundlessness, and ultimacy (45). Certainly, it is not the objective of mental health professionals to verify the ontological reality of those experiences but to provide an open respectful setting to encourage patients to freely express those experiences in psychotherapy (46).

Religious denomination, although relevant, is not necessarily a central issue in addressing spirituality in psychotherapy. Many theoretical contributions provide pathways to understand and deal with religious or spiritual questions and the psychological domains regardless of religious affiliation (19, 45, 46).

Conclusions

SBNR individuals represent a heterogeneous group of people worldwide, especially in secularized societies. Available evidence supports that religious affiliation and religious attendance seem to be protective factors to mental health. More research, in different cultural backgrounds, is required to recognize and understand SBNR individuals. An openminded, interested, and respectful approach to SBNR individuals is essential for addressing their R/S needs in mental health practice, thereby increasing therapeutic engagement and adherence.

References

1. **Willard AK, Norenzayan A.** 'Spiritual but not religious': cognition, schizotypy, and conversion in alternative beliefs. *Cognition.* 2017;**165**:137–46.

2. **Pew Research Center.** *A report on the size and distribution of the world's major religious groups as of 2010.* Washington, DC: Pew Research Center; 2012.

3. **Lipka M, Gecewicz C.** *More Americans now say they're spiritual but not religious.* Washington, DC: Pew Research Center; 2017.

4. **King M, Marston L, McManus S, Brugha T, Meltzer H, Bebbington P.** Religion, spirituality and mental health: results from a national study of English households. *British Journal of Psychiatry.* 2013;**202**(1):68–73.

5. **Mosqueiro B, Messinger M, Bauer F, Barcelos W, Uequed M, Possebon M,** et al. Interest in religion, spirituality, and spiritually integrated psychotherapy among Brazilian depressed patients. *Psychotherapy and Psychosomatics.* 2019;**88**:1–152.

6. **King MB, Koenig HG.** Conceptualising spirituality for medical research and health service provision. *BMC Health Services Research.* 2009;**9**:116.

7. **Lucchetti G, Lucchetti AL, Vallada H.** Measuring spirituality and religiosity in clinical research: a systematic review of instruments available in the Portuguese language. *Sao Paulo Medical Journal.* 2013;**131**(2):112–22.

8. **Melo W, Resende PHC.** The impact of James's varieties of religious experience on Jung's work. *History of Psychology.* 2020;**23**(1):62–76.

9. **James W.** *The varieties of religious experiences.* New York: Barnes and Noble; 2004, orig. 1902.

10. **Fowler JW.** *Stages of faith: the psychology of human development and the quest for meaning.* New York: Harper & Row; 1981.

11. **Koenig HG, King DE, Carson VB.** *Handbook of religion and health.* New York: Oxford University Press; 2012.

12. **Castella T.** Spiritual, but not religious. *BBC News Magazine*; 3 January 2013.

13. **Mercadante L.** Good news about the spiritual but not religious. United States: CNN Belief blog; 2014.

14. **Burton T.** Spiritual but not religious: inside America's rapidly growing faith group. United States: Vox; 2017.

15. **Curcio CSS.** Investigação dos conceitos de 'religiosidade e espiritualidade em amostra clínica e não-clínica em contexto brasileiro: um estudo quali-quatitativo. Brazil: Universidade Federal de Juiz de Fora; 2018.

16. **Hastings O.** Not a lonely crowd? Social connectedness, religious service attendance, and the spiritual but not religious. *Social Sciences Research.* 2016;57:63–79.

17. **Roof W.** 'Varieties of spiritual quest.' *Spiritual marketplace: baby boomers and the remaking of American religion.* Princeton, NJ: Princeton University Press; 1999.

18. **Bartunek J.** *Spiritual but not religious. The search for meaning in a material world.* Charlotte, NC: TAN Books; 2019.

19. **Wallach H.** *Secular spirituality. The next step towards enlightenment.* NY: Springer; 2015.

20. **Stark R.** *The triumph of faith. Why the world is more religious than ever.* Wilmington, DE: ISI Books; 2015.

21. **Habermas J.** Religion in the public sphere. *European Journal of Philosophy.* 2006;14:1–25.

22. **Pedersen HF, Birkeland MH, Jensen JS, Schnell T, Hvidt NC, Sørensen T,** et al. What brings meaning to life in a highly secular society? A study on sources of meaning among Danes. *Scandinavian Journal of Psychology.* 2018;59(6):678–90.

23. **John Hedley B.** Myth 25. That Modern Science Has Secularized Western Culture. In: **Numbers R** (ed.), *Galileo goes to jail and other myths about science and religion.* United States: Harvard University Press; 2009.

24. **Pew Research Center.** *A closer look at how religious restrictions have risen around the world.* Washington, DC: Pew Research Centre; 2019.

25. **Maraldi EDO, Toniol RF, Swerts DB, Lucchetti G, Leão FC, Peres MFP.** The dynamics of religious mobility: investigating the patterns and sociodemographic characteristics of religious affiliation and disaffiliation in a Brazilian sample. *International Journal of Latin American Religions.* 2020. https://doi.org/10.1007/s41603-020-00107-1

26. **Moreira-Almeida A, Pinsky I, Zaleski M, Laranjeira R.** Religious involvement and sociodemographic factors: a Brazilian national survey. *Revista de Psiquiatria Clínica.* 2010;37:12–5.

27. **Hwang K, Hammer JH, Cragun RT.** Extending religion-health research to secular minorities: issues and concerns. *Journal of Religion and Health.* 2011;50(3):608–22.

28. **Braam AW, Koenig HG.** Religion, spirituality and depression in prospective studies: a systematic review. *Journal of Affective Disorders.* 2019;257:428–38.

29. **VanderWeele TJ, Li S, Tsai AC, Kawachi I.** Association between religious service attendance and lower suicide rates among US women. *JAMA Psychiatry.* 2016;73(8):845–51.

30. **VanderWeele TJ, Balboni TA, Koh HK.** Health and spirituality. *JAMA.* 2017;**318**(6):519–20.

31. **Li S, Okereke OI, Chang S-C, Kawachi I, VanderWeele TJ.** Religious service attendance and lower depression among women—a prospective cohort study. *Annals of Behavioral Medicine.* 2016;**50**(6):876–84.

32. **VanderWeele TJ, McNeely E, Koh HK.** Reimagining health-flourishing. *JAMA.* 2019;**321**(17):1667–8.

33. **Hayward RD, Krause N, Ironson G, Hill PC, Emmons R.** Health and well-being among the non-religious: atheists, agnostics, and no preference compared with religious group members. *Journal of Religion and Health.* 2016;**55**(3):1024–37.

34. **Baker JO, Stroope S, Walker MH.** Secularity, religiosity, and health: physical and mental health differences between atheists, agnostics, and nonaffiliated theists compared to religiously affiliated individuals. *Social Science Research.* 2018;**75**:44–57.

35. **Vitorino LM, Lucchetti G, Leao FC, Vallada H, Peres MFP.** The association between spirituality and religiousness and mental health. *Scientific Reports.* 2018;**8**(1):17233.

36. **Wong KM, Cloninger CR.** A person-centered approach to clinical practice. *Focus* (American Psychiatric Publishing). 2010;**8**(2):199–215.

37. **Moreira-Almeida A, Sharma A, van Rensburg BJ, Verhagen PJ, Cook CC.** WPA position statement on spirituality and religion in psychiatry. *World Psychiatry.* 2016;**15**(1):87–8.

38. **Steinhorn DM, Din J, Johnson A.** Healing, spirituality and integrative medicine. *Annals of Palliative Medicine.* 2017;**6**(3):237–47.

39. **Moreira-Almeida A, Koenig HG, Lucchetti G.** Clinical implications of spirituality to mental health: review of evidence and practical guidelines. *Revista Brasileira de Psiquiatria.* 2014;**36**(2):176–82.

40. **Pargament KI, Lomax JW.** Understanding and addressing religion among people with mental illness. *World Psychiatry.* 2013;**12**(1):26–32.

41. **Allport GW.** *The individual and his religion. A classic study of the function of religious sentiment in the personality of the individual.* New York: Macmillan Company; 1950.

42. **Zimpel RR, Panzini RG, Bandeira DR, Fleck MP, da Rocha NS.** Psychometric properties of the WHOQOL-SRPB BREF, Brazilian Portuguese version. *Brazilian Journal of Psychiatry.* 2019;**41**(5):411–8.

43. **Rosmarin DH, Forester BP, Shassian DM, Webb CA, Björgvinsson T.** Interest in spiritually integrated psychotherapy among acute psychiatric patients. *Journal of Consulting and Clinical Psychology.* 2015;**83**(6):1149–53.

44. Andrew Powell, Christopher MacKenna. Psychotherapy. In: Chris Cook, Andrew Powell and Andrew Sims (eds), *Spirituality and psychiatry.* London: RCPsych Publications; 2009, pp. 101–19. https://www.cambridge.org/core/books/spirituality-and-psychiatry/DA5475A8B3957E3284F8951CDB8E4781

45. **Lomax JW, Kripal JJ, Pargament KI.** Perspectives on 'sacred moments' in psychotherapy. *American Journal of Psychiatry.* 2011;**168**(1):12–18. https://doi.org/10.1176/appi.ajp.2010.10050739

46. **Corbett L.** *Psyche and the sacred: spirituality beyond religion.* New York: Routledge; 2020.

Section III

Clinical practice

Chapter 18

Principles of integrating religion and spirituality in mental health care and the World Psychiatric Association's position statement

Christopher C.H. Cook and
Alexander Moreira-Almeida

Introduction

Increasing interest in religion and spirituality (R/S) in clinical practice in mental health care over the past four decades has led to debate about the nature of good practice. This debate has reflected the concerns of both patients and service users on the one hand and mental health professionals on the other. While most of the research has been positive about the potential benefits of addressing R/S concerns in clinical practice, concern has also been expressed about the potential for abuse, and for the intentional or unintentional breaching of the boundaries of good professional practice. It is also clear that R/S influences, while generally positive, can sometimes be harmful. The need arises, therefore, for clinical guidelines and policies that are supportive of good practice and make clear where the boundaries lay.

A number of national psychiatric associations have addressed this need, beginning with guidance issued by the Committee on Religion and Psychiatry of the American Psychiatric Association (APA) in 1990, followed by a position statement of the UK Royal College of Psychiatrists (RCPsych) in 2011. Since then, policies and guidance for psychiatrists have appeared in Australia and New Zealand, Canada, South Africa, and Germany (1). An international position statement on R/S in psychiatry was approved by the Executive Committee of the World Psychiatric Association (WPA) in 2015 (2). Originally written in English, this position statement has since been translated into Portuguese (3) and Spanish (4), and translations into other languages are on the way. As position statements multiply, concern has been expressed that policy documents do not always sufficiently clarify professional boundaries and that rules alone are often not adequate to the task (5). A broad range of contextual factors need to be taken into account in practice. While some things are clearly accepted as good practice, and others widely recognized as lying outside the scope of good practice, there is still much ambiguity and difference of opinion in relation to some issues.

It has been found that psychologists and psychiatrists commonly acknowledge the potential importance of R/S to mental health practice. However, this acknowledgement often does not translate into actual clinical practice. The barriers to implementation most cited are lack of training, lack of time, and fear of trespassing professional boundaries (6–9). The provision of practical guidelines has the potential to significantly ameliorate these obstacles. The WPA position statement does not provide any detailed guidance. In order to facilitate its translation into practice, and to further debate and discussion, this chapter will present and expand upon the practical implications of its seven proposals. While the views expressed here are ours alone, and do not represent WPA policy, we hope that a commentary on the proposals, and an exploration of some of the key issues raised by each one, will encourage and facilitate their translation into practice, as well as further debate. We believe that such debate is an important tool for further clarification of the nature and scope of good professional practice.

A tactful consideration of patients' religious beliefs and practices as well as their spirituality should be considered routinely and will sometimes be an essential component of psychiatric history taking

It has been acknowledged that taking a patient's spiritual history is the first and most consensual step regarding integrating R/S into clinical practice (10). There is now a large literature on assessment of R/S in clinical practice (9, 11–13), and evidence that it may improve patient compliance, satisfaction with care, and health outcomes. Yet, many psychiatrists do not enquire about these matters (10). Failure to consider or undertake such an assessment may arise for a variety of reasons, as discussed above (14).

There is consistent evidence from different countries around the globe that most patients are not only open to being questioned about R/S but actually think it should be approached in the clinical encounter and complain if it has not been addressed (10, 15).

As the RCPsych has indicated in the preamble to its recommendations (16), it is impossible to know in advance how an enquiry about R/S might be received, but there are essentially four possible attitudes that might be anticipated:

+ Identification with a particular social or historical tradition (or traditions).
+ Adoption of a personally defined, or personal but undefined, spirituality.
+ Disinterest.
+ Antagonism.

Any initial inquiry concerning R/S beliefs and practices must be framed in such a way as to work well for all four groups. It should imply neither that patients 'ought' to have such interests, nor should it hint in any way at the possibility of a negative attitude towards them on the part of the clinician making the enquiry. As the WPA position statement makes clear, this initial inquiry should be 'tactful'.

Given that clinicians are busy people and that there is a need to order clinical priorities, it may sometimes be judged within a brief initial assessment that it is not a priority to make such an enquiry, or else that it should be left until a subsequent appointment. However, given the importance of the insights into the patient's world view and self-understanding that it might yield, it should 'routinely be considered' and it may sometimes be 'essential'. Clinicians often ask when, during a consultation, is the right point at which to enquire about R/S. There is no universally 'right moment', but there are two common opportunities. One is when the patient raises the topic of R/S themselves. Another is while taking the patient's personal history, especially when asking about their social activities or interests, beliefs, and values. Usually, a brief and non-directive initial enquiry evokes a response that indicates whether or not this is a topic worthy of further discussion. For example:

CLINICIAN: 'Is religion or spirituality important to you?'

PATIENT 1: 'No—not really—I've never cared much about that kind of thing.'

On the other hand, the identical question can sometimes yield very different responses:

PATIENT 2: 'Yes—I'm a Christian. It's the most important thing in my life.'

PATIENT 3: 'No—my father was religious and he abused me every day. They're all hypocrites. It makes me angry!'

In other cases, the question would have to be worded differently. It would not be appropriate, for example, to ask the question in this way when a patient is wearing a Sikh turban, a Jewish kippah, or a Muslim hijab, or when they had already made clear that they had strong views on such things. In such circumstances, an interested enquiry concerning what is already evident would be more helpful. For example, 'I see that you are Jewish. Can you tell me more about what that means to you ... ?' demonstrates interest and at least some basic awareness of religious sensibilities, which makes it easier for the patient to talk about the topic.

Having opened up the topic, there are many possible ways to proceed and it is beyond the scope of this chapter to explore these in any detail. However, the general principle should be to adopt a patient-centred approach, within which the clinician shows willingness to explore non-judgementally, and with genuine interest, things that are important to the person whom they are seeking to help. This is as true in the case of the atheist patient who has no time for religion as it is in the case of the religious person whose life is completely shaped by it.

The various cultural contexts within which such enquiries are conducted may require different approaches. The most appropriate approach in Western secular societies may not be the best in an Islamic country such as Saudi Arabia, or in a very religious but plural country such as India. The general rule should be to make the consultation a safe space within which to discuss things that the patient considers important. Even if the patient says R/S is not relevant to them at that moment, just by asking about the topic the clinician sends a message that they are open to the subject if it becomes relevant to the patient in the future. More details on taking a spiritual history are provided in the present volume by Kao and Peteet in Chapter 19.

An understanding of religion and spirituality and their relationship to the diagnosis, etiology, and treatment of psychiatric disorders should be considered as essential components of both psychiatric training and continuing professional development

This proposal asserts both that the clinician should have an understanding of R/S and that there is a relationship between R/S and the diagnosis, aetiology, and treatment of psychiatric disorders (see Chapters 1 and 7 in the present volume). Given these two premises, it becomes important that each should be addressed in training and in continuing professional development. The WPA and other national psychiatric associations have included R/S in the core curriculum for the training of psychiatrists (17).

It is clear that most mental health professionals are unlikely to become experts in the study of R/S. Nor is it necessarily helpful if they are. The task is not to form an in-depth understanding of Christianity, or Islam, in the world today but, rather, to understand what Christianity, or Islam, means to the individual person and their family and community. Many religious people have very unorthodox religious beliefs and do not necessarily adhere to all the teachings or practices of their religion. For some, religion is deeply important, and for others it is something to which they adhere very lightly. When patients consider themselves 'spiritual but not religious', as often occurs in Europe and North America, their spirituality is usually very subjective and individual, and may include a rejection of formal religious beliefs. Spirituality of this kind can only be understood by way of interested enquiry concerning the personal beliefs and practices involved. The detailed understanding that is needed of particular spirituality or religious traditions is thus minimal, but an advanced set of skills are required in terms of clinical interviewing. Chapters 10 to 17 cover the implications to mental health of the most prevalent religious traditions in the world.

It is beyond the scope of this chapter to explore in detail the relationships between R/S and 'the diagnosis, etiology, and treatment of psychiatric disorders' (several other chapters cover that). However, it is important to note in passing that R/S themes emerge in psychopathology in various ways and that it is important not to jump to conclusions about their diagnostic significance. 'God told me to stop dating this girl ... ' may be a very normal way of talking about such things in many Christian churches. It does not imply the presence of auditory verbal hallucinations, or of any other psychopathology. Even if the patient is hearing voices, this also does not necessarily imply any psychiatric diagnosis, because many people in the population, especially in certain religious contexts, may hear voices (18, 19). However, if mental state examination reveals that such a statement is part of a more complex picture of beliefs, and perhaps associated with other psychopathology, this clearly needs more careful enquiry. Similarly, belief in djinn as spirits having influence upon human well-being, is normal in most Islamic communities, but this does not mean that no further enquiry should be made when a patient mentions them. It is important to establish a clear picture of exactly what influence they are understood to have by this particular Muslim person, how these beliefs are received by family and community, and what the implications for treatment might be if a medical diagnosis is later also advanced.

The addressing of R/S concerns in treatment is perhaps one of the most contentious aspects of all discussions about R/S in mental health care. However, there are now a variety of specific R/S interventions on offer, and it is important that clinicians are aware of these and of the research evidence base relating to them. Twelve step programmes have become so popular worldwide that it would be almost impossible to work in addictions psychiatry without at least some basic knowledge of the part that spirituality plays within them

(20–22). Mindfulness is a spiritual intervention with a strong evidence base, particularly in relation to the effective management of anxiety and depression, but it is being used increasingly in treatment of a wide range of other psychiatric disorders. It also plays a part in interventions such as compassion focused therapy and dialectical behaviour therapy. Forgiveness therapy, often incorporated within an eclectic approach to psychological therapies and not necessarily identified as a separate intervention, has been shown to be helpful in a wide range of psychiatric disorders (23). A range of other spiritually and religiously integrated forms of psychotherapy are also proving to be both effective and popular (24, 25). See Chapter 22 (Costa and Rosmarin) for a more in-depth discussion of evidence available and the strategies used to integrate R/S in psychotherapy.

The place of prayer in clinical practice remains particularly contentious (26), and is the subject of wide geographical and cultural variation in practice, some of which is culturally normative—often being welcomed by patients— and some of which is coercive and may even contravene patients' human rights (27).

Local psychiatric training schemes and programmes of continuing professional development are very variable in the extent to which they do or do not address these issues. Given the complexities of the issues that they raise for good practice and the possible breaching of professional boundaries, not to mention the potential benefits for patients, there is a need that this should change. R/S should be considered essential components of the curriculum. Examples of topics that may helpfully be addressed in continuing professional development may be found in conference programmes of the WPA Section on Religion and Spirituality or the Spirituality & Psychiatry Special Interest Group of the RCPsych (28) and in a recent review of published initiatives of implementation of a R/S curriculum in psychiatric residencies (29).

There is a need for more research on both religion and spirituality in psychiatry, especially on their clinical applications. These studies should cover a wide diversity of cultural and geographical backgrounds

There are now thousands of published studies investigating the associations of R/S with health, most of them related to mental health (30, 31). We now have evidence that R/S is usually associated with lower depression, suicide, use/ abuse of alcohol and other drugs, and higher well-being and quality of life.

Despite this, much more research is needed. There are still many unanswered research questions. Among the current challenges are understanding the mechanisms of these associations and the impact of integrating R/S in clinical and public health interventions (32, 33). There is a need for much more interdisciplinary research, not least including theology and anthropology (34). Much of the published research focuses on primarily Judeo-Christian populations. Earlier research has also made generic assumptions about the nature of spirituality, within which there is confounding between measures of spirituality and positive mental health outcome variables such as meaning in life, peacefulness, and general well-being (35). Future research either needs to develop new measures of spirituality (unconfounded by psychological variables) or else should focus on religiosity rather than spirituality (see also Chapter 1 by Moreira-Almeida).

Koenig has identified 20 broad research questions, answers to which would significantly advance understanding of the relationship between religion and mental health (30). These questions concern the following:

1. Causality.
2. Religious struggles.
3. Religiosity as a marker for mental distress.
4. Better measures of religiosity.
5. Effects across the lifespan.
6. Chronic mental illness.
7. Prevention of substance abuse.
8. Instilling human virtues.
9. Influences on physical health and neuropsychiatric functioning.
10. Caregiver adaptation.
11. Aspects of religion (or the individual).
12. Impact on relationship with God.
13. Religious transformation.
14. Religious transmission.
15. Negative effects of religion.
16. Mental health of atheists.
17. Genetic and epigenetic influences.
18. Interaction with drug treatment.
19. Efficacy of religiously integrated treatments.
20. Spiritual integration and outcomes.

The approach to religion and spirituality should be person centred. Psychiatrists should not use their professional position for proselytizing for spiritual or secular world view. Psychiatrists should be expected always to respect and be sensitive to the spiritual/religious beliefs and practices of their patients, and of the families and carers of their patients

One of the greatest concerns expressed in relation to greater attention to R/S in psychiatry is that professionals will, either intentionally or inadvertently, end up using the clinical encounter as an opportunity to promote their own faith or world view. It was this concern particularly that led to the introduction of the APA guidelines in 1990 (36). This should never happen if psychiatrists adopt a truly person-centred approach (37, 38). Clinicians should address what is relevant and meaningful to the patient, not to the clinician personally (10). When problems do arise, they may be concerned as much with the imposition of a secular world view as with proselytizing for a religious one. Patients and carers often do not feel that their spiritual/religious views are properly understood or respected by health professionals (39). There is evidence that physicians' political views have an impact on their clinical decisions (40) and that it is common for patients in psychotherapy convert to therapists' values (41, 42).

One example of inadvertently and surreptitiously imposing anti-spiritual views is when clinicians give feedback to patients implicitly interpreting religious thoughts or coping strategies as necessarily immature defences. Patients may also read negative non-verbal cues provided by clinicians when they bring some R/S content into the conversation. In some religious communities, this problem is so severe as to discourage patients from seeking help from mental health professionals at all. On the other side, clinicians need also to avoid the other extreme, imposing R/S views. For example, suggesting a religious practice or interpretation that is not part of a patient's life will rarely, if ever, be appropriate. Active engagement in pursuing a patient-centred approach, and avoiding imposing clinicians' own values, should be a constant principle of good practice.

Psychiatrists, whatever their personal beliefs, should be willing to work with leaders/members of faith communities, chaplains and pastoral workers, and others in the community, in support of the well-being of their patients, and should encourage their multidisciplinary colleagues to do likewise

It is often difficult to know how to evaluate patients' beliefs and practices without intimate knowledge of the faith community to which they belong. Information gained from a conversation with a priest, imam, or rabbi of their congregation can yield invaluable information about what is understood locally as 'normal'. Equally, adherence to treatment plans may be poor where there are conflicts or misunderstandings regarding compatibility with R/S beliefs. Many of these misunderstandings can be avoided when a trusted chaplain or religious leader can explain, or affirm, the treatments on offer.

In our experience, when there are religious disagreements regarding treatment, it is very useful to ask patients for permission to contact one of their religious leaders or clergy. Rather than assuming a confrontative posture, it is then possible to stress how the religious community has been important to the patient and to invite the religious leader to join as a partner to help the patient in achieving a full and stable recovery. This approach is often very useful in transforming opposition into collaboration with treatment. However, it is important to be clear that the religious leader is someone in whom the patient has confidence, and that they will not simply provide an additional source of pressure to change legitimately held R/S beliefs.

Mental health chaplains bring a different, if also ambiguous and often misunderstood, perspective to clinical care than do other mental health professionals (43). While they are usually (not always) anchored in a particular religious tradition with which they self-identify, most are willing to offer care to people of all faiths and none. Having a better understanding of religion than most mental health professionals, and a better understanding of mental health than most clergy, they sit somewhere on the margins of the structures of both the health service and the community of faith. This enables them to have conversations with patients that others—such as psychiatrists or other clergy—are not so easily able to have.

A successful initiative of the APA, in collaboration with the APA Foundation and the Interfaith Disability Advocacy Coalition (a programme of the American Association of People with Disabilities), is the Mental Health and Faith Community Partnership that aims to foster collaboration and mutual education between psychiatrists and clergy.[1]

---

[1] www.psychiatry.org/faith

In addition, faith communities have provided a large proportion of health care worldwide and have been successfully involved in preventive programmes in public health (44). Preventive campaigns for suicide and substance abuse are two examples of potentially effective partnerships between faith communities and public mental health providers. A few years ago, *The Lancet* published a series of articles on the potential of faith-based health care for global health and discussed several related opportunities, challenges, and proposals (45, 46).

Psychiatrists should demonstrate awareness, respect and sensitivity to the important part that spirituality and religion play for many staff and volunteers in forming a vocation to work in the field of mental health care

It may be easy to imagine that R/S is only a patient-facing issue. In fact, a person-centred approach should properly pervade the work of the whole mental health team, with mutual respect shown between colleagues of strongly differing religious or spiritual perspectives. Historically, mental health professionals have been more likely to be agnostic or atheist than their patients (47), but this should not obscure the extent to which many do have strong R/S convictions. Many staff and volunteers work in the healthcare setting because they understand it as a part of their spiritual or religious vocation to do so (48). A large study in the US found that religious psychiatrists reported a stronger sense of calling in the practice of medicine (49) and that this sense of calling related to higher levels of career satisfaction and lower burnout (50). We may expect that these findings would apply also to other mental health professionals. Mutual respect between members of the mental health team with strongly differing views is likely to have an indirect benefit in encouraging mutual respect between clinicians and patients.

Psychiatrists' own R/S beliefs influence their attitudes to R/S in clinical practice, and clinical practice in turn may have an impact on their beliefs (7, 14). It is therefore helpful for psychiatrists to have the opportunity to discuss these interrelationships in a safe environment, with others who are exploring similar concerns. The Spirituality and Psychiatry Special Interest Group of the RCPsych has sought to provide such support in the UK since 1999 (28, 51).

Psychiatrists should be knowledgeable concerning the potential for both benefit and harm of religious, spiritual, and secular world views and practices, and be willing to share this information in a critical but impartial way with the wider community in support of the promotion of health and well-being

Religious, spiritual, and secular world views and practices are all potentially associated, in the mental healthcare context and in wider society, with both benefits and harms. The responsibility of the psychiatrist is to be knowledgeable about these harms and benefits, and to take an objective and impartial view of them, playing a part in the education of both patients and the wider community concerning them (52).

Whilst it is sometimes difficult to make distinctions between 'healthy' and 'unhealthy' spirituality, it is undoubtedly the case that some forms of R/S can be harmful to mental wellbeing (53). In this sense, William James's pragmatic approach may be very useful: 'In the end it had to come to our empiricist criterion: By their fruits ye shall know them, not by their roots' (54, p. 20). How is R/S having an impact on a person's life? Is it promoting flourishing or stagnation (55), constructive or destructive behaviours? While there is extensive evidence for the mental health benefits of intrinsic religiosity and positive religious coping, extrinsic religiosity is not conducive to mental well-being and negative religious coping may be positively harmful (56). For more details on negative religious coping, see Chapter 24 (Pargament).

In an age of global terrorism and radicalization, psychiatrists are sometimes called upon to comment on the relationships between religion, mental illness, and acts of terror. The relationships are complex (57, 58) and not easily reduced to sound bites. Whatever the psychiatrist's own beliefs, it is important to be able to discuss these complex connections objectively, critically, and with a view to the good of the whole community, including those who belong to faith communities appalled at the atrocities perpetrated in their name.

Elsewhere (52) Moreira-Almeida et al. have provided guidelines for public dissemination of information regarding R/S in relation to mental health:

◆ It should be possible to back up whatever is said with solid research data.

◆ Simplistic explanations for the effects of R/S on health should be avoided.

- When interpreting findings, it is important to be careful always to mention the limitations and alternative explanations.
- Stereotyping, or fostering competition or animosity between religious groups, should be avoided.

Conclusions

Spirituality and religion are powerful factors shaping human beliefs and self-understanding. They usually tend to be supportive of mental well-being, but can also have adverse effects on mental health. In clinical practice, these potential harms and benefits can easily be managed, or mismanaged, in a variety of ways, many of which are contextual and may be difficult to understand across religious, spiritual, or cultural boundaries. Proposals such as those provided by the WPA position statement, are thus helpful and important as a guide to consensus on good practice. However, they do not substitute for (on the contrary, they were designed to foster) ongoing professional debate, and they further highlight the need for inclusion of spirituality and religion as important topics in psychiatric training and in programmes of continuing professional development.

References

1. **Cook CCH.** Spirituality and religion in psychiatry: the impact of policy. *Mental Health, Religion & Culture.* 2017;**20**(6):589–94.
2. **Moreira-Almeida A, Sharma A, van Rensburg BJ, Verhagen PJ, Cook CCH.** WPA position statement on spirituality and religion in psychiatry. *World Psychiatry.* 2016;**15**(1):87–8.
3. **Moreira-Almeida A, Sharma A, van Rensburg BJ, Verhagen PJ, Cook CCH.** WPA position statement on spirituality and religion in psychiatry. *Revista Debates em Psiquiatria.* 2018;**15**(Mar/Apr):6–8.
4. **Moreira-Almeida A, Sharma A, Van Rensburg BJ, Verhagen PJ, Cook CCH.** Declaración de la posición de la WPA sobre la espiritualidad y la religión en la psiquiatría. *Actas Españolas de Psiquiatría* . 2018;**46**:246–8.
5. **Poole R, Cook CCH, Higgo R.** Psychiatrists, spirituality and religion. *The British Journal of Psychiatry.* 2019;**214**:181–2.
6. **Lee E, Baumann K.** German psychiatrists' observation and interpretation of religiosity/spirituality. *Evidence-Based Complementary and Alternative Medicine: eCAM.* 2013;**2013**:280168.
7. **Menegatti-Chequini MC, Goncalves JP, Leao FC, Peres MF, Vallada H.** A preliminary survey on the religious profile of Brazilian psychiatrists and their approach to patients' religiosity in clinical practice. *BJPsych Open.* 2016;**2**(6):346–52.

8. **Rosmarin DH, Green D, Pirutinsky S, McKay D.** Attitudes toward spirituality/religion among members of the Association for Behavioral and Cognitive Therapies. *Professional Psychology: Research and Practice.* 2013;**44**(6):424–33.

9. **Lucchetti G, Bassi RM, Lucchetti AL.** Taking spiritual history in clinical practice: a systematic review of instruments. *Explore (NY).* 2013;**9**(3):159–70.

10. **Moreira-Almeida A, Koenig HG, Lucchetti G.** Clinical implications of spirituality to mental health: review of evidence and practical guidelines. *Revista Brasileira de Psiquiatria.* 2014;**36**(2):176–82.

11. **Gomi S, Starnino VR, Canda ER.** Spiritual assessment in mental health recovery. *Community Mental Health Journal.* 2014;**50**(4):447–53.

12. **Payman V.** The importance of taking a religious and spiritual history. *Australasian Psychiatry.* 2016;**24**(5):434–6.

13. **Culliford L, Eagger S.** Assessing spiritual needs. In: **Cook C, Powell A, Sims A,** (eds), *Spirituality and psychiatry.* London: Royal College of Psychiatrists Press; 2009, pp. 16–38.

14. **Menegatti-Chequini MC, Maraldi EO, Peres MFP, Leao FC, Vallada H.** How psychiatrists think about religious and spiritual beliefs in clinical practice: findings from a university hospital in Sao Paulo, Brazil. *Brazilian Journal of Psychiatry.* 2019;**41**(1):58–65.

15. **Best M, Butow P, Olver I.** Do patients want doctors to talk about spirituality? A systematic literature review. *Patient Education and Counseling.* 2015.

16. **Cook CCH.** *Recommendations for psychiatrists on spirituality and religion.* London: Royal College of Psychiatrists; 2013. Report No.: PS03/2013.

17. **López-Ibor JJ, Okasha A, Ruiz P, Katona C, Mak FL.** *World Psychiatric Association institutional program on the core training curriculum for psychiatry.* Yokohama, Japan: World Psychiatric Association; 2002.

18. **Cook CCH.** *Hearing voices, demonic and divine: scientific and theological perspectives.* London: Routledge; 2018.

19. **Moreira-Almeida A, Cardeña E.** Differential diagnosis between non-pathological psychotic and spiritual experiences and mental disorders: a contribution from Latin American studies to the ICD-11. *Revista Brasileira de Psiquiatria.* 2011;**33**(Suppl. 1):S29–S36.

20. **Dermatis H, Galanter M.** The role of twelve-step-related spirituality in addiction recovery. *Journal of Religion and Health.* 2016;**55**(2):510–21.

21. **Cook CCH.** Addiction and spirituality. *Addiction.* 2004;**99**:539–51.

22. **Cook CCH.** Substance misuse. In: **Cook C, Powell A, Sims A,** (eds), *Spirituality and psychiatry.* London: Royal College of Psychiatrists Press; 2009, pp. 139–68.

23. **Enright RD, Fitzgibbons RP.** *Forgiveness therapy: an empirical guide for resolving anger and restoring hope.* Washington, DC: American Psychological Association; 2015.

24. **Pargament KI.** *Spiritually integrated psychotherapy.* New York: Guilford Press; 2011.

25. **Rosmarin DH.** *Spirituality, religion, and cognitive-behavioral therapy.* New York: Guilford Press; 2018. 230 p.

26. **Poole R, Cook CCH.** Praying with a patient constitutes a breach of professional boundaries in psychiatric practice. *British Journal of Psychiatry.* 2011;**199**(2):94–8.

27. **Ofori-Atta A, Attafuah J, Jack H, Baning F, Rosenheck R,** Joining Forces Research C. Joining psychiatric care and faith healing in a prayer camp in Ghana: randomised trial. *The British Journal of Psychiatry*. 2018;**212**(1):34–41.

28. **Powell A, Cook CCH.** Spirituality and Psychiatry Special Interest Group of the Royal College of Psychiatrists. *Reaching the spirit*. Social perspectives network study day, paper 9. London: Social Perspectives Network; 2006. p. 33.

29. **Hathaway, David B**, de Oliveira e Oliveira, Fabrício H. A, Mirhom, Mena, Moreira-Almeida, Alexander, Fung, Wai Lun Alan, Peteet, John R. Teaching spiritual and religious competencies to psychiatry residents. *Academic Medicine*. 2021. Publish Ahead of Print. doi: 10.1097/ACM.0000000000004167.

30. **Koenig HG.** *Religion and mental health: research and clinical applications*. Academic Press: London; 2018. 363 p.

31. **Koenig HG.** Research on religion, spirituality, and mental health: a review. *Canadian Journal of Psychiatry*. 2009;**54**(5):283–91.

32. **Moreira-Almeida A.** Religion and health: the more we know the more we need to know. *World Psychiatry*. 2013;**12**(1):37–8.

33. **Idler E, Levin J, VanderWeele TJ, Khan A.** Partnerships between public health agencies and faith communities. *American Journal of Public Health*. 2019;**109**(3):346–7.

34. **Dein S, Cook CCH, Koenig H.** Religion, spirituality, and mental health. *Journal of Nervous and Mental Disease*. 2012;**200**(10):852–5.

35. **Koenig HG.** Concerns about measuring 'spirituality' in research. *Journal of Nervous and Mental Disease*. 2008;**196**(5):349–55.

36. **Committee on Religion and Psychiatry.** Guidelines regarding possible conflict between psychiatrists' religious commitments and psychiatric practice. *American Journal of Psychiatry*. 1990;**147**(4):542.

37. **Royal College of Psychiatrists.** *Person-centred care: implications for training in psychiatry*. London: Royal College of Psychiatrists; 2018. 46 p.

38. **RCPsych Person-Centred Training and Curriculum Scoping Group.** Training in psychiatry: making person-centred care a reality. *BJPsych Bulletin*. 2019;**43**(3):136–40.

39. **Foskett J, Marriott J, Wilson-Rudd F.** Mental health, religion and spirituality: attitudes, experience and expertise among mental health professionals and religious leaders in Somerset. *Mental Health, Religion & Culture*. 2004;**7**(1):5–22.

40. **Peteet JR, Rodriguez VB, Herschkopf MD, McCarthy A, Betts J, Romo S,** et al. Does a therapist's world view matter? *Journal of Religion and Health*. 2016;**55**(3):1097–1106.

41. **Kelly TA, Strupp HH.** Patient and therapist values in psychotherapy: perceived changes, assimilation, similarity, and outcome. *Journal of Consulting and Clinical Psychology*. 1992;**60**:34–40.

42. **Tjeltveit AC.** The ethics of value conversion in psychotherapy: appropriate and inappropriate therapist influence on client values. *Clinical Psychology Review*. 1986;**6**:515–37.

43. **Harrison S.** What is a mental health chaplain *for*? In: **Fletcher J,** (ed.), *Chaplaincy and spiritual care in mental health settings*. London: Jessica Kingsley; 2019, pp. 19–30.

44. **Schumann C, Stroppa A, Moreira-Almeida A.** The contribution of faith-based health organisations to public health. *International Psychiatry*. 2011;**8**(3):62–4.

45. **Summerskill W, Horton R.** Faith-based delivery of science-based care. *Lancet.* 2015;**386**(10005):1709–10.

46. **Duff JF, Buckingham WW.** Strengthening of partnerships between the public sector and faith-based groups. *Lancet.* 2015;**386**(10005):1786–94.

47. **Cook CCH.** The faith of the psychiatrist. *Mental Health, Religion & Culture.* 2011;**14**(1):9–17.

48. **Carson VB, Koenig HG.** *Spiritual caregiving: healthcare as ministry.* Philadelphia, PA: Templeton Press; 2004. 242 p.

49. **Yoon JD, Shin JH, Nian AL, Curlin FA.** Religion, sense of calling, and the practice of medicine: findings from a national survey of primary care physicians and psychiatrists. *Southern Medical Journal.* 2015;**108**(3):189–95.

50. **Yoon JD, Daley BM, Curlin FA.** The association between a sense of calling and physician well-being: a national study of primary care physicians and psychiatrists. *Academic Psychiatry.* 2017;**41**(2):167–73.

51. **Powell A.** The spirituality and psychiatry special interest group of the Royal College of Psychiatrists. In: **Cook C, Powell A, Sims A,** (eds), *Spirituality and psychiatry.* London: RCPsych Press; 2009, pp. xv–xviii.

52. **Moreira-Almeida A, Cordeiro Q, Koenig HG.** Ethical considerations regarding religion/spirituality in psychiatric research. In: **Peteet J, Dell ML, Fung WLA,** (eds), *Ethical considerations at the intersection of psychiatry and religion.* New York: Oxford University Press; 2018, pp. 247–58.

53. **Crowley N, Jenkinson G.** Pathological spirituality. In: **Cook C, Powell A, Sims A,** (eds), *Spirituality and psychiatry.* London: Royal College of Psychiatrists Press; 2009, pp. 254–72.

54. **James W.** *The varieties of religious experience.* Harmondsworth, UK: Penguin; 1985.

55. **VanderWeele TJ.** On the promotion of human flourishing. *Proceedings of the National Academy of Sciences of the USA.* 2017;**114**(31):8148–56.

56. **Pargament KI, Smith BW, Koenig HG, Perez L.** Patterns of positive and negative religious coping with major life stressors. *Journal for the Scientific Study of Religion.* 1998;**37**(4):710–24.

57. **Coid JW, Bhui K, MacManus D, Kallis C, Bebbington P, Ullrich S.** Extremism, religion and psychiatric morbidity in a population-based sample of young men. *The British Journal of Psychiatry.* 2016;**209**(6):491–7.

58. **Bhui K, James A, Wessely S.** Mental illness and terrorism. *BMJ.* 2016;**354**:i4869.

Chapter 19

Spiritually and culturally sensitive evidence-based approaches to taking a spiritual history

Larkin Kao and John Peteet

Introduction

Given the demonstrated relationship between religion and spirituality (R/S) and mental health, and the recommendations from the World Psychiatric Association to take a spiritual history (1), the question arises of how mental health clinicians should integrate patients' R/S into clinical care. Answering this question relies on the clinician understanding both the patient's R/S, as well as the patient's preferences on whether and how they would like R/S included in his care. The process of gathering this information is known as 'taking a spiritual history'—the first, and most basic, step in incorporating R/S into clinical practice (1–4).

In this chapter, we address reasons to take a spiritual history, the question of whether mental health professionals gather this information, and commonly cited barriers to taking a spiritual history. We then describe various methods of taking a spiritual history, along with a discussion of challenges and nuances that may arise in different clinical and cultural scenarios. The chapter concludes with a summary of areas for future study.

Why take a spiritual history?

To understand the patient as a whole person

In caring for the patient as a whole person, mental health clinicians seek to understand not only a patient's presenting symptoms, sometimes referred to as 'what's the matter', but also what is important to the patient, or 'what matters'. Given the high proportion of the world's population who describe R/S as important (5), inquiring about spirituality can be an important way for the clinician to understand what matters to the patient, while also learning mental health information.

For example, hearing about a patient's relationship with a higher power may reveal not only their spirituality, but also their object relations (6) and/or attachment style (7–9). A patient's difficulty trusting a religious group may expose broader issues with trust, and their description of their prayer life may reveal an otherwise hidden source of strength amidst suffering. For patients who describe their mental health in spiritual rather than clinical language, the R/S history can elucidate symptoms that would otherwise go unnoticed. Consider a devout Catholic patient who denies feeling depressed when asked directly, but describes intense guilt and dysphoria due to feeling separated from God when asked about spirituality. These are a few of many potential examples of R/S information providing clinicians with key details regarding patients' relationships, development, coping skills, and mental health history.

To aid diagnosis and treatment

These details become particularly important when patients present with symptoms that may represent either a psychiatric disorder or a culturally normative experience. For example, if a patient reports hearing religious omens, it is important to know if this is common in the patient's community or belief system, or if these occurrences began abruptly or with other symptoms, possibly suggesting mania or psychosis (10–12). This knowledge can help the clinician to bolster a patient's coping resources and avoid inaccurately pathologizing R/S beliefs. As one example, some Muslim patients attribute negative medical symptoms to *jinn*, invisible spirits that may be evil in nature (13). A thorough R/S history would clarify that a patient's description of a physical symptom arising from *jinn* need not represent a somatic delusion, and may instead reveal sources of meaning and support for the patient. In a study of patients with religious delusions in Switzerland and Canada, its authors note that even delusional religious beliefs may provide potential coping resources for patients (12). By taking a spiritual history, providers can understand the complexity of a patient's views and avoid dismissing or stigmatizing beliefs (12).

Spiritual histories can similarly aid in treatment planning. For a patient who shares that they find support and healing through prayer or attending religious services, these activities can be encouraged to enhance recovery. For a patient who feels that mental health care should come exclusively from a religious leader, or that spiritual healing is preferred over a psychiatric medication, clinicians can better advise the patient if these preferences are known. Patients' beliefs can also guide clinicians as to whether to recommend interventions whose origins overlap with spiritual traditions. For example, Marsha Linehan's dialectical behaviour therapy is heavily influenced by Zen Buddhism (14, 15). Depending on a patient's views towards Buddhism, this treatment could be perceived as either helpful or unacceptable. Similarly, the emphasis of Alcoholics Anonymous (AA) on a higher power carries R/S connotations for some patients (16–18). When recommending a group treatment for alcohol use disorder, understanding the patient's R/S can help a clinician choose whether to recommend AA or a more secular programme.

Even more attention to patients' beliefs and preferences is needed when considering interventions with unambiguous R/S content, such as referral to pastoral counselling or spiritually integrated therapy (19, 20). These treatments can be extraordinarily helpful to some patients, as discussed in other chapters. However, assuming that a patient wants these interventions or others based on incomplete information can lead to therapeutic ruptures or boundary transgressions. For example, consider a clinician recommending that a patient attend synagogue as behavioural activation, or see a rabbi for Jewish counselling, after the patient identifies as Jewish on an intake form. However, the patient considers themself secularly Jewish and associates organized religion with coercion. Gathering a full spiritual history allows clinicians to recommend interventions without assumptions, minimizing the possibility of unwanted or otherwise harmful R/S recommendations.

To respect patients' preferences

Though patients may be reticent to bring up R/S beliefs, many wish for R/S questions to be asked in healthcare settings (21, 22), particularly when discussing mental illness (23). In a US study of internal medicine patients aged 55 and older diagnosed with depression or anxiety, 83% described discussing spiritual issues as either somewhat or extremely important when receiving counselling for a mental disorder. No patient in this survey described discussing R/S as not important at all (24). In a study of patients with schizophrenia in Switzerland, one-quarter of the patients reported wishing very much to discuss R/S issues with their respective psychiatrists (25). In a sample of all psychiatric outpatients and inpatients in a hospital in Australia, 82% of patients reported belief that therapists should be aware of patients' R/S beliefs, and 69% reported that patients' spiritual needs should be considered by providers when treating mental illness (26). Two systematic literature reviews of patients' preferences with physicians in general (not limited to psychiatrists) similarly identified themes of patients desiring spiritual discussion to promote holistic care (27, 28), strengthen the doctor–patient relationship (29), allow the doctor to consider religious preferences in treatment recommendations (30, 31), and provide opportunities for chaplaincy referral (28, 32, 33). While clinicians seek to know what matters to their patients, patients appreciate feeling known and understood by their providers.

In line with these themes, inclusion of R/S discussions with patients has been shown to correlate with enhanced trust and better treatment adherence. In a US survey of general medical patients, 66%–81% stated they would trust a physician more if the physician asked about R/S (22). In a randomized controlled study of outpatients with schizophrenia in Switzerland, patients received either care as usual, or had a spiritual history gathered by a psychiatrist. At three-month follow-up, the control group and spiritual history groups did not differ regarding patient satisfaction or medication adherence, but the spiritual history group showed significantly better appointment attendance, with only 8% missing appointments as compared with 26% in the control group (25). Though this is a small study that does not show causation, the results suggest that taking a spiritual history could enhance mental health care access and engagement.

To directly benefit patients

The evidence above focuses on why clinicians should take a R/S history to better understand and respect patients, leading to better care. In some instances, the spiritual history appears to be therapeutic in itself. In a Brazilian study in which 50 healthcare students interviewed 362 patients with a spiritual history instrument, 85.1% of participants reported that their patients appeared to have appreciated the spiritual approach, and 47.5% reported that the patients appeared to feel better after the interview (34). Similar and enduring results were found when patients were surveyed in the OASIS study. In this study, out of 118 consecutive patients in a US oncology clinic, every second patient had a spiritual history gathered. After three weeks, those for whom a spiritual history had been gathered reported a greater sense of interpersonal caring from their physicians, less depression, and better quality of life (35). Though many clinicians fear that the spiritual history will make patients uncomfortable, these studies suggest that the opposite may be true.

Do mental health clinicians take spiritual histories?

Based on the above reasons to take a spiritual history, it is not surprising that healthcare professionals and students report interest in incorporating R/S into care (36, 37). This interest is even higher in mental health professionals. Compared with other US physicians, US psychiatrists are more likely to report that they inquire about patients' R/S (reported by 87% of psychiatrists compared with 49% of other physicians), and more likely to believe that it is appropriate to ask patients about R/S (93% of psychiatrists vs 53% of other physicians) (38).

In countries where the general population's emphasis on R/S is higher than that in the US, one would predict that an even larger proportion of mental health professionals consider patients' R/S important.

Unfortunately, there is a gap between this acknowledgment of the importance of R/S and actual practice. Most physicians report that they have never addressed R/S in practice (39) and patients continue to have undetected R/S needs (40). One hypothesized reason for the lack of incorporation of R/S into care is the relative dearth of training provided on how to take a spiritual history. Only 7% of US medical schools (41) and 10% of Brazilian medical schools (42) have specific courses on R/S and health. Other commonly cited barriers to taking spiritual histories include lack of time, discomfort with the topic, and fear of imposing R/S views on patients (34, 36, 43, 44). Popular perceptions of mental health care have been proposed as another obstacle. Although R/S groups were often historically the sole purveyors of mental health care (45), and continue to play this role in some cultures today, in other contexts, mental health care and R/S are viewed as antithetical (see Chapter 3). This view may affect clinicians' willingness or interest to bring up R/S topics, as well as patients' inclination to share beliefs with clinicians. These effects of patients' and clinicians' attitudes towards R/S likely vary across cultures, and have not been formally studied.

In summary, despite the potential benefits of the spiritual history to both patients and clinicians, most health professionals do not gather a spiritual history. To address some of the proposed barriers of lack of training, lack of time, and fear of boundary violations, the next section focuses on practical, time-effective, ethical techniques of taking a spiritual history.

How to take a spiritual history

General principles

While questionnaires and mnemonic devices exist to help clinicians take a spiritual history, as Culliford eloquently describes, 'Taking a spiritual history is best thought of as a clinical skill to acquire and hone, rather than an activity to be performed by recipe or rote. It is a skill that requires empathic engagement with the patient, which therefore sanctions the judicious use of both intuition and initiative on the part of the assessor' (46). Here we describe four principles to aid assessment.

1. *Create an open environment.* A study of psychiatric patients in England describing key elements of spiritual care revealed the importance to patients of sympathetic and confidential listening, feeling valued and trusted, and being treated with respect and dignity (47). These principles are important

in any type of clinical encounter but can be particularly critical when speaking about R/S, a topic that may feel especially private to vulnerable patients. Moreira-Almeida and colleagues emphasize the importance of being open-minded and person-centred to convey appreciation of all aspects of the patient's life, including R/S (2).

Practically speaking, achieving an open environment can be aided by gathering the spiritual history in a confidential, quiet space. While this is often expected in a private clinic room, adjustments may be needed in a crowded emergency room or shared hospital room. In any setting, clinicians are encouraged to use a gentle, unhurried manner. As time constraints often exist in clinical care, it can be helpful to acknowledge these constraints and share with patients that the spiritual history may require conversations across several visits (46). This approach also allows trust to develop as the history is gathered iteratively (48, 49).

2. *Reflect on one's own R/S history prior to interviewing patients*. The goal of this reflection is to minimize potential negative effects of countertransference (50). While most clinicians aim to listen to patients with curiosity rather than judgement, this is not always the natural reaction to hearing about a patient's R/S. Consider a patient who identifies strongly as Buddhist and explains to their clinician how much they value Buddhist meditation. However, they share that they do not believe in samsara, the Buddhist conception of a cycle of life and afterlife. For a Buddhist clinician who believes in samsara, this could seem blasphemous, eliciting feelings that the patient is undermining their shared belief system. For a non-Buddhist provider, hearing about this or other beliefs could provoke feelings that the patient's thinking is magical or delusional on the one hand, or limited and concrete on the other. Either situation could harm the therapeutic alliance. Positive countertransference may arise as well, especially if a patient shares the clinician's world view. This has the potential to be equally harmful if the clinician crosses therapeutic boundaries or otherwise strays from standard care. Being grounded in one's own R/S can help clinicians to be attuned to their reactions to patients' histories, fostering unbiased, non-judgemental care.

3. *Listen actively*. The clinician must listen carefully to the patient's responses to R/S questions, and should also attend to clues to R/S information elsewhere in the interview and in the patient's body language. Some have referred to the latter as the implicit spiritual history, contrasted with the explicit history (51). A patient's hunch in posture at the mention of a religious institution, or a decrease in speech volume upon speaking of prayer content, are examples of the non-verbal implicit history. A patient who rejects the terms

'spirituality' or 'religion' may speak of finding peace in nature, or feeling comforted by the meaning found in sharing wisdom with his grandchildren. These parts of the patient's life may relate to R/S in a manner comparable to another patient's synagogue attendance or prayers (51). Other patients may wish to describe an aspect of their R/S, only to find the experience difficult to articulate in words. Spirituality is at times inchoate, even if the clinician is open-minded and the patient wants to share. As Griffith states, part of the clinician's job is 'to listen for that which has not yet been expressed' (51, 52). Hodge suggests that a clinician's 'spiritual radar' must function throughout all sections of the patient's interview, emphasizing the importance of active listening and observation (48).

4. *Take a spiritual history routinely.* While many patients wish for clinicians to discuss R/S, prior to broaching the topic, there is no way to tell who will desire or eschew this discussion. Given the power dynamic in clinician–patient relationships, and the common patient fear that clinicians will react to R/S information with judgement or disinterest, the clinician should initiate the conversation.

Specific guidelines

With the above principles in mind, several tools are available to aid clinicians with the spiritual history. First, a distinction may be made between screening and assessment questions. In many cases, one to two brief screening questions can help determine whether a patient wants further discussion of his R/S. Culliford suggests asking the patient either if he is religious or spiritual, or where he finds strength in difficult circumstances (46). These open-ended prompts invite the patient into conversation and allow the clinician to tailor subsequent discussion to patient preferences. Consider a patient who responds to screening questions by stating that they identify as Christian. The clinician might then ask about the importance of Christianity to this patient, and what beliefs and practices are important to them or have affected their mental health. Alternatively, when asked if they are religious or spiritual, another patient may reply that they identify as Christian culturally, but do not view themself as spiritual or religious. A simple prompt regarding where this patient finds strength could allow them to share about how secular meditation helps them to cope with stress, or might reveal their interest or ambivalence about exploring other faiths. In any of these scenarios, screening questions provide the clinician with information to guide the interview.

Especially for patients who share during screening that their sense of meaning, hope, or strength may not fit with the terms 'spiritual' or 'religious', prompts focused on the implicit spiritual history can be useful. For example, one might ask about a patient's sense of meaning in life, to whom or what a patient is grateful or devoted, or what stands in the way of a patient living their fullest life. In difficult times, the clinician might ask about sources of peace during prior difficult times, or for whom or what a patient perseveres. These and other prompts are described in more detail in Griffith and Griffith's *Encountering the Sacred* in psychotherapy (51). As patients respond to these and other implicit prompts, a nuanced vocabulary may become apparent. A patient may use terms such as 'religion' in a manner unique to their own beliefs, such as referring to his secular soccer league as their church. Other patients may share terms specific to their respective backgrounds, such as alluding to the Word of Wisdom regarding health practices encouraged in the Church of Latter Day Saints. Culliford emphasizes the importance of clinicians avoiding jargon or potentially ambiguous terms, opting for ordinary language instead (46). As the patient shares their own terms, the clinician can ask the patient to clarify what each term means to them.

Using the above implicit history prompts has the advantage of flexibility. In other cases, clinicians may wish to have more guidance following the initial R/S screening. In a 2013 systematic review of the literature, Lucchetti and colleagues found 25 instruments for taking a spiritual history, and evaluated each one based on 16 criteria including ease of memorization, validation, and aspects of R/S covered (4). Two instruments were developed specifically for mental health: The Royal College of Psychiatrists (RCP) assessment (53) and the spiritual assessment interview (54). The highest-ranked instrument was the FICA Spiritual History Tool (3), followed by the SPIRITual history (55), FAITH (56), HOPE (57), and the RCP's assessment (53). Each clinician may find one instrument more helpful than another, based on his comfort discussing R/S, the time available during patient interviews, and each patient's background and preferences (4, 46).

The FICA Spiritual History Tool is time-efficient (taking an average of 4–5 minutes) and easy to remember, because its name contains a mnemonic for the four domains assessed by this tool (Faith and belief, Importance and Influence of this faith and belief, whether a patient is in an R/S Community, and how the patient would like R/S Addressed in care). The FICA tool is designed for use by any healthcare practitioner, and is one of the few instruments that has been validated for clinical assessment (58). The SPIRITual history, FAITH, and HOPE instruments are similarly acronyms. These three instruments have not been validated and take slightly longer to administer compared with the FICA. They were originally developed for use by physicians, though contain prompts relevant to many clinicians. The RCP's assessment was developed specifically for mental health clinicians. This instrument takes longer than the others to administer, but assesses R/S in more depth. The RCP examines a patient's R/S in the past, present, and future, and includes questions exploring loss, fear, and spiritual resources (53). The spiritual assessment interview was similarly developed primarily for mental health professionals. This instrument is more succinct than the RCP assessment, but covers fewer R/S topics, and focuses less on R/S in relation to clinical care (4).

Another structured method that a mental health clinician may find helpful is the DSM-5 (59) cultural formulation interview (CFI). This is an interview designed to gather a wide range of cultural information to aid in mental health formulation and treatment planning. It can provide a framework for hearing about a patient's R/S background and determining whether some of a patient's psychiatric symptoms may be better characterized by culturally normative practices or cultural idioms of distress. For example, the CFI emphasizes the patient's explanatory model of his symptoms, and also asks the patient how others in their community might characterize the cause of their symptoms. The CFI recognizes that some patients may have sought alternative sources of mental health care outside Westernized medicine, including R/S healers as one example.

Nuances of taking a spiritual history

With the aforementioned principles and guidelines in mind, it is crucial that clinicians tailor the spiritual history interview for each unique patient. For example, it may be necessary to focus on different aspects of the history depending on one's differential diagnosis of a patient's mental health issue. For a patient who describes a compulsive need to engage in specific religious behaviours, one may inquire about a sense of relief following the behaviours, or distress endured if the behaviours cannot be completed, to distinguish R/S from an obsessive–compulsive disorder. For patients with developmental or intellectual disabilities who have higher vulnerability to abuse and coercion, the clinician may focus more attention on the patient's relationships with others within an R/S community to help ensure the patient's safety.

The style of interview and approach to the patient may also need to be adjusted based on personality traits, defences, and the patient's comfort with the clinician. For example, patients whose cultural backgrounds differ from those of the clinician may be more reticent in initial interviews. These patients may require a more guided approach to the interview, with a higher proportion of closed-ended questions than would be recommended for others (60). If these patients' cultural backgrounds are not taken into consideration, their behaviour may be misinterpreted as guarded or paranoid. This can often occur when patients from more traditional or orthodox traditions speak with clinicians of the opposite gender, but can be seen with any patient who is unfamiliar with the mental health system or who senses that his cultural background differs from that of his clinician. A patient's personality traits can similarly inform the clinician's choice of interview style. For example, with a patient with prominent narcissistic traits, the spiritual history may devolve due to tangents about the patient's own achievements. Gently guiding the patient back to the topic, while allowing their narcissism, can aid both the clinician and the patient. This is one example of a general mental health interview technique that can be applied to the R/S history (60).

The clinical situation and life phase of the patient can also guide the clinician's approach to the spiritual history. For a patient with an estimate of days left to live, more emphasis may be placed on their overarching life narrative, or their beliefs as to what happens after death. If a clinician meets a young patient in the emergency room with a new medical diagnosis, the patient may interpret R/S questions catastrophically, thinking the clinician is suggesting that death is imminent. In these situations, it can be particularly helpful for the clinician to explain that they ask about R/S routinely, and to explain how R/S may help patients to cope with acute illness. Similarly, while a discussion of R/S coping resources and general beliefs may be helpful in this situation, it would generally not be prudent for a clinician who will meet the patient only once to delve into extensive detail during the R/S history. Doing so may be confusing for the patient and frustrating when they must subsequently repeat a very personal and vulnerable story to their long-term provider.

While this chapter has often focused on patients being surprised by a mental health clinician gathering a spiritual history, some individuals may expect and benefit from an earlier, stronger focus on R/S issues. For example, consider a Hindu patient who attributes their depression and anxiety to being a victim of witchcraft, who sees a psychiatrist after visiting several spiritual healers. The psychiatrist would likely benefit from discussing the patient's explanatory model of their illness early in the interview, along with asking about their experience with faith healers. This approach could help convey to the patient that the provider is open to helping the patient according to the patient's unique view of their symptoms. Similarly, a Christian patient from the Southern United States may expect a clinician to discuss R/S in a conversation about grief, and may feel uncared for if the issue never arises. The clinician cannot be clairvoyant about these preferences, but can ascertain them through screening and being flexible in how and when R/S is incorporated into each patient's visit.

Finally, a growing number of patients describe themselves as SBNR and many (particularly modern Europeans) would not describe themselves as spiritual. Nevertheless, they may be struggling to find answers to existential questions regarding identity, hope, meaning/purpose, morality, or ultimate connection. Without explicitly calling this a spiritual quest, clinicians can explore these patients' experiences by actively listening for such questions, and by probing for more detail when hearing the patient use words such as courage, despair, comfort, suffering, and peace.

Hesitance to engage in the spiritual history

Many clinicians and patients remain hesitant to discuss R/S in the mental health setting. For patients, the topic may seem either too personal or irrelevant to the medical interview, particularly if there is limited time. Other patients may prefer to discuss R/S in settings that feel more familiar and/or confidential. For example, hospital chaplains are held to less stringent requirements regarding chart documentation when compared with requirements for physicians or nurses. Finally, patients may fear judgement or proselytization.

Clinicians can help address a patient's concerns by explaining the reasons behind the R/S history and providing an open environment, as discussed earlier in this chapter. However, some patients will still decline to speak about R/S beyond or even during the screening questions. This is not necessarily a failure of the interview but rather a patient choice that should be respected. The clinician can convey respect by closing the subject, while reassuring the patient that they can change his mind in the future. On rare occasions when R/S appears closely related to an acute psychiatric illness or safety risk, the clinician may need to gently probe further after a patient declines to discuss the topic. This is the exception rather than the rule, and should be undertaken with great sensitivity.

As well as patients' fears about discussing R/S, clinicians may also have doubts. Many clinicians fear upsetting or offending a patient, inducing guilt, or reminding patients of traumatic memories by asking about R/S (43). Some question whether consent should be obtained prior to asking about R/S. Though the topic can be private and vulnerable, the consensus remains that there is no special consent required to ask R/S screening questions in a mental health interview. To go beyond R/S screening questions to discuss R/S topics in more detail, the provider should obtain verbal consent and ensure that the patient's decision is educated, without coercion. Formal or written consent is not required (43).

Another challenge that clinicians cite for not asking about R/S is fear of not knowing how to reply if a patient asks about the clinician's faith, or asks the clinician to pray together. When this occurs, the clinician should discuss with the patient their reason for asking the questions. In some cases, it may be appropriate for the clinician to speak briefly about their background. To make this decision, the clinician should consider the likely effects on the patient of any disclosure, and should continue only if it appears that such sharing would be beneficial to the patient without violating boundaries or distracting from treatment.

An example of when provider disclosure might be appropriate is a patient requesting prayer under the assumption that the clinician shares their faith, when in fact this is not the case and the clinician thus feels unable to fulfil the request. Explaining to the patient the reason for declining his request might include sharing that their faiths differ. Beyond that detail, the clinician would not need to share further. Alternatively, for a patient discussing feeling judged by their religious community for living with their partner before marriage, and who asks the clinician their beliefs, it would likely not be wise or relevant for the provider to disclose that they come from a more conservative background that prohibits the practice. These examples highlight the importance of taking a full R/S history to understand the patient's background before making a decision on what may be appropriate to disclose when asked. Even when self-disclosure is appropriate, it is important for clinicians to remember that it is never appropriate to debate with patients or to prescribe or proscribe specific beliefs or practices. Further principles on how to integrate R/S into patient care are discussed in Chapter 20.

Conclusion

This chapter provides information on why to take a spiritual history, along with methods of how to gather a spiritual history. A key caveat is that the spiritual history must be tailored to each individual. Clinical examples allude to potential challenges of the spiritual history, but cannot cover the multitude of nuances that can arise while discussing R/S with patients across cultures. Learning about specific R/S groups can be helpful. However, there is no substitute for speaking with each patient about their unique R/S.

An additional limitation is the need for further research. Future study of how mental health professionals view the R/S history, and their comfort in taking a spiritual history, could help to inform areas of need for training programmes. Though anecdotally, mental health professionals receive minimal training on the spiritual history, a formal study of existing curricula would be useful. There is also a need for further examination of patients' views on the spiritual history. Do patients wish that clinicians had more training on the spiritual history? If so, what training or end skills would be helpful? Finally, though many tools exist for gathering the spiritual history, most are not validated. Is one superior for certain clinicians, patients, or clinical settings? Are these instruments helpful cross-culturally, or would alternative phrasing or questions be useful depending on a patient's cultural background? How should these instruments be shared with clinicians while still emphasizing that the spiritual history should be a conversation rather than a list of questions? Beyond these tools, how can clinicians be best reminded of the many nuances that arise in taking a spiritual history?

While these and similar questions have yet to be fully studied, clinicians can begin to provide more culturally competent care by routinely and openly asking patients about R/S. Further research on the above topics has the potential to inform best practices for taking a spiritual history in a culturally sensitive manner.

References

1. Moreira-Almeida A, Sharma A, van Rensburg BJ, Verhagen PJ, Cook CC. WPA position statement on spirituality and religion in psychiatry. *World Psychiatry.* 2016;**15**(1):87–8.

2. Moreira-Almeida A, Koenig HG, Lucchetti G. Clinical implications of spirituality to mental health: review of evidence and practical guidelines. *Revista Brasileira de Psiquiatria.* 2014;**36**(2):176–82.

3. Puchalski C, Romer AL. Taking a spiritual history allows clinicians to understand patients more fully. *Journal of Palliative Medicine.* 2000;**3**(1):129–37.

4. Lucchetti G, Bassi RM, Lucchetti AL. Taking spiritual history in clinical practice: a systematic review of instruments. *Explore (NY).* 2013;**9**(3):159–70.

5. Koenig HG. Research on religion, spirituality, and mental health: a review. *Canadian Journal of Psychiatry.* 2009;**54**(5):283–91.

6. Finn ME. *Object relations theory and religion: clinical applications.* Westport, CT: Praeger: 1992.

7. Kaufman GD. *The theological imagination: constructing the concept of God.* Westminster, UK: John Knox Press; 1981.

8. Kirkpatrick LA. Attachment theory and religious experience. In: RW Hood Jr, (ed.), *Handbook of religious experience.* Birmingham, AL: Religious Education Press; 1995, pp. 446–75.

9. Hill PC, Pargament KI. Advances in the conceptualization and measurement of religion and spirituality. Implications for physical and mental health research. *American Psychologist.* 2003;**58**(1):64–74.

10. Menezes A, Moreira-Almeida A. Religion, spirituality, and psychosis. *Current Psychiatry Reports.* 2010;**12**(3):174–9.

11. Pierre JM. Faith or delusion? At the crossroads of religion and psychosis. *Journal of Psychiatric Practice.* 2001;**7**(3):163–72.

12. Mohr S, Borras L, Betrisey C, Pierre-Yves B, Gilliéron C, Huguelet P. Delusions with religious content in patients with psychosis: how they interact with spiritual coping. *Psychiatry.* 2010;**73**(2):158–72.

13. **Lim A, Hoek HW, Blom JD.** The attribution of psychotic symptoms to jinn in Islamic patients. *Transcultural Psychiatry.* 2015;**52**(1):18–32.

14. **Johnson DR, Westermeyer J.** Psychiatric therapies influenced by religious movements. In: **JK Boehnlein,** (ed.), *Psychiatry and religion: the convergence of mind and spirit.* Washington, DC: American Psychiatric Press; 2000, pp. 87–108.

15. **Linehan MM.** *Skill training manual for treating borderline personality disorder.* New York: Guilford Press; 1993.

16. **Borman PD, Dixon DN.** Spirituality and the 12 steps of substance abuse recovery. *Journal of Psychology and Theology.* 1998;**26**(3):287–91.

17. **Galanter M.** Spirituality and recovery in 12-step programs: an empirical model. *Journal of Substance Abuse Treatment.* 2007;**33**(3):265–72.

18. **Peteet JR.** A closer look at the role of a spiritual approach in addictions treatment. *Journal of Substance Abuse Treatment.* 1993;**10**(3):263–7.

19. **Worthington EL, Hook JN, Davis DE, McDaniel MA.** Religion and spirituality. *Journal of Clinical Psychology.* 2011;**67**(2):204–14.

20. **McCullough ME.** Research on religion-accomodative counseling: review and meta-analysis. *Journal of Counseling Psychology.* 1999;**46**(1):92–8.

21. **Banin LB, Suzart NB, Guimarães FA, Lucchetti AL, de Jesus MA, Lucchetti G.** Religious beliefs or physicians' behavior: what makes a patient more prone to accept a physician to address his/her spiritual issues? *Journal of Religion and Health.* 2014;**53**(3):917–28.

22. **Ehman JW, Ott BB, Short TH, Ciampa RC, Hansen-Flaschen J.** Do patients want physicians to inquire about their spiritual or religious beliefs if they become gravely ill? *Archives of Internal Medicine.* 1999;**159**(15):1803–6.

23. **Panzini RG, Bandeira DR.** Coping (enfrentamento) religioso/espiritual. *Archives of Clinical Psychiatry.* 2007;**34**:126–35.

24. **Stanley MA.** Older adults' preferences for religion/spirituality in treatment for anxiety and depression. *Aging & Mental Health.* 2011;**15**:334–43.

25. **Huguelet P, Mohr S, Betrisey C, Borras L, Gillieron C, Marie AM,** et al. A randomized trial of spiritual assessment of outpatients with schizophrenia: patients' and clinicians' experience. *Psychiatric Services.* 2011;**62**(1):79–86.

26. **D'Souza R.** Do patients expect psychiatrists to be interested in spiritual issues? *Australasian Psychiatry.* 2002;**10**(1):44–7.

27. **Grant E, Murray SA, Kendall M, Boyd K, Tilley S, Ryan D.** Spiritual issues and needs: perspectives from patients with advanced cancer and nonmalignant disease. A qualitative study. *Palliative Support Care.* 2004;**2**(4):371–8.

28. **Hart A, Kohlwes RJ, Deyo R, Rhodes LA, Bowen DJ.** Hospice patients' attitudes regarding spiritual discussions with their doctors. *American Journal of Hospice and Palliatve Care.* 2003;**20**(2):135–9.

29. **Best M, Butow P, Olver I.** Spiritual support of cancer patients and the role of the doctor. *Support Care Cancer.* 2014;**22**(5):1333–9.

30. **Padela AI, Killawi A, Forman J, DeMonner S, Heisler M.** American Muslim perceptions of healing: key agents in healing, and their roles. *Qualitative Health Research.* 2012;**22**(6):846–58.

31. **Pathy R, Mills KE, Gazeley S, Ridgley A, Kiran T.** Health is a spiritual thing: perspectives of health care professionals and female Somali and Bangladeshi women on the health impacts of fasting during Ramadan. *Ethnicity & Health.* 2011;**16**(1):43–56.

32. **Best M, Butow P, Olver I.** Doctors discussing religion and spirituality: a systematic literature review. *Palliative Medicine.* 2016;**30**(4):327–37.

33. **Best M, Butow P, Olver I.** Do patients want doctors to talk about spirituality? A systematic literature review. *Patient Education and Counseling.* 2015;**98**(11):1320–8.

34. **Gonçalves LM, Osório IHS, Oliveira LL, Simonetti LR, Dos Reis E, Lucchetti G.** Learning from listening: helping healthcare students to understand spiritual assessment in clinical practice. *Journal of Religion and Health.* 2016;**55**(3):986–99.

35. **Kristeller JL, Rhodes M, Cripe LD, Sheets V.** Oncologist assisted spiritual intervention study (OASIS): patient acceptability and initial evidence of effects. *International Journal of Psychiatry in Medicine* 2005;**35**(4):329–47.

36. **Anandarajah G, Stumpff J.** Integrating spirituality into medical practice: a survey of FM clerkship students. *Family Medicine.* 2004;**36**(3):160–1.

37. **Lucchetti G, de Oliveira LR, Koenig HG, Leite JR, Lucchetti AL.** Medical students, spirituality and religiosity—results from the multicenter study SBRAME. *BMC Medical Education.* 2013;**13**:162.

38. **Curlin FA, Lawrence RE, Odell S, Chin MH, Lantos JD, Koenig HG, et al.** Religion, spirituality, and medicine: psychiatrists' and other physicians' differing observations, interpretations, and clinical approaches. *American Journal of Psychiatry.* 2007;**164**(12):1825–31.

39. **Lucchetti G, Lucchetti AG, Badan-Neto AM, Peres PT, Peres MF, Moreira-Almeida A, et al.** Religiousness affects mental health, pain and quality of life in older people in an outpatient rehabilitation setting. *Journal of Rehabilitation Medicine.* 2011;**43**(4):316–22.

40. **Clark PA, Drain M, Malone MP.** Addressing patients' emotional and spiritual needs. *Joint Commission Journal on Quality and Safety.* 2003;**29**(12):659–70.

41. **Koenig HG, Hooten EG, Lindsay-Calkins E, Meador KG.** Spirituality in medical school curricula: findings from a national survey. *International Journal of Psychiatry in Medicine.* 2010;**40**(4):391–8.

42. **Lucchetti G, Lucchetti AL, Espinha DC, de Oliveira LR, Leite JR, Koenig HG.** Spirituality and health in the curricula of medical schools in Brazil. *BMC Medical Education.* 2012;**12**:78.

43. **Koenig H.** *Spirituality in patient care: why, how, when, and what.* Third edition. West Conshohocken, PA: Templeton Press; 2013.

44. **Sloan RP, Bagiella E, Powell T.** Religion, spirituality, and medicine. *Lancet.* 1999;**353**(9153):664–7.

45. **Koenig HG, McCullough ME, Larson DB.** A history of religion, science and medicine. In: **Koenig HGM, McCullough ME, Larson DB** (eds), *Handbook of religion and health.* New York: Oxford University Press; 2001, pp. 24–49.

46. **Culliford L.** Taking a spiritual history. *Advances in Psychiatric Treatment.* 2007;**13**:212–9.

47. **Nathan M.** *A study of spiritual care in mental health practice: patients' and nurses' perceptions.* Enfield, UK: Middlesex University; 1997.

48. **Hodge DR.** Implicit spiritual assessment: an alternative approach for assessing client spirituality. *Social Work.* 2013;**58**(3):223–30.

49. **Canda ER, Furman LD.** *Spiritual diversity in social work practice: the heart of helping.* Oxford: Oxford University Press; 2009.

50. **Josephson AM, Peteet JR.** Talking with patients about spirituality and worldview. *Psychiatric Clinics of North America.* 2007;**30**:181–97.

51. **Griffith JL, Griffith ME.** *Encountering the sacred: how to talk with people about their spiritual lives.* New York: Guilford Press; 2002.

52. **Kao LE, Shah SB, Pargament KI, Griffith JL, Peteet JR.** 'Gambling with God': A self-inflicted gunshot wound with religious motivation in the context of a mixed-mood episode. *Harvard Review of Psychiatry.* 2019;**27**(1):65–72.

53. **Culliford L, Powell A.** Spirituality and mental health. 2006. Available from: http://www.rcpsych.ac.uk/mentalhealthinformation/therapies/spiritualityandmentalhealth.aspx

54. **Spiritual Competency Resource Center**: Spiritual assessment interview 2009 Available from: http://www.spiritualcompetency.com/recovery/lesson7.html

55. **Maugans TA.** The SPIRITual history. *Archives of Family Medicine.* 1996;**5**(1):11–6.

56. **Neely D, Minford E.** FAITH: spiritual history-taking made easy. *The Clinical Teacher.* 2009;**6**(3):181–5.

57. **Anandarajah G, Hight E.** Spirituality and medical practice: using the HOPE questions as a practical tool for spiritual assessment. *American Family Physician.* 2001;**63**(1):81–9.

58. **Borneman T, Ferrell B, Puchalski CM.** Evaluation of the FICA tool for spiritual assessment. *Journal of Pain and Symptom Management.* 2010;**40**(2):163–73.

59. **American Psychiatric Association.** *Diagnostic and statistical manual of mental disorders (DSM-5).* American Psychiatric Publishing; 2013.

60. **MacKinnon RA, Michaels R, Buckley PJ.** *The psychiatric interview in clinical practice.* Second edition. Washington, DC: American Psychiatric Publishing Inc; 2009.

Chapter 20

Religion and spirituality in prevention and promotion in mental health

Arjan W. Braam

Introduction

Almost 40 years ago, Brown and Prudo carried out their pioneering research on the epidemiology of depression (1). On the Isle of Lewis (Outer Hebrides, Scotland), they described the associations of several social factors with depression in a community-based sample of working-class women. They identified 'lack of regular church going' as a vulnerability factor for depression. Although hardly noticed at the time, religiousness entered the stage of psychiatric epidemiology. At present, a substantial body of research with origins in very different disciplines, ranging from the religion sciences, social sciences, and psychiatry to clinical epidemiology, has emerged on the association between religion/spirituality (R/S) and mental illness. Research overviews—for example, by Koenig et al.—show evidence of many associations and connections between R/S and multifarious mental health problems (2, 3). In addition, a highly relevant aspect pertains to the significant association between R/S and lower suicide rates, an association that can clearly be interpreted as protective, as is apparent from meta-analytic work by Wu et al. (4).

It remains uncertain whether protective aspects of R/S are perhaps inherent to mental health or represent an independent predictor of mental health outcomes. Similarly, other aspects of R/S that reflect an individual's strenuous relationship with R/S themes, generally coined as 'religious struggle', are likely to relate to mental health problems. Meticulous, lifetime studies are required to elucidate the underlying dynamics of these relationships. The evidence nonetheless suggests that R/S may deserve the careful scrutiny of clinicians and therapists to evaluate its impact on individuals who exhibit mental disorders or are at risk of them. Sometimes, positive aspects of R/S in terms of coping with stress may emerge, sometimes religious struggle, sometimes both. So one might wonder whether and how R/S relate to the prevention of mental illness and promotion of mental health.

This chapter offers a theoretical, epidemiological approach to the principles and possible main venues regarding how R/S can be understood in the context of the prevention of mental illness and promotion of mental health. These principles and main venues are likely to depend on cultural factors and worldwide value patterns (5).[1] For example, certain principles may feel superfluous to anyone used to living and working in countries with a predominantly religious tradition. Perhaps without even being very explicit about religion, here mental healthcare professionals may have a clear or at any rate sufficient affinity with the religiousness and spirituality of their patients.

However, to mental healthcare professionals in countries or regions with a predominantly secularized cultural climate, some principles and venues regarding R/S and the prevention of mental illness may feel over-emphasized. These R/S themes may need further translation in terms of meaning in life, purpose in life, sense of coherence, significance, or existential questions. Research insights are less available on these themes and, whenever possible, hypotheses need to be developed.

General principles of prevention and promotion in mental health

As the World Health Organization (WHO) notes, mental disorders are common, account for high levels of disability, lead to enormous emotional suffering and a diminished quality of life, and contribute to alienation, stigma, and discrimination (6). This affects society as a whole and can take a tremendous toll on the emotional and socio-economic well-being of the relatives who take care of people with mental disorders. WHO recommends devoting more attention to prevention and promotion in mental health.

Prevention can pertain to the incidence of a disorder, its relapses, or the disabilities and risks associated with it (6). In general, three levels of prevention are distinguished (7): primary (preventing the illness, reducing its incidence), secondary (reducing its severity and duration, and thus its prevalence), and tertiary (preventing relapses and reducing associated disabilities). Primary prevention can involve the general population or a population group (universal prevention), or target subgroups at risk of developing a specific disorder

---

[1] With respect to value patterns all across the globe, sociological research has followed a two-axis approach (5). The first axis is about traditional values (with an emphasis on religion, parent–child ties, and authority) and secular–rational values (with less emphasis on these themes). The second axis pertains to survival values (emphasizing economic and physical security) and self-expression values (emphasizing subjective well-being, self-expression, and quality of life).

(selective prevention), or subgroups at high risk for mental illness (indicated prevention) (6).

Conceptually, the *prevention* of mental illness and *promotion* of mental health may have different meanings, but can involve similar activities or supplement each other (6). In individuals, families, groups, or communities, mental health promotion can enhance coping capacities and reduce vulnerability or morbidity. The parallels of primary, secondary, and tertiary prevention are evident.

The WHO document on prevention and promotion in mental health does not refer to R/S (6). It does however emphasize the relevance of mental health 'on the scale of values of individuals, families or communities' (p. 8). It recognizes how preventive practices may depend on 'the community needs, values and ideology' (p. 12). The document frequently refers to communities, which may be related to religious institutions. Lastly, especially in countries with limited research capacity and programme development regarding prevention, the WHO document underlines the relevance of cultural background.

In order to arrive at the greatest probability of effectiveness in mental health, prevention and promotion interventions and programmes should be evidence-based. Good evidence requires a thorough methodological design, such as a randomized control trial or a times series design. Sometimes, however, 'best practices' are only available as examples for a prevention or promotion intervention.

Early approaches

In the 1980s, Mildred Reynolds describes how religious institutions can play a role in the prevention of mental illness in the United States (8). She refers to the President's Commission on Mental Health (PCMH, installed by President Carter), with a Task Panel on Prevention. This Task Panel examined how the social and community support system represented a critical factor in coping with the major stresses in life such as bereavement, divorce, illness, job loss, and retirement. The PCMH recommended strengthening the natural community support networks such as families, religious institutions, and self-help groups.

Religious organizations can provide support, also on a regular basis, and are likely to represent an enduring (throughout the life cycle), integrative, and community-based resource for mental health (8). At least, this may be the case in countries with substantial adherence to religious institutions such as the United States. Reynolds refers to the PCMH Task Panel on Community Support Systems, which presented some of the types of programmes sponsored by religious institutions to provide support. Table 20.1 shows eight types, with examples given by Reynolds. To give an impression of the variety of preventive interventions, the type of prevention (primary, secondary, tertiary) has been added.

Table 20.1 An early example of prevention and promotion in mental health and religion: eight types of prevention/promotion interventions provided by religious institutions as suggested by the President's Commission on Mental Health's Task Panel on Prevention working group on religious support systems

	Type of programme	Example	Type of prevention [a]
1	Lay care teams in congregations	Support to the sick, bereaved, aged, disabled; weekly visits	II + III
2	Congregation-based sharing groups	Groups about: grief, divorce, alcohol abuse, handicapped children, children with anorexia	II + III
3	Marriage enrichment groups	Strengthening the marital relationship	I
4	Church-related counselling and growth centres	Pastoral counseling (charge according to ability to pay)	II
5	Use of pastoral counselling by community agencies	E.g. counselling for staff members	I
6	Neighbourhood social and civic action	Supporting initiatives for:	
		◆ runaways	III
		◆ mentally retarded	III
		◆ mentally ill	III
		◆ nutrition programmes	I
		◆ elderly people	I
		◆ youth employment	I
7	Holistic health centres in churches	Providing total healthcare, looking at 'the whole person' and total needs, e.g. yoga, weight-watching, cardiopulmonary resuscitation training	I + II
8	Publication programme	Books, pamphlets, tapes about coping with problematic situations:	I + II + III
		◆ divorce	
		◆ death and dying	
		◆ suicide	

Notes:

[a] I: primary prevention: preventing the disease itself (reducing risk factors)

II: secondary prevention: protecting against the severity of the disease, reducing the prevalence

III: tertiary prevention: reducing the associated disability and preventing relapses

Source: Data from Reynolds, M. M. (1982). Religious institutions and the prevention of mental illness. *J Relig Health*. 21(3):245–53.

In 1992, Pargament, Maton, and Hess edited a book on religion and prevention in mental health. In the introduction of this book, Maton and Pargament admit that the topic of religion and prevention may seem far-fetched (9). Religion is often a resource to people after they encounter problems (9, p. 1). However, religion offers 'an overarching framework for living, one which carries with it implications for anticipating, avoiding, or modifying problems before they develop' (9). Maton and Pargament point to differences between the approaches of religious institutions and the human service community. The religious world generally emphasizes the limits of personal control and individual agency,[2] whereas the human service community stresses the power of people to make changes in their lives. Nevertheless, religious institutions have greater natural access to people and offer specific services to minorities, the disenfranchised, and marginal groups. Overlooking the chapters of their book, with a variety of psychological and theological approaches, Maton and Pargament do not overstate the possibilities of prevention. Instead, they advise authors to be humble and precise on this subject, as is apparent from their ten commandments for prevention and promotion in religious settings summarized in Table 20.2 (9).

Epidemiology and religion/spirituality: points of departure

Epidemiology represents one of the foundations of prevention. In essence, this also pertains to psychiatric epidemiology. What mental disorders or vulnerabilities to mental illness prevail? In what age groups? What causal determinants can be identified? What stressors trigger episodes of mental illness and what maintaining factors can be identified? In the epidemiology of R/S and mental illness, at least five assumptions can be made.

First, aspects of R/S may act as epidemiological determinants—that is, as causal factors, provoking factors (triggers, stressors), or maintaining factors. Here, the stress-vulnerability model formulated by Brown (the same as who identified a lack of religious practice as a correlate of emerging depression on the Isle of Lewis, as described in the introduction of this chapter) and Harris serves as a point of departure (11).

Second, in line with the stress-vulnerability model, aspects of R/S can be protective, but can also add to the risk of mental illness. Table 20.3 summarizes

---

[2] In the chapter on the theological perspective on religion and prevention, Spilka and Bridges suppose that, from a traditional theological (probably Calvinist) orientation, primary prevention is a theological impossibility (10). A chaotic state of affairs (including mental problems) is regarded as an existential given—the world and all humanity would exist within a state of *sin*.

Table 20.2 Summary of the 'Ten commandments for prevention and promotion in religious settings'

I	Know the phenomenon	When examined closely, religion and prevention are diverse, complex, rich, and variegated.
II	Know the local setting	Settings of preventive actions have their own distinctive traditions, histories, ideologies, goals, and norms.
III	Know the level of analysis	Religion is a multi-level phenomenon, expressed through individuals, groups, congregations, and society.
IV	Know oneself	As human service professionals, we carry along our own world view and attitude (and biases!) towards religion.
V	Do not worship false gods	Traditional ideas of science may impede research on religion; acknowledge the centrality of values.
VI	Do not disempower	Enhance resources, avoid harming sources we do not understand, respect the spiritual dimension of life.
VII	Seek out new forms and means of collaboration and partnership	Create shared narratives, reciprocal ministry and empowerment, participant research, and action.
VIII	Be humble	There are few grounds for arrogance; appreciation of what we *do not know* is an essential guide.
IX	Seek wisdom	Learn to ask the most important questions about individuals, communities, health, and well-being.
X	Celebrate paradox and diversity	Understand and appreciate different, even contradictory, forms of religion and spirituality in the lives of individuals and communities.

Source: Data from Pargament, K and Maton, K. I., Hess, R. (eds). (1992). *Religion and prevention in mental health: Research, vision, and action*. Binghamtom, NY:: The Haworth Press, 1–15.

Table 20.3 Assumptions to conceive of religion and spirituality as epidemiological factors with positive and negative effects on mental illness and mental health

	↑ **Mental illness** ↓ **Mental health**	↓ **Mental illness** ↑ **Mental health**
Origins	Causal/vulnerability	Protective
Acute	Provoking	Coping/stress buffering
Prediction	Persistence/relapses	Recovery promoting
Absent/ Counterbalancing Outcome in itself	Neutral	Neutral

the range of possible associations. It should be noted that, though R/S may be relevant in life, it may be unrelated to mental illness. An absence of associations deserves attention because it may reflect different patterns. Apart from a simple absence of a relationship between aspects of R/S and mental illness, there can be counterbalancing effects of supportive aspects of R/S against burdening effects due to R/S struggle. Irrespective of the presence or absence of an association, R/S can also be an *outcome in itself*, such as spiritual well-being, access to the resource of contemplation, or an existential source of values about life, death, identity, relationships with others, goals, and destinations.

Third, the variety of aspects of R/S exhibits a wide but meaningful hetero-geneity in their possible links to mental illness. R/S can be understood as a multi-dimensional concept involving beliefs (that can vary widely), public or private practices, cognitive processes (intrinsic religious motivation or import-ance), and various psychological aspects such as religious coping and attach-ment styles. A positive attachment is reflected, for example, by the perception of a positive or supportive image of God or the deity. In addition, some aspects of R/S reflect a troubled relationship with the deity or religious community, called 'religious struggle' or 'negative religious coping' (12). This can reflect anxious or detached attachment styles—for example, involving pessimistic interpretations of punishment or abandonment by God. So one aspect of R/S may clearly relate to a specific type of disorder, whereas another may not reveal any association at all.

Fourth, the type of population is highly relevant to whether aspects of R/S are important in their epidemiological impact on mental illness. Studies in the general population may show different patterns of association between R/S and mental health from those in samples of hospitalized patients with a somatic dis-ease or serious psychiatric symptoms (13).

Fifth, aspects of R/S may have very different effects in different cultures. The contents of religious or spiritual beliefs connect with cultural or sub-cultural heritage. Some types of religious pious behaviour, however, such as private prayer, can have fairly universal traits. *How* people conceive of mental illness depends on the three levels of explanatory models formulated by Kleinman (14): (1) individual and existential, based on personal meaning making and per-sonal experience, (2) medical, following scientific or empirical insights, and (3) cultural, including institutional, political, and economic aspects of health care.

Religion and spirituality embedded in the stress-vulnerability model

If aspects of R/S relate to mental illness, what types of relationships can play a role and how are we to understand them? As is noted earlier, aspects of R/S can be examined as factors in a psychiatric epidemiological model following lines of causality, or at least a temporal sequence as supportive, non-supportive, or neutral/indifferent. Supportive would indicate that R/S decreases vulnerability to mental illness, helps prevent mental disorders (coping, buffering against other stress factors), or promotes recovery. Non-supportive would imply adding to vulnerability and provoking episodes or relapses of mental illness.

As is shown in Fig. 20.1, R/S can be mapped into the vulnerability-stress model, as defined by Brown and Harris (11). In addition to aspects of R/S, two stages have been added. First, some individual origins of R/S are included with three factors: (1) attachment style as an element of personality structure (as theorized by Kirkpatrick (15)), (2) personal affinity with R/S as a constitutional factor (including sensitivity to R/S experiences up to schizotypical traits), and (3) cultural tradition as a factor influencing the types of R/S beliefs and behaviour. At the end of the pathway to psychopathology, the course over time is added, because epidemiology is not only about the onset of mental disorders but also about their persistence, recovery, and risk of relapse.

Aspects of R/S can be assumed to be protective, such as a potential meaning in life framework, a sense of basic trust in relation to a deity, healthy lifestyles advised or inspired by R/S, and social and emotional support exchanged with other members of an R/S community. The potential for coping with stress is positively related to these protective aspects as well. Here, more complex associations can be expected since stressors in life may lead to emotional distress and symptoms of mental illness. In cross-sectional research, aspects of R/S likely to respond to stress, such as frequency of prayer and positive religious coping, may emerge simultaneously with *higher* levels of symptoms of mental distress and disorders. Meticulous longitudinal studies are required to show whether

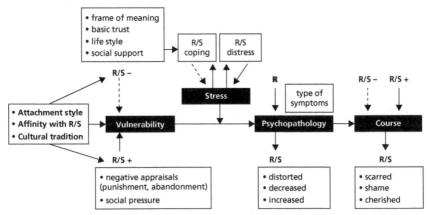

Fig. 20.1 Religion/spirituality embedded in the stress–vulnerability model. Solid lines represent an increasing effect, dotted lines a decreasing effect.

these aspects of R/S would predict a better outcome. Ai and colleagues once provided support for this suggestion. In patients who had coronary bypass surgery, prayer was associated with higher levels of distress in the period of surgery, but lower levels of distress a year later (16). However, the same research group did not entirely confirm their results in a replication study (17).

Other aspects of R/S may contribute to vulnerability, probably related to extremely strict beliefs, an over-emphasis on moral issues, or social pressure from an R/S community. Factors that can contribute to vulnerability are closely related to R/S struggle, as is noted on page 347 as the third epidemiological assumption.

When symptoms of a mental disorder develop, the type and severity of some symptoms are likely to be influenced by R/S. In depression, R/S may contribute to guilt feelings, and, in psychosis, R/S is likely to contribute to the risk of delusions with a religious or spiritual content (18, 19). Brown and Harris categorize this type of effect as symptom-formation factor or pathoplastic factor (11).

And, vice versa, psychopathology can affect R/S. A notorious example is how depression eliminates a depressed patient's sense of meaning and sense of presence, including the perceived proximity of God or a deity. Another example pertains to manic episodes, when patients may feel very close to, or even one with, God, which can derail into a delusion of grandeur—that is, the patient's conviction that he is God, Jesus, or another important religious person, agent, or entity. These feelings may be perceived by patients as *simultaneously* pathological and authentic, as is described by Ouwehand et al. (20). In the course of mental disorders, ideas and feelings about R/S may change. If someone cherishes the R/S experiences that occurred during a psychotic episode, the experiences may still be meaningful. But a patient might also be disillusioned about R/S if R/S coping fails to buffer major stressors or prevent the emergence or recurrence of episodes of mental illness. This last pathway can be characterized as the scarring hypothesis, with episodes of mental illness seriously affecting R/S. Although more research is called for, this pathway may present options for intervention.

With respect to associations between R/S and the course of mental disorders, the evidence mainly pertains to depression. In a recent systematic review of 152 prospective studies, Braam and Koenig note that measures of R/S such as religious attendance or importance of religion in personal life exhibit a weak association with less depression over time (effect size $d = -0.18$) (13). There is, however, a somewhat stronger association between measures of religious struggle and more depression over time (effect size $d = 0.30$). Another mental health outcome over time is suicide. The meta-analysis by Wu, Wang, and Jia, based on nine studies on religiosity and suicide, suggests an overall protective effect of religiosity from suicide (with a pooled odds ratio of 0.38, which would correspond with an effect size d = −0.53) (4). Another study, by Vanderweele et al. in a very large sample of nurses in the US, confirms this possibly protective effect against suicide for religious service attendance (hazard ratio 0.16, corresponding with an effect size d = −1.0) (21).

Prevention and promotion: targets

Research considerations

As R/S connect with culturally determined value patterns, it is not very likely that prevention and promotion activities regarding mental health would always exhibit the normally required scientific evidence. Without ethically sound conditions for the control condition or the R/S intervention, experimental situations are hard to create. Maton and Pargament address this apparent shortcoming in their fifth commandment (Table 20.2: Do not worship false gods) (9). Apart from circumstantial evidence, there is some systematic research evidence though about the use of R/S-based cognitive behavioural therapy. In a systematic review and meta-analysis, Anderson et al. show that faith-adapted cognitive behavioural therapy is equally effective and perhaps even outperforms standard cognitive behavioural therapies (22).

To justify prevention and promotion interventions, scientific evidence remains an important requirement. Since quantitative studies with a more or less experimental design (randomized controlled trials, time series) are not or not yet feasible, careful attention should be devoted to other studies to at least detect *best practices* and, if possible, to connect with value-based practices as defined by Fulford (23).

Primary prevention: contributing to mental hygiene?

Given the state of scientific knowledge, targets for *primary* prevention may not be obvious in the field of R/S and mental health. Numerous community studies, although usually cross-sectional, have nonetheless revealed modest but positive associations between R/S and positive mental health outcomes (2, 3). It can be hypothesized that R/S contributes to *mental hygiene*, provided that two conditions are fulfilled:

(1) In the individual patient, R/S does not clearly provoke or complicate mental disorders.

(2) R/S does more or less coincide with people's cultural traditions, sub-cultural expectations, social networks, and individual interests.

An R/S contribution to mental hygiene would imply the positive elements outlined in Fig. 20.1. The cultural environment is highly relevant but, in the context of mental health, professionals may not always be aware of the potential preventive and health-promoting capacity of R/S. Mental health professionals tend to have less affinity with R/S than their patients—a discrepancy referred to as the 'religiosity gap' (24). A recent qualitative study carried out in the Netherlands at a Protestant mental health clinic and a secular one shows that patients prefer a religious match at both clinics. Patients who have a religiosity gap with their mental health professional report disappointing experiences and are apt to expect to be misunderstood by the professional (25).

Primary universal prevention can aim to *educate* the public about how R/S generally contributes to mental equilibrium and is considered relevant in coping with stress. Primary selective prevention can aim to *teach* the same principles, including the main epidemiological findings, to mental health professionals and students in medicine, nursing, and psychology as well as to peer support workers and spiritual counsellors. In training programmes, mental health professionals devote attention to the relation between their own views on R/S, philosophy of life, personal value patterns, and their professional and ethical values. The prevention and promotion aims of education and teaching are clearly addressed in the concise World Psychiatric Association (WPA) position statement on spirituality and religion in psychiatry (26). Sometimes, simple acronyms can be helpful in instructing students and professionals, although their application deserves further research. Koenig and Pritchett (p. 327) use the acronym 'FICA' to assess R/S on the following points: Faith important—Influenced your life—Community—Spiritual needs to Address (27).

In the US, examples are available of how religious institutions operate in the field of public health, a field of medicine where prevention serves as a key principle (28). As described by Long et al., collaboration between religious leaders and healthcare professionals may feel like *boundary crossing* (29). They suggest four ways healthcare professionals and public health scholars can cooperate with R/S institutions: (1) opting for academic and intellectual humility (reminiscent of Maton and Pargament's commandments) (9), (2) engaging with a wider range of literature (e.g. on history, philosophy, and religion), (3) building relations and networks with people of faith, and (4) acknowledging that the goals and ends of religious communities include but extend far beyond *physical health*.

The advice with respect to primary prevention and mental health promotion pertains to a cultural context as long as public and health professionals sufficiently recognize the relevance and proximity of religious traditions, narratives, and values. There could be collaboration here between conventional medicine and traditional and complementary medicine (30). In middle- and low- income countries, widely available traditional medicine generally applies explanatory models emphasizing a supernatural origin of mental illness. In wealthy countries, the variety of complementary and alternative medical practices utilize holism and meaning as essential principles. Exchange, education, and even the integration of services have been suggested to improve the prevention of mental illness (30).

The research insights on prevention and promotion with attention devoted to R/S generally come from studies carried out in the United States. Although cross-cultural replication and refinement of the findings are called for, these insights can be generalized to many other regions in the world. Currently, such studies are gradually becoming available.

However, some regions such as Western Europe are undergoing processes of secularization. This secularization gives rise to far more individualized lifestyles with less religious institutions or traditions and probably more spirituality: either religiously inspired or non-religious. Research into relations between non-religious spirituality and mental health is still at an early stage. Definitions of non-religious spirituality often include elements such as spiritual well-being that overlaps with mental health (31). The same overlap with mental health is evident in other secularized approaches to the contemplative dimension in life, such as *meaning in life* or *existential concerns*. Definitions and conceptualizations of these approaches do not sufficiently align with aspects of religiousness. The generalization of findings on religiousness and mental health cannot be carried forward towards their secularised alternatives. Nevertheless, underlying patterns can be assumed where elements of spirituality, meaning in life, and existential concern may play a role in relations between R/S and mental health. A fascinating research area is opening up.

Indicated primary and secondary prevention: contributing to compliance?

As is also the case in prospective studies, meta-analyses and systematic reviews show that R/S struggle is associated with higher levels of mental distress and depressive symptoms (32, 33, 13). The concept of R/S struggle includes psychological as well as relational or social issues. The psychological issues can include an overemphasis on attributions about guilt and interpretations of abandonment (12). These negative religious coping strategies may parallel other psychological traits such as an unsafe attachment style, as has been noted before (15). Negative religious coping may closely coincide or even overlap with symptoms of mental distress. Relational and social issues can pertain to disagreements (or even perceived social pressure) on differing ideas about religious doctrines, but can also involve disappointment due to a perceived lack of support from the R/S community.

How can these signs of R/S struggle be relevant to prevention and promotion? Issues of R/S struggle might be subject to treatment—for example, in faith-adapted cognitive behavioural therapy. For individuals prone to mental illness, especially with a clear overlap between symptoms of a disorder and R/S struggle, faith-adapted cognitive behavioural therapy, on face value, can be valuable. *Psycho-education* about a possible overlap between R/S struggle and psychiatric symptomatology can be an essential component of the intervention.

However, if there is no clear overlap or the patient or mental health care consumer does not feel comfortable with the interpretation of an overlap, the ethical issue of *not-harming* (nonmaleficence) is relevant (34). Research evidence about this type of intervention falls short. Only indirect approaches to R/S struggle seem to be justified—that is, addressing R/S, or R/S struggle, and listening as the only interventions. Here, the single goal is to invest in the therapeutic relationship and aim for *compliance with treatment* as the patient may notice a more holistic approach and perceive a sense of attentiveness or *presence* on the part of the practitioner, therapist, or nurse (35). More research on the possible positive effects of addressing R/S in prevention or early treatment is called for.

The ethical line of thought needs to be taken one step further. R/S struggle qualifies as a risk factor for mental illness and deserves clinical attention, but positive as well as negative elements of R/S may still simultaneously relate to mental illness, as has been shown in late life depression for positive, fearful, and critical feelings towards God (36). Selectively addressing the negative aspects of R/S can involve a risk of over-emphasizing the patient's expectations that the practitioner, therapist, or nurse has a limited connection with R/S. Because this can add to pessimistic expectations of a religious gap, positive elements of R/S deserve gentle assessment as well.

Tertiary prevention: caring for religion and spirituality in times of suffering?

At this stage of prevention and health promotion, the arrows of causality change direction. Aspects of R/S are no longer mainly protective or provoking determinants of mental disorders. Facing a mental illness may arouse a need to make sense of the suffering with the core questions about *meaning and meaninglessness*: *Why? Why me?* How does the R/S background help the patient to interpret or explain the causes and course of a disorder? And, similarly, do aspects of R/S, including R/S experiences during episodes of mental illness, provide an outlook on recovery, rehabilitation, security, and hope? Here, issues about one's *existential position* come to the fore. The relation between R/S and mental illness may touch the key ultimate existential concerns as formulated by Yalom

(37)—death, lack of freedom, isolation, and meaninglessness. The last con-cern, meaninglessness (*Why? Why me?*), is addressed above. With respect to *death and dying*, questions may relate to the prospect of recurrent episodes, further suffering, loss of health, loss of mental health, or even suicide. Could R/S offer consolation? Furthermore, in mental illness episodes, one may have less control over one's own decisions and even be subjected to the unavoid-able decisions of others—for example, imposing involuntary admission or treatment or involving guilt, shame, and even victimhood, clearly mirroring a *lack of freedom*. This may also give rise to questions about a lack of personal competence and identity. R/S may provide cognitive cues—for example, con-victions that one deserves punishment. R/S may also, or even simultaneously, provide confidence about one's uniqueness, including a sense of acceptance. Lastly, mental illness episodes can lead to a profound sense of *isolation* caused by symptoms of the disorder—for example, alienation from oneself, others, so-ciety as a whole; misunderstandings, and stigmatization. R/S can then offer a sense of spiritual connection and acceptance.

During recovery, the role of R/S may become even clearer and R/S may in-spire the recovery journey, the personal narrative of recovery. Leamy et al. de-scribe a conceptual framework of psychiatric recovery based on a systematic review (38). This framework includes five elements of recovery processes de-fined by the acronym 'CHIME': Connectedness, Hope, Identity, Meaning, and Empowerment. The thematic overlap with the existential concerns discussed above is evident. Leamy et al. conclude that 'for clinical practice, the CHIME recovery processes support reflective practice'. Interventions that can support these recovery processes, and utilize or develop R/S, call for further research.

An important limitation is that the literature on R/S and mental illness is at an early stage. There are nonetheless accurate qualitative studies on the role of R/S during and after episodes of psychosis in patients with schizophrenia and bi-polar disorder (39, 40). Here, R/S may no longer fit the regular epidemiological model as a determinant of mental illness. Following the suggestion of arrows in the opposite direction, the role of R/S in tertiary prevention may become similar to that of R/S in palliative medicine (41). R/S is not primarily relevant for avoiding further symptomatology, but has become a *subject of care* itself. *Caring for R/S* may involve accommodating R/S in patients who may need to face existential concerns due to the severe impact of episodes of mental illness. For some, R/S may even be a last resort. Mental health care professionals can try to help patients with R/S needs fulfil these needs. Or at least: they can try to avoid obstructing patients heading for this last resort.

Table 20.4 offers a concise overview of some possible prevention and promo-tion targets in the field of mental health where R/S play a role. From an ethical

Table 20.4 Overview of targets and main themes of prevention and religion/spirituality in mental health care

Category of prevention	Target	Main themes
Primary	Mental hygiene	Educating the public Teaching professionals [a]
Secondary	Compliance	Psycho-education Addressing religion/spirituality (R/S) struggle: ◆ Ethical: do not harm R/S ◆ Explore positive elements of R/S
Tertiary	Caring for R/S in times of suffering	Existential concerns ◆ Meaning: 'Why?' 'Why me?' ◆ Death: loss, suicide ◆ Lack of freedom: stigmatization ◆ Isolation Recovery processes ◆ Reflective practice ◆ Narratives ◆ R/S as last resort

Note: [a] Including mental health professionals; students in the medical, nursing, and psychological disciplines; peer support workers, spiritual counsellors, and practitioners in traditional and complementary medicine.

and professional point of view and in accordance with the WPA position statement on spirituality and religion in psychiatry, these targets do not proselytize for either R/S or secular world views. The *contents* of R/S are thus, so far, hardly the subject of interventions. Other prevention or promotion options can be presented and depend on the professional position. Based on the epidemiological literature, clergy, religious leaders, spiritual counsellors or mental health chaplains can offer interventions other than those currently suggested. The multidisciplinary area can be a complication in this field of expertise, but simultaneously harbours wisdom and opportunities for collaboration. This point is reminiscent of Maton's and Pargament's seventh commandment: 'Seek out new forms and means of collaboration and partnership' (Table 20.2).

Conclusion

The epidemiology of R/S and mental health offers multifarious possible relations between R/S and mental illness, and ways they can affect an individual's life course. Several general options for prevention and promotion in mental health are suggested, such as educating people on how R/S and mental hygiene are intertwined, investing in compliance to treatment by addressing R/

S and religious struggle, and devoting attention (care) to R/S in times of suffering. Research on R/S and prevention and promotion initiatives—for example, bridging the religiosity gap and making R/S teaching programmes more effective—will gradually appear, along with efforts to implement the key points of the WPA position statement on spirituality and religion in psychiatry. The current chapter emphasizes the ethical requirements that largely depend on the cultural setting.

In an effort to provide a first design for a guideline on R/S and psychiatry in the Netherlands, an acronym is proposed that also applies to the current exploration of the role of R/S in prevention and promotion in mental health (42). First, a positive message relating R/S to mental health is that R/S and existential questions constitute a normal element in life. It is better to adopt an *easy* (E), inviting, humble attitude than to act over-seriously. Second, from an ethical point of view, discussing the tenacity of certain themes (e.g. the contents of religious and spiritual beliefs) is a bridge too far (43). The best option is thus *listening* (L), and exhibiting professional and personal presence. Third, the main question pertains to the *meaning* (M) of R/S, the search for meaning in general, and the professional's recognition that meaning in life is normal. Verhagen clearly advises integrating a meaning-centred approach when applying the biopsychosocial model in daily practice (44). Fourth, if a professional feels a patient needs further R/S consideration or guidance but lacks the affinity or connection, the best option is to ask *others* (O) for consultation or cooperation. The acronym is thus 'ELMO', reminiscent of Jim Henson's charming, harmless, but not over-sophisticated character on *Sesame Street*. So keep the issue of R/S in mental health easy, listen (do not influence R/S), consider meaning normal, or ask others. These principles can facilitate prevention and promotion in mental health as well.

References

1. **Brown GW, Prudo R.** Psychiatric disorder in a rural and an urban population: 1. Aetiology of depression. *Psychological Medicine.* 1981;11(3):581–95.

2. **Koenig HG, McCullough ME, Larson, DB.** *Handbook of religion and health.* Oxford and New York: Oxford University Press; 2001.

3. **Koenig HG, King DE, Benner Carson V.** *Handbook of religion and health.* Second edition. Oxford and New York: Oxford University Press; 2012.

4. **Wu A, Wang J-Y, Jia C-X.** Religion and completed suicide: a meta-analysis. *PloS ONE.* 2015;10(6):e0131715. doi: 10.1371/journal.pone.0131715.

5. **Inglehart R, Welzel C.** Changing mass priorities: the link between modernization and democracy. *Perspectives on Politics.* 2010;8(2):551–67. doi: 10.1017/S1537592710001258.

6. **World Health Organization (WHO); Saxena S, Maulik PK.** *Prevention and promotion in mental health.* Geneva: WHO; 2002.

7. **Caplan G.** *Principles of preventive psychiatry.* New York: Basic Books, Inc; 1964. pp. 16–17.

8. **Reynolds MM.** Religious institutions and the prevention of mental illness. *Journal of Religion and Health.* 1982;**21**(3):245–53.

9. **Maton KI, Pargament KI.** Religion as a resource for preventive action: an introduction. In: **KI Pargament, KI Maton, RE Hess** (eds), *Religion and prevention in mental health: research, vision, and action.* Binghamton, NY: Haworth Press; 1992, pp. 1–15.

10. **Spilka B, Bridges RA.** Religious perspectives on prevention: the role of theology. In: **KI Pargament, KI Maton, RE Hess** (eds), *Religion and prevention in mental health: research, vision, and action.* Binghamton, NY: Haworth Press; 1992, pp. 19–35.

11. **Brown GW, Harris TO.** *Social origins of depression; a study of psychiatric disorder in women.* London: Tavistock; 1978.

12. **Pargament KI, Smith BW, Koenig HG, Perez L.** Patterns of positive and negative religious coping with major life stressors. *Journal for the Scientific Study of Religion.* 1998;**37**(4):710–24.

13. **Braam AW, Koenig HG.** Religion, spirituality and depression in prospective studies: a systematic review. *Journal of Affective Disorders.* 2019;**257**:428–38. doi: 10.1016/j.jad.2019.06063.

14. **Kleinman A.** *The illness narratives: suffering, healing, and the human condition.* New York: Basic Books; 1988.

15. **Kirkpatrick LA.** *Attachment, evolution, and the psychology of religion.* New York: Guilford Press; 2005.

16. **Ai AL, Dunkle RE, Peterson C, Bolling SF.** The role of private prayer in psychological recovery among midlife and aged patients following cardiac surgery. *Gerontologist.* 1998;**38**(5):591–601.

17. **Ai AL, Ladd KL, Peterson C, Cook CA, Shearer M, Koenig HG.** Long-term adjustment after surviving open heart surgery: the effect of using prayer for coping replicated in a prospective design. *Gerontologist.* 2010;**50**(6):798–809. doi: 10.1093/geront/gnq046.

18. **Braam AW, Sonnenberg CM, Beekman ATF, Deeg DJH,** van **Tilburg W.** Religious denomination as a symptom-formation factor of depression in older Dutch citizens. *Int J Geriatric Psychiatry.* 2000;**15**(5):458–66.

19. **Cook CCH.** Religious psychopathology: the prevalence of religious content of delusions and hallucinations in mental disorder. *International Journal of Social Psychiatry.* 2015;**61**(4):404–25. doi: 10.1177/0020764015573089.

20. **Ouwehand E, Zock TH, Muthert JK, Boeije HR, Braam AW.** 'The awful rowing toward God': interpretation of religious experiences by individuals with bipolar disorder. *Pastoral Psychology.* 2019;**68**(4):437–62. doi: 10.1007/s11089-019-00875-4.

21. **VanderWeele TJ, Li S, Tsai AC, Kawachi, I.** Association between religious service attendance and lower suicide rates among US women. *JAMA Psychiatry.* 2016;**73**(8):845–51. doi: 10.1001/jamapsychiatry.2016.1243.

22. **Anderson N, Heywood-Everett S, Siddiqi N, Wright J, Meredith J, McMillan D.** Faith-adapted psychological therapies for depression and anxiety: systematic review and meta-analysis. *Journal of Affect Disorders.* 2015;**176**:183–96. doi: 10.1016/j.jad.2015.01.019.

23. **Fulford KWM.** Values-based practice: a new partner to evidence-based practice and a first for psychiatry? [Editorial]. In: **AR Singh, SA Singh** (eds), *Medicine, mental health, science, religion, and well-being. Mens Sana Monographs.* 2008;**6**(1):10–21. doi: 10.4103/0973-1229.40565.

24. **Bergin AE, Jensen JP.** Religiosity of psychotherapists: a national survey. *Psychotherapy.* 1990;**27**(1):3–7.

25. **van Nieuw Amerongen-Meeuse JC, Schaap-Jonker J, Schuhmann C, Anbeek C, Braam AW.** The 'religiosity gap' in a clinical setting: experiences of mental health care consumers and professionals. *Mental Health, Religion & Culture.* 2019; **21**(7):737–52. doi: 10.1080/13674676.2018.1553029.

26. **Moreira-Almeida A, Sharma A, Janse van Rensburg B, Verhagen PJ, Cook CCH.** WPA position statement on spirituality and religion in psychiatry. *World Psychiatry.* 2016;**15**(1):87–8. doi: 10.1002/wps.20304.

27. **Koenig HG, Pritchett J.** Religion and psychotherapy. In: **HG Koenig** (ed.), *Handbook of religion and mental health.* San Diego, CA, Academic Press; 1998, pp. 323–36.

28. **Idler E, Levin J, VanderWeele TJ, Khan A.** Partnerships between public health agencies and faith communities. *American Journal of Public Health.* 2019;**109**(3):346–47. doi: 10.2105/AJPH.2018.304941.

29. **Long KNG, Gregg RJ, VanderWeele TJ, Oman D, Laird LD.** Boundary crossing: meaningfully engaging religious traditions and religious institutions in public health. *Religions.* 2019;**10**(7):412. doi: 10.3390/rel10070412.

30. **Gureje O, Nortje G, Makanjuola V, Oladeji BD, Seedat S, Jenkins R.** The role of global traditional and complementary systems of medicine in the treatment of mental health disorders. *Lancet Psychiatry.* 2015;**2**(2):168–77. doi: 10.1016/s2215-0366(15)00013-9.

31. **Koenig HG.** Concerns about measuring 'spirituality' in research. *Journal of Nervous and Mental Disease.* 2008;**196**:349–55. doi: 10.1097/NMD.0b013e31816ff796.

32. **Ano GG, Vasconselles EB.** Religious coping and psychological adjustment to stress: a meta-analysis. *Journal of Clinical Psychology.* 2005;**61**(4):461–80. doi: 10.1002/jclp.20049.

33. **Smith TB, McCullough ME, Poll J.** Religiousness and depression: evidence for a main effect and the moderating influence of stressful life events. *Psychological Bulletin.* 2003;**129**(4):614–36. doi: 10.1037/0033-2909.129.4.614.

34. **Beauchamp TL, Childress JF.** *Principles of biomedical ethics.* Fourth edition. Oxford: Oxford University Press; 1994, pp. 6–10.

35. **Baart A, Vosman F.** Relationship based care and recognition. Part one: Sketching good care from the theory of presence and five entries. In: **C Leget, C Gastman, M Verkerk** (eds), *Care, compassion and recognition: an ethical discussion.* Series: Ethics of care, volume 1. Leuven: Peters; 2011, pp. 183–200.

36. **Braam AW, Schaap-Jonker J, van der Horst MHL, Steunenberg B, Beekman ATF, Tilburg W van, Deeg DJH.** Twelve year history of late life depression and subsequent feelings to God. *American Journal of Geriatric Psychiatry.* 2014;**22**(11):1272–81. doi: 10.1016/j.jagp.2013.04.016.

37. **Yalom ID.** *Existential psychotherapy.* New York, Basic Books; 1980.

38. **Leamy M, Bird V, Le Boutillier C, Williams J, Slade M.** Conceptual framework for personal recovery in mental health: systematic review and narrative synthesis. *British Journal of Psychiatry.* 2011;**199**(6):445–52. doi: 10.1192/bjp.bp.110.083733.

39. **Rieben I, Mohr S, Borras L, Gillieron C, Brandt P-Y, Perroud N, Huguelet P.** A thematic analysis of delusion with religious contents in schizophrenia. *J Nerv Ment Dis.* 2013;**201**(8):665–73. doi: 10.1097/NMD.0b013e31829c5073.

40. **Ouwehand E, Braam AW, Renes JW, Muthert JK, Stolp HA, Garritsen HH, Zock TH.** Prevalence of religious and spiritual experiences and the perceived lasting influence thereof in patients with bipolar disorder in a Dutch specialist out-patient center. *Journal of Nervous and Mental Disease.* 2019;**207**(4):291–9. doi: 10.1097/ NMD.0000000000000965.

41. **Leget C.** and taskforce guideline revision. Spiritual care guideline [Spirituele zorg; Landelijke richtlijn, Versie 2.0]. Utrecht, Netherlands: Vereniging van Integrale Kankercentra; 2018. Available from: www.oncoline.nl/richtlijn/item/index. php?pagina=/richtlijn/item/pagina.php&richtlijn_id=1081.

42. **Braam AW.** Towards a multidisciplinary guideline religiousness, spirituality and psychiatry: what do we need? *Mental Health, Religion and Culture.* 2017;**20**(6):579–88. doi: 10.1080/13674676.2017.1377949.

43. **Cook CCH.** *RCPsych recommendations on spirituality and religion. Position statement PS03.* London: Royal College of Psychiatrists; 2013.

44. **Verhagen PJ.** Psychiatry and religion: consensus reached! *Mental Health, Religion and Culture.* 2017;**20**(6):516–27. doi: 10.1080/13674676.2017.1334195.

Chapter 21

The key role of spirituality in positive psychiatry and psychology

Simone Hauck and C. Robert Cloninger

Introduction

The field of positive psychology and psychiatry has the goal of helping people to achieve an above-average or optimal level of functioning and greater happiness (1). Positive psychology emerged from the perception that, since World War II, psychology has become largely about treating mental disorders, while what makes life worth living has been disregarded. In their paper, 'Positive psychology: an Introduction', Martin E. P. Seligman and Mihaly Csikzentmihalyi (2) two of the main proponents of positive psychology comment on how psychology has become a science largely about healing sickness in the second half of the past century, concentrating its efforts on repairing damage within a disease model of human functioning. There was great progress in understanding how people survive and endure adversity, and many mental diseases turned out to be successfully treatable or at least ameliorated. Nevertheless, very little was known about how normal people flourish under benign conditions, nor was there a substantial literature on how to improve individual and social conditions to better face adversity, aiming at prevention and flourishing (2, 3). Positive psychology is the study of what is 'right' about people—their positive attributes, psychological assets, and strengths. Its aim is to understand and foster the factors that allow individuals, communities, and societies to thrive (4).

In 2004, based on the analysis of different religious, cultural, and legal texts from around the world, Peterson and Seligman proposed a hierarchy of positive psychological character strengths, composed of 24 specific human qualities (5). The effort was based on the assumption that human beings have dispositions to behave consistently over time and situation, and that there are 'preferred traits' that are regarded as 'positives' and are common to different cultures and traditions. The criteria for a strength were the following: valuing a quality in and of itself (not as a means to an end); the existence of paragons and prodigies of the strength but also people who are egregiously devoid of it; being endorsed universally (or at least ubiquitously); and a consensus that the quality contributed to fulfilment in life (5, 6). These strengths were organized under the helm of six virtues that supposedly were situated at a higher level of abstraction and were linked to constructs proposed by philosophers and religious figures over many centuries (Table 1) (5).

To measure and assess the 24 character strengths, Peterson and Seligman developed the Virtues In Action Inventory of Strengths (VIA-IS), a self-assessment measure whereby respondents rate how likely they are to participate in certain behaviours that are representative of the different character strengths (5). According to Seligman (6), it is very important to emphasize that positive psychology does not prescribe good character, but rather it describes, studies, and asks how to build what is 'prescribed' within the culture. Also, he states that positive psychology is an attempt to help cultures and individuals better achieve what they already value (6).

Along with other authors who have been emphasizing the importance of well-being and human development beyond the absence of suffering, diseases, and materialistic thinking, positive psychology gives voice to an urgent and essential matter upon which may depend the continuity of the human existence. Efforts to better understand the paths that can lead humanity to a healthier attitude, not only towards itself but also towards the planet, are essential and urgent (7–9).

However, empirical studies evaluating the structure of the VIA-IS yielded different results, and no two VIA-IS studies produced identical results, even in similar populations (10–12). Peterson and Seligman's theoretical model describing the 24 strengths as the 'ingredients' that make up the six 'virtues' did not hold up in factor analytic studies of the VIA-IS scale. Therefore, although the role of positive psychology in bringing to the fore aspects that lead to a meaningful life and a flourishing society is undeniable, the theoretical framework that lies behind its concepts need to be further developed.

In the same direction, advocates of a 'Positive psychiatry' (13) call attention to the fact that many psychiatrists tend to consider only the 'sick' aspect of the patient, disregarding the possibility of assessing the other half of the sky: resources, skills, and potential of those people who are too often viewed exclusively as carriers of pathological signs and symptoms and, therefore, summarily catalogued. Psychological states such as optimism and hope, positive views of life, and the ability to feel united and 'socially engaged' with other persons, make people—and especially people with mental difficulties—stronger and more accessible to psychotherapeutic techniques, psychosocial interventions, and psychoeducational strategies (13–17).

Growing biomedical research supports the understanding that positive emotions are not simply the opposite of negative emotions, but may be independent dimensions that have been associated with many benefits related to health, work, family, and economic status (4, 18). Positive emotions are present in most mammals and have been experimentally shown to help humans behave communally and to learn more quickly (19). Furthermore, fostering psychological resilience and leading individuals to a healthier attitude towards themselves and their communities certainly can bring many benefits to our society, and, at the end, for mankind as a whole. In opposition to the dominant materialistic thinking that has led our planet and many sectors of our societies to harm, poverty, and suffering, well-being and positive emotion paradigms can help us to shift towards a better (and safer) path (8, 9).

Positive psychology, psychiatry, and spirituality

Spirituality is one of the 24 character strengths in the positive psychology model proposed by Peterson and Seligman, even though they describe themselves as agnostics who specifically deny any faith in the Divine. They accommodate the whole of faith by recognizing it as an alternative to hope. However, empirical findings show that the character traits that measure faith, hope, and charity are highly interdependent and synergistic, and only weakly dissociable. This casts doubt on the agnostic view that hope and faith are simple alternative paths for well-being. Their limited approach to faith and spirituality might indeed be one of the major weaknesses of their model, by limiting the potential of growing in awareness. Without faith, hope and love, a person cannot reach a transcendental level that is spontaneous and unconditional. When faced with adversity or death, one realizes that the agnostic moral level of intellect and virtue is incomplete and falls short of what is needed (7, 20).

When it comes to psychiatry, the potential advantages of spiritually oriented well-being therapies are also a promising and much-needed field. Cultivation of spirituality provides an inexpensive and powerful way to enhance well-being, as shown by recent randomized controlled trials and clinical studies of spiritual treatment methods (21–23). The introduction of many medications and psychotherapy techniques led to acute benefits in randomized controlled trials, but those treatments work for only a limited number of cases and are unfortunately associated with frequent drop-out, relapse, and recurrence of illness in the long run (24, 25). On the other hand, growth in well-being reduces vulnerability to depressive relapses and recurrences (21).

The awakening of the spiritual dimension in human life can provide meaning and purpose even when people face disturbing adversities, thereby preventing the emergence of, and facilitating recovery from, mental illness. Several studies have provided evidence for an inverse relationship between religiosity and depression over past decades (26, 27). Spiritually augmented therapy is more effective than CBT in activating feelings of hope and life satisfaction. It is also shown in randomized controlled trials to reduce relapse rates and enhance the quality of functional recovery (28–30). Recently, a study has found an association between high intrinsic religiosity and higher levels of brain-derived neurotropic factor (BDNF), a widely studied brain neurotrophin responsible for synaptic plasticity, dendritic and neuronal fibre growth, and neuronal survival. This finding points to a potential pathway to help understand the protective effect of religiosity in depressive disorders (31).

Spirituality is the search for something beyond human existence, creating a sense of connectedness with the world and with the unifying source of all life—an expression of a profound need of people for coherent meaning, love, and happiness. A spiritual attitude towards oneself and towards life and others often prevents stress and lifestyle imbalances that lead to physical and mental disorders, and can be particularly crucial for people facing existential crises, which can appear along with suicidal thoughts. Though not always obvious, patients are often searching for answers to questions about their existence, including he meaning of life, sickness and suffering, and happiness. If, on the one hand, this questioning can lead to the feeling of an existential vacuum (e.g. emptiness and despair), on the other hand, a spiritual approach to these questions can bring a liberating perspective creating an awareness of our inseparable participation in a universal unity of being. Due to their materialistic approach, psychiatry and psychology have been neglecting this dimension, refraining from helping patients to use this perspective in their favour and in favour of their communities (9, 21, 32).

The bio-pycho-social model

The bio-psycho-social model developed by Cloninger and colleagues is an empirically based model of personality that considers the importance of spirituality in the human constitution and development. To better contextualize the role of spirituality, we will take the view of positive psychiatry in valuing aspects related to growth and well-being, and develop the idea according to the bio-psycho-social model and its applications. Mental health has been described as a state of well-being in which the person realizes and uses their own abilities, can cope with the normal stresses of life, can work productively and fruitfully, and is able to contribute to his or her community (33). An understanding of the mechanisms of personality development provides a systematic way to promote health as an integrated state of physical, mental, social, and spiritual well-being, rather than merely the absence of disease or infirmity (18, 34).

Personality has been defined as the dynamic organization within an individual of the psychobiological systems by which a person shapes and adapts to ever-changing internal and external influences. In other words, it is a way to describe the person as a being who learns and adapts to situations in life (35, 36). This includes metacognitive patterns and systems that regulate cognition, emotion, mood, personal impulse control, and social relations. In this context, personality traits are enduring patterns of perceiving, relating to, and thinking about oneself, other people, and the world as a whole (7, 37). These three aspects of being are associated with physical, mental, social, and spiritual heath (7, 9, 16, 38, 39)

The Temperament and Character Inventory (TCI) is a tool for personality assessment that deconstructs personality in seven dimensions. These dimensions represent four temperament and three character traits that vary widely in the general population (Fig. 1—Psychobiological model of temperament and character). The TCI depicts a psychobiological model that considers complex interactions among genetic, psychological, social, cultural, and spiritual variables that interact in a non-linear way so that different traits can lead to the same clinical outcome ('equifinality') and the same traits can lead to different consequences ('multifinality') (18, 40). The test has 240 questions, either true–false or on a 5-point Likert scale, and can be completed by the patient in about 45 minutes. The review and discussion of the patient's personality profile not only informs the clinician but also allows the patient to reflect, creating a shared language for discussion. This allows an effort to understand strengths and vulnerabilities, unfolding possible paths towards recovery and well-being (36).

Temperament refers to individual differences in the strength of drives underlying basic emotions, such as fear, anger, disgust, and surprise, which are moderately stable throughout life. In contrast, character refers to individual differences in a person's goals and values that develop in a step-like manner as a person matures in insight through experiences over his or her lifespan (41). All seven dimensions have been found to have unique genetic determinations (42–44), and to be regulated by different brain systems as measured by functional brain imaging (7, 39, 45).

While temperament traits are biases in emotional responses that are fully developed early in life and moderately stable thereafter, character involves higher cognitive processes that develop in a stepwise manner over the life course to enable a person to regulate emotions, achieve certain goals, and express particular values. The key difference between them is the underlying type of learning involved. Procedural learning of habits and skills influences the conditioning of temperament so temperament remains stable through life, except in response to behavioural conditioning that is unique for each individual. Propositional or semantic learning of goals and values influences the development of character, so profiles are pulled toward the norm favoured in the person's culture. Likewise, parental role models and attachments have a greater influence on character than on temperament, in addition to the effects attributable to genetic inheritance. Both temperament and character interact, allowing a self-aware consciousness that gives a personal sense of continuity (identity) as life unfolds (36).

The differences between people in their emotional style can be reliably measured by four traits of 'temperament' measured by the TCI (35). The identification of configurations is useful because they are stable in the absence of major trauma or behavioural conditioning (36). The four temperament traits are Harm Avoidance, Novelty Seeking, Reward Dependence, and Persistence—they are linked to procedural learning and constitute the habit systems (see Fig. 21.1). Generally speaking, these four temperaments correspond to people with anxiety proneness (high harm avoidance), impulsivity, and anger proneness (high novelty seeking), social detachment (low reward dependence) and perseverance or obsessionality (high persistence). Each trait varies in intensity, and each can be present in any combination. However, even though groups of temperament profiles differ in maturity on average, and people with particular combinations are much more likely to be immature than others, some people are mature and responsible regardless of their temperament configuration (7, 36).

Hence, temperament alone is not adequate to determine whether an individual does or does not have a personality disorder, or his or her level of well-being. The development of character traits, cognitive sets linked to propositional learning, allow people to regulate their emotional impulses and conflicts in such a way that they are mature and healthy regardless of their temperament.

The TCI measures three character traits named Self-directedness, Cooperativeness, and Self-Transcendence. Initially, it was thought that character was less heritable than temperament but empirical studies have shown that both are moderately heritable (36, 44). Character traits provide a description of a person's goals and values, and also correspond to key functions of a person's mental self-government. A self-directed person is responsible, purposeful, and resourceful in dealing with life's challenges. As a result, it is an important indicator of reality testing, maturity, and vulnerability to mood disturbance. Cooperativeness provides a clinical measure of a person's ability to get along well with others. A cooperative person is tolerant, empathic, helpful, compassionate, and principled. Self-transcendent people are described as self-forgetful (intuitive and engaged), transpersonal (altruistic and joyful), and spiritual in perspective, whereas those who are low in self-transcendence are self-striving (controlling), individualistic (defensive), and secular (materialistic and non-religious). High character development is desirable for each of the TCI dimensions, although the development of self-transcendence may seem countercultural in Western societies. However, despite Western ambivalence about spirituality and self-transcendence, available data strongly indicate that this dimension is extremely important for emotional well-being, especially when a person faces suffering or death (26, 27, 36, 46–48). A psychobiological approach to the cultivation of well-being must take into account the three branches of self-government, and excessive development of one of them, without the balance of the other two, can lead to an imbalance and particular pathologies (36).

Evolution of spiritual awareness and the three memory systems

The human brain has evolved in a series of steps over millions of years. Each step in this evolutionary hierarchy contributed to advances in the ability of our ancestors to adapt, survive, and reproduce. Three major systems of learning and memory are still recognizable in a human being. The earliest regulating procedural learning or associative conditioning of habits is shared with all animals; the brain circuitry varies through phylogeny so, in humans, the limbic system, particularly the cortico-striatal system, serves as our 'emotional brain'—regulating procedural learning of habits and skills. The second system to evolve was the propositional or declarative learning system of reasoning about goals and social interactions, which begins to develop in hominids, including great apes and pre-modern humans; it constitutes the 'rational brain' with prominent development of the pre-frontal cortex. The last system to evolve is exclusive to the modern human species and is expressed by episodic memories that allow self-awareness for recollection and introspection about events that happen throughout our lives, from an autobiographical perspective.

The first learning system is related to the temperament traits, providing the person's emotional style. The second one relates to the ability to be self-directed and cooperative, and the third one allows human beings to grow in awareness of what influences our body, our emotions, our thoughts, and even the initial perspectives that are present before we formulate words with our rational brain or automatic responses with our emotional brain. The emergence of the modern human brain was characterized by the development of the capacity for art, science, and spirituality (32).

Recent studies, using data-driven analysis, yielded nearly 1,000 genes that influence temperament and character. More specifically, about 700 genes influence human temperament, while again about 700 genes influence how well people are able to self-regulate their emotions. About 33% of the genes influence both temperament and character, while 67% are specific. The method used in these studies allowed identification of clusters of genes that interact with each other and with the environment to influence profiles of traits that describe the person as a whole (39, 49, 50). Further analysis was able to recognize that genes encode temperament profiles and character profiles separately, and then these are integrated by genetic–environment interactions into complex adaptive networks. Furthermore, the three memory and learning systems mentioned above were mapped and related to phenotypic networks (integrated temperament–character networks) made up of people who express the prototypical features of each of the three major systems of learning and memory present in modern human beings: associative conditioning for emotional reactivity (emotional-unreliable network), intentional self-regulation (organized-reliable network), and self-awareness of autobiographical memory (creative-reliable network). The emotional-unreliable profile was consistently associated with less wellness and more illness, and the creative-reliable profile was associated with the highest levels of physical, mental, and social well-being. Another important finding is that the genes for personality are expressed in most organ systems, not only in the brain, so the physical, mental, and social aspects of health are expected to be strongly interdependent. Due to the reciprocal interactions, physical, mental, social, and spiritual aspects of health cannot be separated. Consequently, norms for healthy functioning need to consider the importance of self-transcendent functions, such as spontaneous creativity, altruism, and generosity, which are sometimes neglected (51, 52).

Therefore, the path to well-being has to take into account the complex interaction and function of the three memory learning systems that are involved in different stages of self-awareness (Table 2, Stages of self-awareness) (32). The absence of self-awareness occurs in severe personality disorders and psychoses in which there is little or no insightful awareness of the preverbal outlook or beliefs and interpretations that automatically influence emotional drives and actions. The first stage of self-awareness is typical of most adults today, whereby ordinary cognition permits delayed gratification to attain personal goals but in an egocentric way with frequent distress when attachments and desires are frustrated. The second stage of self-awareness is typical in adults operating as 'good parents', being allocentric in perspective and capable of calmly considering the perspective and needs of the children and other people in a balanced way that leads to satisfaction and harmony. This state implies the capacity of observing one's own subconscious thoughts and considering the thoughts of others in an understanding non-judgemental way. This stage can be described as 'meta-cognitive', mindfulness, or 'mentalizing'. The ability of mind to observe itself allows for more flexibility in action by reducing dichotomous thinking (32, 53). The third stage of self-awareness is called contemplation because it is direct perception of one's initial perspective—that is, the preverbal outlook of schemas that direct one's attention and which provide the framework that organizes our expectations, attitudes, and interpretation of events. It allows access to unconscious material directly, enlarging consciousness (32). The third stage of self-awareness can also be described as 'soulful', because of the awareness of deep preverbal feelings that emerge spontaneously from a unitive perspective, such as hope, compassion, and reverence. Soulfulness is much more powerful in transforming personality than is mindfulness, which often fails to reduce feelings of hopelessness. However, most people experience contemplation in transient peak experiences but are rarely able to maintain a stable contemplation state in contemporary societies, which are replete with materialistic and anti-spiritual messages (7, 21).

Character develops through growth in self-awareness as we try to find meaning and satisfaction by learning ever-more coherent perspectives on our lives. Self-transcendence, a spiritual trait that is unique to human beings allows us to reach the higher levels of awareness that are associated with the highest levels of positive emotions and the lowest levels of negative emotions (34). A spiritual perspective allows us to see that we often live our lives in division—split between contradictory desires that create conflict and dissatisfaction. Growing in awareness of this division helps a person transcend problems and rediscover a sense of unity, not only within her/himself but also potentially with nature and the world, or even with all of life (32).

A psychobiological approach to the cultivation of well-being

Psychological suffering and mental illness are widely prevalent, and are still leading causes of disability (21, 54). According to recent studies, they represent heterogeneous disorders that depend on complex interactions among many genes and environmental variables; therefore, it is difficult or impossible to design interventions that are broadly effective and well tolerated. Effective treatments must be tailored for each individual in a person-centred manner (34, 51). Furthermore, there is extensive evidence that treatments are most effective when they address all three systems of learning and memory in a coordinated manner: behaviour conditioning, intentional self-control, and self-aware evaluation need to be integrated in order to be strongly and consistently effective in promoting well-being. Additionally, relating a person's current well-being to both his or her temperament and character provides powerful motivation for a person to change (36).

Being person-centred is a key to an effective treatment or well-being programme, and the use of a tool such as TCI facilitates non-stigmatization while patient and clinician are assessing the patient's personality. A deep knowledge about one's self is required to lead someone to authentic awareness, calm, and realistic 'acceptance' that underlines a peaceful state of mind and a creative joyful way of living. The promotion of well-being must begin with a recognition regarding what brings health and lasting satisfaction, considering her or his particular emotional style.

Discussing and reflecting about the way the patient describes him or herself promotes a person-centred therapeutic dialogue in which the strengths and weakness in regulating emotions in accord with goals and values can be explored, serving as the basis for change and growth (34, 36, 55). However, additional methods need to be integrated with personality assessment to promote character development and well-being in a systematic way.

Know yourself programme

As a practical example, we will describe a multi-model psychoeducational course developed by C.R. Cloninger in consultation with the Anthropedia Foundation for the purpose of promoting growth in self-awareness as described in this chapter. The course integrates evidenced-based techniques from a variety of therapeutic approaches (CBT, person-centred, psychodynamic, logotherapy, well-being therapy, positive psychology, and others) (Anthropedia, http://anthropedia.org). It comprises 16 modules (50 minutes each), suitable for use in consultation with a trained well-being coach or therapist or as an adjunct to individual or group therapy. It is designed to be a universal intervention for anyone who has the reading comprehension of a 14 year old, regardless of physical or mental health level (21, 34, 36).

The therapeutic sequence corresponds to the natural sequence by which a person grows in self-awareness (Table 3—The Know Yourself Course—Anthropedia). In the first module (exploring personality), a patient takes the TCI along with other brief life satisfaction and emotionality measures to provide a baseline and stimulate reflection. The patient reflects on what has provided lasting personal satisfaction in the past, improving self-knowledge and fostering motivation towards the experiences, while facilitating the establishment of a therapeutic alliance (55, 56). Exercises that promote satisfaction, such as acts of kindness, are suggested (7, 57–59). The second part of the course aims at understanding the processes of thought that can lead to greater life satisfaction—for example, cognitive-behaviour descriptions of thought and the three major systems of learning and memory (34, 40). Once what is satisfying and the current habits of thinking that may interfere with health and happiness are identified, modules three to five provide exercises and meditations to help patients to activate their prefrontal cortex so that they can be more aware. Each exercise builds on the other but focuses on a different aspect of being and a different system of learning. At first, there is a simple meditation for relaxing the body and calming the emotional brain; then observing one's own thoughts to understand without judging or blaming—this aims at experiencing mindfulness in a non-judgemental state (7, 34, 60, 61). The next two modules help to enhance this natural ability by facilitating the perception of unity and harmony through the practice of integrative sensory awareness with the activation of the respective brain areas (62). The practices lead to the perception of unity and connectedness while acting spontaneously, and reduce feelings of loneliness and isolation. The final meditation focuses on deepening awareness of one's outlook of life—the backdrop that colours a person's perceptions. The ability to shift outlook on situations or temporal viewpoint is a function of contextual 'mental time travel' that depends on self-awareness (7, 34, 63). A crucial feature of the course is that exercises, information, and activities are directed to all three aspects of a person (i.e. physical, mental, and spiritual) so that the person develops the plasticity, virtue, and creativity to integrate all aspects of their being so that they are functioning in harmony. The TCI provides a baseline, as well as an outcome measure, as the person works at their own pace toward self-actualization.

Following the 'Know Yourself' course, a person-centered, interdisciplinary, and bio-psycho-social one-year specialized training was developed by the Anthropedia Foundation in collaboration with the Center for Well-Being at Washington University in St. Louis. Subjective well-being measures and the TCI were applied before and after the training for 50 trainees, showing an increase in subjective well-being as well as in self-directedness (self-acceptance), cooperativeness (empathy and moral reasoning), and self-transcendence after the training. These results reinforce developing and testing interventions following this model as a promising resource to increase sustainable global health resilience and psychological well-being that take into account both personality and cultural conditions (64).

The dynamics of cultural change in unstable world conditions

In developing a flexible positive approach to clinical therapeutics in different countries and cultural subgroups, we have recognized that individual well-being and collective well-being are highly interdependent because our survival and safety, as well as ability for self-expression and self-actualization, depend on the culture in which we participate and on the planetary habitat in which we live (65). What is most important to recognize is that both personalities and cultures are constantly self-organizing and evolving. We can recognize the same key variables to target for promotion of well-being in recent research on individual personality development and on cultural evolution of societies.

The three networks of human learning and memory that we identified for personality development correspond to three clusters of people in cultural subgroups that have been identified in longitudinal studies of cultural development around the world: traditionals, moderns, and post-materialists/cultural creatives (65–68). People in the traditionalist subculture have the features typical of the emotional-unreliable personality profiles: they usually act by habit and custom with little self-awareness (Stage 0 in Table 2), they are fearful for their survival and cling to security provided by traditional habits and conventions and by authorities who promise to take good care of them. Consequently, they highly value religious and political authorities that are conservative in depending on their old habits, traditions, and beliefs, even when these are no longer adaptive and realistic. Traditionalists are hostile toward outsiders and intolerant of people with diverse ideas and preferences, particularly when their fears of scarcity and change are provoked.

People in the modernist subculture have the features typical of organized-reliable personality profiles: they are usually in Stage 1 of self-awareness (Table 2), so they are highly materialistic and secular, seeking individual enhancement through achievement and quest for power and wealth, using their analytical intelligence and personal hard work with little concern for social justice or other communal and spiritual virtues. They are individualistic and self-centred, seeking dominance and mastery in top-down hierarchies rather than egalitarian democracy (68). They are prosocial to the degree of being tribal and sectarian, considering the needs of others only to the extent that it is also to their own benefit.

People in the post-materialist subculture have been also been called 'cultural creatives' (66) and 'self-transcendent' rather than self-interested like modern materialists (66) (Schwartz, 1999, (67)). They are often intermittently in Stage 3 and may occasionally reach a stable unitive level of self-awareness

(Table 2). They have the features of creative-reliable personalities manifest by their questioning the value of reliance on external authority, and by emphasizing the value of freedom of self-expression and self-actualization. They place high value on self-transcendence, service to others, creativity, and openness to change. Longitudinal studies show that the proportion of people with creative profiles is increasing while traditionalists and modern materialists are decreasing in most parts of the world, except in some parts of the world where there is existential insecurity, and/or oppressive and self-serving authoritarian regimes (e.g. Africa, China, Russia) (65, 69). In North American and Western Europe, traditionalists and modernists are engaged in a hateful and divisive culture war pitting liberty rights against social duties, but actually both groups are shrinking in numbers because they do not effectively promote a sustainable and satisfying life for most people by an approach that unifies individual liberties with social duties in equitable ways that address current crises related to collective well-being, such as universal health care, safety and security, ecological sustainability, and the scope and quality of educational opportunities. Materialists and traditionalists dominate media communications, and control legislatures and military activity through economic forces. In contrast, the creative post-materialist subculture has been remarkably silent because materialists and traditionalists control much of the media and the creatives quietly go their own way to serve others in peace while preparing to step up to help if and when society begins to collapse when others fail to address critical problems effectively. Although they have been called the 'silent revolution' until recently, cultural creatives are increasingly active and vocal in major protests around the world because of frustration with the resistance, denial, or ineffectiveness of political leaders regarding their responsibility to reduce the exploitation and inequities that jeopardize and hinder human development around the world (70).

Values are strongly developed prior to adulthood, so cultural change depends largely on replacement of older generations by younger generations except when individuals or cultures face existential threats they cannot control, such as the ultimate situations like death and suffering that are currently very clear, at least to the dominantly post-materialist generation of people (i.e. born after 1965). As the younger post-materialist generations replace the older generations, they are preparing to adapt to the real needs of most people to change their values and priorities for meaningful action to improve the quality of life and health of people and the planet as a whole. For example, democracies in Latin American countries have had only weakly effective democratic governments when millennials were adolescents, but post-materialist values for self-expression, social justice, and autonomy are now replacing materialistic and authority-based values; these democratic values for freedom of self-expression and self-actualization are consistently closely linked to greater collective well-being, as is prominently displayed in Scandinavian countries (65, Fig. 2.4, p. 32). However, the potential of the younger generations can be stagnated, as has been seen recently in the USA and Western Europe, as a result of the insecurities created by their current culture wars, militarism, terrorism, and socio-economic inequity. As a result, in these countries where respect for democratic ideals is stagnating, there is increasing social and emotional discontent, and decreasing health and longevity in the absence of effective programmes for promotion of individual and collective well-being.

Key elements of positive clinical therapeutics for health promotion

Now that the world has many interdependent crises that have been created by the unrestrained excesses of the secular materialistic subculture (9, 16), it is essential for people to be aware of how their own community is functioning in relation to what are meaningful, satisfying, and health-promoting values. In order to promote health, we have found it necessary to be aware of the strengths and weaknesses of different people with distinct clusters of personality features, and the distinct subcultures and communities that they comprise and inhabit. Otherwise, it is not possible for people to understand their own motivation and how it relates to those of their workplace and country, both of which are needed to identify values that are meaningful and satisfying for them. In order to serve others selflessly, we need to understand ourselves in relationship to them and our living habitat, Mother Earth, who currently is sick and febrile. With that awareness of both the person and his/her community and habitat, we can begin to address all human needs in a balanced and integrated way, including needs for security and safety, healthy nutrition and exercise, human and ecological relationships, culture and art, and spirituality.

Addressing all human needs in a coordinated way rather than *ad seriatum* means that effective clinical therapeutics addresses each of the following elements needed for promotion of physical, emotional, social, ecological, and spiritual well-being: 1) safety and security, so that people feel calm enough to be open to change, and can think realistically and impartially; 2) resilience and plasticity, including physical, mental, social, and spiritual flexibility, so that we experience the satisfaction of accepting and coping with adversity and disappointment, adapting in flexible and resourceful ways, rather than giving into our fears with rigid avoidance or aggressive defences; 3) building mutually respectful and satisfying relationships by compassionate and selfless service to others, and by expression of gratitude when we are fortunate enough to receive such kindness ourselves; 4) building understanding and respect for ecological balance in our planetary habitat, including modifying patterns of consumption, pollution, and environmental degradation, by recognizing that the planet has limits beyond which it cannot heal itself; and 5) working creatively on self-transcendence and self-actualization by increased introspection of who we are really, what we find satisfying and meaningful, and what satisfies our need for coherence, unity, and participation in something greater than our individual self. Therapists benefit from doing such work themselves or they cannot really help others to do so optimally. When they engage in self-actualization themselves, clinicians have the good fortune to grow along with the people they serve.

There are many ways to address each of these therapeutic targets. What to do and in what order to do them in depends on the individual people involved (i.e. both treating and treated in co-active person-centred work). Safety and security can be addressed by the quality of the working alliance itself (respectful, regular, encouraging work on common goals) and use of physiological interventions that address the molecular biology of temperament (like cryotherapy, breathing techniques to enhance autonomic balance, physical exercise, and sometimes use of medications for anxiety and depression) (17, 71).

Resilience and plasticity require joint attention to anxiety, frustration, and goal setting, such as help in exploring alternative goals that are specific, measurable, attainable, relevant, and timed (SMART) and coping with intermittent and partial success by hierarchies of goals that balance difficulty and importance by insight into values and motivation. This always requires work on body awareness, especially among intellectuals: it is crucial to learn to tolerate trying to do things that are physically challenging for the particular individual, as well as to work on goal setting, acceptance of responsibility, and letting go of control, with awareness of what is personally meaningful and valued, as in many third-wave psychotherapies (72).

The cultivation of social relationships always recognizes that we cannot make others love and respect us, but we can always serve others selflessly. Service to others is healing to every aspect of a person's being, whereas seeking self-interests only is a self-defeating and insatiable quest, as is well demonstrated by the current crises of the materialistic phase of the Anthropocene and long recognized in all wisdom traditions, such as the Bagavad Gita (7, 73). The search for happiness and subjective well-being is filled with such paradoxes: we cannot be truly joyful and happy when we seek happiness for ourselves at the expense of others, but we are satisfied when we let go of expectations for personal benefit from the fruits of our work to serve others.

Improving awareness and respect in human relationships by increasing social intelligence can be extended to work on ecological intelligence by greater engagement and experience with nature, and awareness that the earth is actually our sacred mother and beyond our control, not something to be exploited like we were gods of infinite power. Even some materialists recognize that nature has finite resources and it is practical to limit consumption to sustainable levels that do not degrade our only habitat irreversibly (74). However, full development of ecological intelligence generally requires work on self-transcendence that most traditionalists and materialists resist, so it is implemented in clinical work while cultivating virtue and willingness to make selfless sacrifices for the good of future generations more generally.

Selfish, cruel, and controlling people are obviously not virtuous, but neither are they really happy or healthy in the long run (49). Only the creative profile with high self-transcendence activates the mechanisms that support healthy longevity, altruism, and creativity, so effective health promotion requires work on mindfulness and then contemplation and prayer. Such work on mindfulness and contemplation is crucial for awakening self-transcendence and the spiritual aspects of well-being that go beyond dogmatic beliefs and logical reasoning to awaken insight (i.e. immediate, deep intuitive understanding) (17).

The process of health promotion is complex so that, as progress or resistance occur, there is an iterative cycle to understand the new-found strengths and weaknesses. Ultimately, people begin to realize that they have enormous potential for change and development in creative ways that allow them to recognize the unconscious biases of repressed traumas, to let go of the resulting struggles, and to vividly recollect the painful past so that they can also vividly image a healthy future. When that is done, archaic memories and epigenetic marks are changed, allowing illumination, creativity, flourishing, and wisdom to emerge in the way people function. Dark times like the world today provides us with are opportunities to learn how to realize the natural human potential for good. Clinicians need to prepare themselves to do what they can to be healthy, flexible, and virtuous so that they can serve others and help individuals and communities to be healthier too.

Conclusion

Recent work in psychology and psychiatry has now produced a solid empirical foundation for an integrative and effective approach to the promotion of health and well-being. Personality development depends on the creative process of integration of three aspects of the person through three complex adaptive systems of learning and memory involving associative conditioning of habits, intentional self-control, and creative processes of self-awareness. Well-being depends on such integration in order for a person to cultivate an outlook of unity and connectedness about their life, which is essential for healthy longevity, positive emotionality, and prosocial behaviour. The physical, mental, and spiritual aspects of human life are interdependent, so must be addressed jointly in order for a person to self-actualize a healthy, happy, and good life. By extension, individual well-being and collective well-being are interdependent because we are social beings who must grow, learn, and live in the world.

Future perspectives

At present, the world and our planet are in crisis with major planetary changes in climate from excessive exploitation of finite resources. People feel stressed by the dehumanization of civil institutions that treat people as objects, consumers, and employees without respect for the intrinsic dignity of all people, without understanding the need to function in harmony with nature, and without awareness that we cannot be healthy, happy, or good without working to live with moderation and humility in harmony with all people and things. Fortunately life is a great, relentless, and fair teacher so, in order to be healthy, happy, and good, each of us will discover what is required to live well at our own individual pace and in our own way. The world situation is urgent, but we can only begin by each of us learning to help ourselves by doing what we can to be healthy. Each of us will discover that our individual well-being depends on collective well-being and vice versa. Therefore, each of us can begin to contribute in an important and meaningful way to addressing the current world crisis by learning to know who we are really. Even though the challenges are vast and may feel overwhelming, each of us can make a meaningful difference, even if we only change our own life because that will also have an impact on the way we affect other people and the planet on which we all live.

References

1. Gable SL, Haidt J. What (and why) is positive psychology? *General Review of Psychology*. 2005;9(2):103–10.
2. Seligman MEP, Csikszentmihalyi M. Positive psychology: an introduction. *American Psychologist*. 2000;55(1):5–14.
3. Gillham JE, Seligman ME. Footsteps on the road to a positive psychology. *Behaviour Research and Therapy* 1999;37(Suppl. 1):S163–73.
4. Kobau R, Seligman ME, Peterson C, Diener E, Zack MM, Chapman D, et al. Mental health promotion in public health: perspectives and strategies from positive psychology. *American Journal of Public Health*. 2011;101(8):e1–9.
5. Peterson C, Seligman MEP. *Character strengths and virtues*. New York: Oxford; 2004.
6. Seligman MEP. Positive psychology: a personal history. *Annual Review of Clinical Psychol*. 2019;15:1–23.
7. Cloninger CR. *Feeling good: the science of well-being*. New York: Oxford; 2004.

8. **Cloninger CR, Salvador-Carulla L, Kirmayer LJ, Schwartz MA, Appleyard J, Goodwin N,** et al. A time for action on health inequities: foundations of the 2014 Geneva declaration on person- and people-centered integrated health care for All. *International Journal of Person Centered Medicine.* 2014;4(2):68–89.

9. **Cloninger CR.** What makes people healthy, happy, and fulfiled in the face of current world challenges? *Mens Sana Monographs.* 2013;11:16–24.

10. **Macdonald C, Bore M, Munro D.** Values in action scale and the Big 5: an empirical indication of structure. *Journal of Research in Personality.* 2008(42):787–99.

11. **Brdar I, Kashdan TB.** Character strengths and well-being in Croatia: an empirical investigation of structure and correlates. *Journal of Research in Personality.* 2010(44):151–4.

12. **Shryack J, Krueger MF, Kallie CS.** The structure of virtue: an empirical investigation of the dimensionality of the virtues in action inventory of strengths. *Personality and Individual Differences.* 2010(48):714–9.

13. **Jeste DV, Palmer BW** (eds). *Positive psychiatry. A clinical handbook.* Washington, DC: American Psychiatric Publishing; 2015.

14. **Vaillant GE.** Adaptive mental mechanisms. Their role in a positive psychology. *Am Psychol.* 2000;55(1):89–98.

15. **Vaillant GE.** Psychiatry, religion, positive emotions and spirituality. *Asian J Psychiatr.* 2013;6(6):590–4.

16. **Cloninger CR, Cloninger KM.** People create health: effective health promotion is a creative process. *International Journal of Person Centered Medicine.* 2013;3(2):114–22.

17. **Cloninger KM, Cloninger CR.** The psychobiology of the path to a joyful life: implications for future research and practice. *Journal of Positive Psychology.* 2019;15(1):74–83.

18. **Cloninger CR, Zohar AH.** Personality and the perception of health and happiness. *Journal of Affective Disorders.* 2011;128(1–2):24–32.

19. **Lyubomirsky S, King L, Diener E.** The benefits of frequent positive affect: does happiness lead to success? *Psychological Bulletin.* 2005;131(6):803–55.

20. **Cloninger CR.** Book review of Peterson and Seligman's Character and Human Virtues. *American Journal of Psychiatry.* 2005;162(4):820–1.

21. **Cloninger CR.** The science of well-being: an integrated approach to mental health and its disorders. *World Psychiatry.* 2006;5(2):71–6.

22. **Chiesa A, Serretti A.** Mindfulness-based stress reduction for stress management in healthy people: a review and meta-analysis. *Journal of Alternative and Complementary Medicine.* 2009;15(5):593–600.

23. **Chiesa A, Serretti A.** A systematic review of neurobiological and clinical features of mindfulness meditations. *Psychological Medicine.* 2010;40(8):1239–52.

24. **Walsh BT, Seidman SN, Sysko R, Gould M.** Placebo response in studies of major depression: variable, substantial, and growing. *JAMA.* 2002;287(14):1840–7.

25. **Fava GA, Rafanelli C, Grandi S, Conti S, Belluardo P.** Prevention of recurrent depression with cognitive behavioral therapy: preliminary findings. *Arch Gen Psychiatry.* 1998;55(9):816–20.

26. **VanderWeele TJ, Li S, Tsai AC, Kawachi I.** Association between religious service attendance and lower suicide rates among US women. *JAMA Psychiatry.* 2016;73(8):845–51.

27. **Miller L, Wickramaratne P, Gameroff MJ, Sage M, Tenke CE, Weissman MM.** Religiosity and major depression in adults at high risk: a ten-year prospective study. *American Journal of Psychiatry.* 2012;**169**(1):89–94.

28. **D'Souza RF, Rodrigo A.** Spiritually augmented cognitive behavioural therapy. *Australasian Psychiatry.* 2004;**12**(2):148–52.

29. **Fava GA, Ruini C.** Development and characteristics of a well-being enhancing psychotherapeutic strategy: well-being therapy. *Journal of Behavior Therapy and Experimental Psychiatry.* 2003;**34**(1):45–63.

30. **Fava GA, Tomba E.** Increasing psychological well-being and resilience by psychotherapeutic methods. *Journal of Personality.* 2009;**77**(6):1903–34.

31. **Mosqueiro BP, Fleck MP, da Rocha NS.** Increased levels of brain-derived neurotrophic factor are associated with high intrinsic religiosity among depressed inpatients. *Frontiers in Psychiatry.* 2019;**10**:671.

32. **Cloninger CR.** Spirituality and the science of feeling good. *Southern Medical Association.* 2007;**100**(7):740–3.

33. **World Health Organization (WHO).** *Mental health: new understanding, new hope.* Geneva,: WHO; 1946.

34. **Cloninger CR, Zohar AH, Cloninger KM.** Promotion of well-being in person-centered mental health care. *Focus.* 2010;**8**(2):165–79.

35. **Cloninger CR, Svrakic DM, Przybeck TR.** A psychobiological model of temperament and character. *Arch Gen Psychiatry.* 1993;**50**(12):975–90.

36. **Cloninger CR, Cloninger KM.** Person-centered therapeutics. *International Journal of Person Centered Medicine.* 2011;**1**(1):43–52.

37. **Cloninger CR.** The psychobiological theory of temperament and character: comment on Farmer and Goldberg (2008). *Psychological Assessment.* 2008;**20**(3):292–9; discussion 300–4.

38. **Cloninger CR.** Person-centered health promotion in chronic disease. *International Journal of Person Centered Medicine.* 2013;**3**(1):5–12.

39. **Garcia D, Cloninger KM, Lester N, Cloninger CR.** The future of personality research and applications: some latest findings. In: D. Garcia, T. Archer, R. Kostrzewa (eds), *Personality and brain disorders, contemporary clinical neuroscience.* Cham, Switzerland: Springer; 2019, pp. 3–24.

40. **Cloninger CR.** Evolution of human brain functions: the functional structure of human consciousness. *Australian and New Zealand Journal of Psychiatry.* 2009;**43**(11):994–1006.

41. **Cloninger CR.** Temperament and personality. *Current Opinion in Neurobiology.* 1994;**4**(2):266–73.

42. **Garcia D, Lundstrom S, Brandstrom S, Rastam M, Cloninger CR, Kerekes N,** et al. Temperament and character in the child and adolescent twin study in Sweden (CATSS): comparison to the general population, and genetic structure analysis. *PLoS One.* 2013;**8**(8):e70475.

43. **Garcia D, Strage A, Lundstrom S, Radovic S, Brandstrom S, Rastam M,** et al. Responsibility and cooperativeness are constrained, not determined. *Frontiers in Psychology.* 2014;**5**:308.

44. **Gillespie NA, Cloninger CR, Heath AC, Martin NG.** The genetic and environmental relationship between Cloninger's dimensions of temperament and character. *Personality and Individual Differences.* 2003;**35**(8):1931–46.

45. **Gusnard DA, Ollinger JM, Shulman GL, Cloninger CR, Price JL, Van Essen DC**, et al. Persistence and brain circuitry. *Proceedings of the National Academy of Sciences of the USA*. 2003;**100**(6):3479–84.

46. **Ellermann CR, Reed PG**. Self-transcendence and depression in middle-age adults. *Western Journal of Nursing Research*. 2001;**23**(7):698–713.

47. **Runquist JJ, Reed PG**. Self-transcendence and well-being in homeless adults. *Journal of Holistic Nursing*. 2007;**25**(1):5–13; discussion 4–5.

48. **Rosmarin DH, Bigda-Peyton JS, Kertz SJ, Smith N, Rauch SL, Bjorgvinsson T**. A test of faith in God and treatment: the relationship of belief in God to psychiatric treatment outcomes. *Journal of Affective Disorders*. 2013;**146**(3):441–6.

49. **Zwir I, Arnedo J, Del-Val C, Pulkki-Raback L, Konte B, Yang SS**, et al. Uncovering the complex genetics of human character. *Molecular Psychiatry*. 2020;**25**(10):2295–312.

50. **Zwir I, Arnedo J, Del-Val C, Pulkki-Raback L, Konte B, Yang SS**, et al. Uncovering the complex genetics of human temperament. *Molecular Psychiatry*. 2020;**25**(10):2275–94.

51. **Cloninger CR, Cloninger KM, Zwir I, Keltikangas-Jarvinen L**. The complex genetics and biology of human temperament: a review of traditional concepts in relation to new molecular findings. *Translational Psychiatry*. 2019;**9**(1):290.

52. **Zwir I, Del-Val C, Arnedo J, Pulkki-Raback L, Konte B, Yang SS**, et al. Three genetic-environmental networks for human personality. *Molecular Psychiatry*. 2019 Nov 21. Online ahead of print. doi:10.1038/s41380-019-0579-x.

53. **Teasdale JD, Moore RG, Hayhurst H, Pope M, Williams S, Segal ZV**. Metacognitive awareness and prevention of relapse in depression: empirical evidence. *Journal of Consulting and Clinical Psychology*. 2002;**70**(2):275–87.

54. **Liu Q, He H, Yang J, Feng X, Zhao F, Lyu J**. Changes in the global burden of depression from 1990 to 2017: findings from the global burden of disease study. *Journal of Psychiatric Research*. 2020;**126**:134–40.

55. **Wong KM, Cloninger CR**. A person-centered approach to clinical practice. *Focus*. 2010;**8**:199–215.

56. **Hilsenroth MJ, Peters EJ, Ackerman SJ**. The development of therapeutic alliance during psychological assessment: patient and therapist perspectives across treatment. *Journal of Personal Assessment*. 2004;**83**(3):332–44.

57. **Limb CJ, Braun AR**. Neural substrates of spontaneous musical performance: an FMRI study of jazz improvisation. *PLoS One*. 2008;**3**(2):e1679.

58. **Gusnard DA, Akbudak E, Shulman GL, Raichle ME**. Medial prefrontal cortex and self-referential mental activity: relation to a default mode of brain function. *Proceedings of the National Academy of Sciences of the USA*. 2001;**98**(7):4259–64.

59. **Koechlin E, Corrado G, Pietrini P, Grafman J**. Dissociating the role of the medial and lateral anterior prefrontal cortex in human planning. *Proceedings of the National Academy of Sciences of the USA*. 2000;**97**(13):7651–6.

60. **Krasner MS, Epstein RM, Beckman H, Suchman AL, Chapman B, Mooney CJ**, et al. Association of an educational program in mindful communication with burnout, empathy, and attitudes among primary care physicians. *JAMA*. 2009;**302**(12):1284–93.

61. **Teasdale JD, Segal ZV, Williams JM, Ridgeway VA, Soulsby JM, Lau MA**. Prevention of relapse/recurrence in major depression by mindfulness-based cognitive therapy. *Journal of Consulting and Clinical Psychology*. 2000;**68**(4):615–23.

62. **Levine B.** Autobiographical memory and the self in time: brain lesion effects, functional neuroanatomy, and lifespan development. *Brain and Cognition.* 2004;**55**(1):54–68.

63. **Tulving E.** Episodic memory: from mind to brain. *Annual Review of Psychology.* 2002;**53**:1–25.

64. **Cloninger KM, Lester N, Muszynski A, Lindskar E, Cloninger CR, Garcia D.** Increases in character development, resilience, and well-being among participants in Anthropedia's well-being coaching training. 30th APS Annual Convention, San Francisco; 24–27 May 2018.

65. **Inglehart RF.** *Cultural evolution: people's motivations are changing, and reshaping the world.* Cambridge, UK: Cambridge University Press; 2018.

66. **Ray PH, Anderson SR.** *The cultural creatives: how 50 million people are changing the world.* New York: Random House; 2000.

67. **Schwartz S.** Basic human values: theory, measurement, and applications. *Revue Française de Sociologie.* 2006;**47**(4):929–68.

68. **Schwartz SH.** A theory of cultural values and some implications for work. *Applied Psychology: An International Review.* 1999;**48**:23–478.

69. **Tibbs H.** Changing cultural values and the transition to sustainability. *Journal of Future Studies.* 2011;**15**(3):13–32.

70. **United Nations Development Program.** United Nations Human Development Report (UNHDR) *Beyond income, beyond average, beyond today: inequities in human development in the 21st century.* New York: United Nations Development Program; 2019.

71. **Cloninger CR, Cloninger KM.** Person-centered psychotherapy. In: **JE Mezzichea** (ed.), *Person-centered psychiatry.* Cham, Switzerland: Springer; 2016, pp. 247–62.

72. **Granjard A,** et al. *Resilience profiles among Swedish long-term unemployed.* Chicago, IL: Association for Psychological Science; 2020.

73. **Gandhi MK.** *The Bhagavad Gita according to Gandhi.* Berkeley, CA: Berkeley Hills Books; 2000.

74. **Stiglitz JE.** *The price of inequality: how today's divided society endangers our future.* First edition. New York: WW Norton & Company; 2013.

Chapter 22

Spiritually integrated psychotherapy

Marianna de Abreu Costa and
David H. Rosmarin

Relevance and available evidence

There is growing recognition of the importance of culturally adapting interventions in order to offer client-centred treatment focused on the needs of the individual (1). Along these lines, there is also growing recognition of the importance of addressing religiosity and spirituality in clinical practice (2, 3). Spiritually integrated psychotherapy (SIP) involves the utilization of spiritual/ religious content in the therapy process. Consistent evidence suggests that SIP can be as effective (4) or even more effective than standard protocols (5), especially for religious clients (6), and effects seem to be independent of therapists' own levels of religiosity. Interestingly, one study found that the spiritually adapted protocol conducted by non-religious therapists was more effective than when conducted by religious therapists (7). Several reviews have found that SIPs are at least as effective as conventional psychotherapy for mental disorders (4, 5, 13–16), and cognitive behavioural therapy (CBT) is the most investigated SIP and has robust evidence of efficacy (17).

The advent and study of SIPs is significant because most individuals are spiritual. Furthermore, religious beliefs and practices are often central to how spiritual clients create meaning in life (8), implement coping resources, and develop resilience (9). However, at times, spirituality can be a struggle and the cause of conflict or suffering, resulting in mental health problems (10). The integration of spirituality into psychotherapy can therefore help clients to harness their religious beliefs and practices as coping resources, and directly address spiritual struggles. Data suggests that SIP can also improve the therapeutic relationship, strengthen adherence to treatment, and improve the individual's capacity to deal with suffering (11). In addition, research also shows that most clients want clinicians to address religiousness-related issues in their general psychiatric care (12) and in psychotherapy (13). These findings are supported by the recent Position Statement on religiosity and spirituality of the World Psychiatric Association, which proposes a careful consideration of clients' religious beliefs and practices, regardless of the professional's belief (2).

Practical clinical implications

First of all, it is important to highlight the ethical aspects of this approach. As already discussed, SIP is part and parcel of client-centred and humanistic care. More broadly though, religion and spirituality are important dimensions of life (8), and delivering treatment without addressing these domains could cause harm to some clients. It is therefore incumbent upon all clinicians to gain the necessary skills to address clients' spirituality/religion in treatment, in order to understand how such beliefs and practices are relevant to clinical care, and to address these dimensions in a sensitive, respectful, and non-proselytizing way. As with any intervention, when providing SIPs, it is important to obtain the client's *informed consent* . This can be done by simple asking the client about their interest in discussing spiritual issues in their treatment (18). Of course, clinicians must respect clients' wishes if they do not wish to address spiritual life. However, the data suggests that most clients would like to address spiritual life in treatment. Chapter 21 of this book gives information about how to take the spiritual history of the client. Beyond informed consent and a spiritual history, CBT clinicians can address spirituality/religion in the context of *assessment, psychoeducation, motivational strategies, behavioural strategies and cognitive strategies*. See Table 22.1 for a summary of adapted techniques.

Assessment

It is important to remember that, even if the therapist is not a religious or spiritual person, they can be effective in assessing and integrating spiritual issues to psychotherapy (7) because spirituality is like other areas of clients' lives, many of which the therapists sometimes do not have experiential familiarity with. Also, it is improbable that the therapist will know nothing about a specific religious tradition because religion is often embedded in our cultural context and different traditions tend to share principles, beliefs, and activities (18). With that said, a basic knowledge of the major religious traditions can be advantageous. The aim of assessment in the practice of SIP is to collect information about the client in order to develop a formulation of the case (19). Also, it is important to identify and use the same religious language and symbols used by the client (6, 20), so that therapists can consult specific literature about the client's religion.

Rosmarin (2018) divides the assessment into four parts (orientation, functional analysis, collaboration, and monitoring). First, in orientation, the

Table 22.1 Summary of adapted techniques

	Techniques	Description
Initial therapy session	Psycho-education about symptoms and mental health disorders	Discussion about religious theories for the causation of symptoms and disorders. Information provided about the impact of spirituality on mental health.
	Psycho-education about cognitive behavioural therapy (CBT) model	Explanation about the relationship between thoughts, behaviours, and emotions using spiritual content.
Motivational strategies		Using spiritual content to motivate clients to engage in treatment.
Behavioural intervention	Religious activities	Explicitly encourage private religious activities (e.g. praying, reading religious texts, meditating) and religious community activities (e.g. religious services, engaging in charity), and religious and spiritual activities as homework tasks. These activities are used for behavioural activation.
	Values	Motivating clients to act according to their values (e.g. forgiveness, generosity, altruism, compassion).
	Coping strategies	Explicitly encourage act using positive spiritual coping instead negative spiritual coping.
Cognitive Intervention	Cognitive restructuring	Modifying distorted automatic thoughts and beliefs using spiritual content.
	Sharing stories	Sharing spiritual stories as metaphors in order to amplifying some issue.
	Religious imagery modification	Combining cognitive restructuring with systematic desensitization. Clients are encouraged to imagine a depressive image while also imagining themselves coping using a spiritual perspective.
	Coping strategies	Encouraging client to reason using positive spiritual coping and reducing the use of negative spiritual coping.

purpose is to obtain informed consent and start collecting information in order to clarify the client's religious/spiritual experiences as well as their involvement in religious activities in the community and private settings (18, 20). Simple questions such as 'Would you mind if I asked you about spirituality or religiosity' (18) and 'What aspect of your religious or spiritual life has been important to you?' can guide this initial approach. The functional assessment intends to explore how spiritual issues are related to clients' symptoms or problems ('How is your spirituality related to your symptoms?') (18). This is the cornerstone of assessment in the practice of spiritually integrated CBT, in that it helps clients and therapists to identify the emotional functions of spirituality within the client's life, and the relevance of this domain to their mental and behavioural health.

In collaboration, the therapist and client explore how religiosity and spirituality are related to symptoms in an experimental way (18). The therapist may ask the client: 'Did you notice any ways in which spirituality or religiosity was relevant to your symptoms over the past week?' or 'Would you like to see whether using any of the following concepts or activities (like reading a religious text, meditating, attending a religious group) has any effect on your symptoms?' Also, the therapist and client can define positive and negative religious and spiritual coping, and identify their own positive spiritual resources (21). Finally, monitoring refers to the part in which therapist and client will analyse the impact of including spiritual and religious issues in treatment (18).

Psychoeducation

Along with assessment, spiritually integrated CBT can provide psychoeducation to clients about the *cognitive behavioural model* of various disorders, which serves as a platform to explain the *treatment rationale*. Adapted psychoeducation involves the utilization of spiritual content for framing CBT. Also, it can include information about the *impact of spirituality on mental health* (6, 20, 21). For example, many religious traditions claim that our thoughts, behaviours, and emotions are interconnected and therefore influence each other (18). Therapists can use this conviction to explain about the *relationship between thoughts, behaviours, and emotions*. One example to elucidate it is the proverb, 'For as he (a person) thinketh in his heart, so is he' (Proverbs 23:7) (22). Also, it is possible to discuss religious theories for the formation of mental health symptoms (21, 23–25). Pecheur and Edwards (1984) reviewed biblical teachings about the self, the world, and the future with Christian clients with depression, for example (23).

Another possibility is to use spiritual beliefs to *frame treatment rationale* (6, 22, 25) as the importance of becoming an observer of one's thoughts, and the idea that thought modification is a therapeutic mechanism, which are concepts found in several world religion's sacred texts. One Christian example is the following (6):

> The ancient Greek word 'metanoia' literally means to 'change your mind' or 'change how you think,' which the Bible translated as 'repent.' Thus, changing the way we think (i.e., repenting in Christian language) is a biblically-based concept (Matthew 4:17).

Another example of biblical verse is (22):

> And be not conformed to this world: but be ye transformed by the renewing of your mind, that ye may prove what is that good, and acceptable, and perfect, will of God (Roman 12:2).

Motivational strategies

Teachings of many religious traditions can help individuals to face their life struggles. To this end, therapists can harness spiritual/religious content to help patients stay motivated to engage in therapy. In monotheistic traditions, for example, it is understood that a loving God asks people to do things they don't necessarily feel like doing but are for their benefit (6):

> The 13th Century in Jewish tradition work 'Sefer HaChinuch' writes, '*Know that a man is* influenced in accordance with his actions. His heart and thoughts follow after his deeds in which he is occupied ... Therefore, look carefully at what you do, for after your actions your heart will be drawn.

Also, the Serenity Prayer in Christian traditions can motivate clients to change what they can change (20): 'God, give me grace to accept with serenity the things that cannot be changed, Courage to change the things which should be changed, and the Wisdom to distinguish the one from the other'.

Besides using spiritual content to motivate clients to better engage in treatment, the adapted motivational strategies can be framed as a test of faith or as exerting heroic effort for God (18) because many traditions understand actions as a form of divine service. So, discussing and understanding relevant spiritual reasons that support treatment can more effectively and consistently engage clients in the treatment.

Behavioural activation

Behavioural activation is a CBT-based treatment involving the scheduling of adaptive and helpful behaviours without restructuring cognitive content. Numerous studies support the efficacy of behavioural activation as a treatment for depression, and other conditions as well. Spiritually integrated behavioural activation consists in *using private and community religious activities* to help clients re-engage with meaningful aspects of their spiritual life. Such approaches can also help motivate clients to act according to *their life values*, which can add a significant meaning to behaviour interventions. It is also noteworthy that there are known protective effects of religious service attendance for mental disorders, especially in suicide (26).

In the context of spiritually integrated behavioural activation, religious activities can be performed privately or in a faith community. These activities can explicitly be suggested for behavioural interventions (6, 20, 21, 24, 25,27). Below is a list of community and private activities:

> *Community activities*: attend a sacred liturgy, minister at a religious service or function, attend bible study, attend a religious social function, attend a group, go and speak with a religious leader, volunteer or engage with a charity.

> *Private activities*: praying, reading religious texts, meditating, reciting psalms or hymns, religious rituals, listening to religious music, seeking clergy support, confession, studies about faith.

Most religions promote values like forgiveness, generosity, altruism, and compassion, and the literature shows that acting in accordance with one's own personal values is an important factor for mental health (28). Also, *value-based intervention* is an underpinning component of the contextual therapies in which clients are invited to clarify their life values and to behave in that direction (29). In spiritual-adapted techniques, values like gratitude, discernment, forgiveness, trust, meaning and purpose, altruism, and social engagement can be assessed (6, 18, 21). So, clients can be invited to identify these values as something that they either had or desired more in their lives, and encouraged to engage in valued exercises (6, 18, 21). The exercises can range from identifying some specific value throughout the day to act according to the value. Also, monitoring changes in mood during this practice can enrich the exercise (18).

Another important set of behaviours to attend to in treatment is the use of *negative spiritual/religious coping*. Although individuals typically use their faith in a positive way, sometimes they engage in negative spiritual/religious coping and use this content in a distorted way, leading to a negative impact on their emotions (9, 21). In the practice of spiritually integrated behavioural activation, clients can be explicitly encouraged to use spiritual positive coping strategies (e.g. spiritual beliefs that give meaning to existential questions and suffering, a secure relationship with a forgiving and acceptant God, a sense of spiritual connection with others) and discouraged to use negative R/S coping strategies (e.g. viewing God as punishing or abandoning them, being unable to forgive) (21, 30). In one therapy manual for generalized anxiety disorder, for example, clients were exposed to Taoism and Confucianism teachings (30):

> a. *'Benefiting without hurting others and acting without striving'; b. 'Restricting selfish desires, learning to be content, and knowing how to let go'; c. 'Being in harmony with others and being humble, using softness to defeat hardness'; and d. 'Person should maintain tranquility, act less, and follow the laws of nature'*. Then, clients were invited to put these principles into practice in their daily life.

Cognitive intervention

Spiritual beliefs can have an impact on emotion in positive and negative ways. Many spiritual beliefs, such as the idea that God is benevolent, or belief in the immortality or reincarnation, or the concept that suffering can have a purpose, can be positively used to facilitate coping with different stressors through life. Conversely, the beliefs that God is malevolent or unfair, or that human beings cannot overcome their challenges, can have a negative impact on mental health and well-being. Adapted cognitive restructuring encompasses modifying distorted automatic thoughts and beliefs using spiritual content as well as restructuring specific distorted spiritual beliefs that have a negative impact on emotion. This can be done by using reflections from spiritual texts to better explore cognitive restructuring, sharing spiritual stories to help clients to gain perspective, and by using religious imagery modification.

In standard cognitive therapy, restructuring automatic negative thoughts and irrational beliefs involves first identifying distorted automatic thoughts and then modifying them using more adaptive perspectives. Spiritually integrated CBT simply uses clients' spiritual rationales and values as resources for cognitive restructuration (6, 7, 22–25). In other words, maladaptive automatic thoughts are identified and then changed using religious values, teachings, and beliefs. Naturally, any scriptural or holy text examples need to be extracted specifically from a client's tradition and need to resonate with their particular belief system. Therapy manuals adapted for Christians often use Biblical scripture (6, 7), while Muslim protocols use the Holy Koran and Hadith (6, 25). Here is an example as to how this can be done in practice by considering the type of congenital distortion and the client's belief:

> Depressive Christian clients with distorted thoughts about the self can be presented with this verse: 'God demonstrates His own love towards us, in that while yet sinners, Christ died for us. (Romans 5:8; i.e. God loves, accepts, and values us just as we are) (23).
>
> Depressive Christian clients with distorted thoughts about the world and future could be presented with this verse: 'In the world you have tribulation but take courage; I (Jesus Christ) have overcome the world (John 16:33b). These things I have spoken to you, so that in Me you may have peace.' (John 16:33a) (22).
>
> Depressive Jewish clients with distorted thoughts about 'should and must' statements may benefit from reflecting on the following: 'I must be thoroughly competent, adequate, and achieving in all possible respects if I am to consider myself worthwhile', would be: 'All of us have become like one who is unclean, and all our righteous acts are like filthy rags (Isaiah 64:6)' (6,17).

Other distorted beliefs can similarly be restructured using spiritual content. Notably, research suggests that belief in a benevolent God can help individuals to deal with intolerance of uncertainty or catastrophizing, for example

(18). As well, devotion to God can help individuals who suffer from fears of negative evaluation from others, as well as perfectionism and body distortions (18). Along these lines, an interesting adaptation to restructuring cognition is found in Koenig et al. (2015, (6)). They adapted an instrument called the 'ABCD(R)E' thought based on Albert Ellis's method for cognitive restructuring. In their protocol, they added a step 'R,' which stands for religious beliefs and resources (6, 17) In step R, clients are invited to challenge their automatic thought with their own religious beliefs, values, and teachings: 'How can your view of God, your religious/spiritual worldview, religious writings, spiritual wisdom, and other sources provide evidence that challenge your automatic negative beliefs and beliefs that you can't cope?'. So, it is important to note that, even if clinicians do not have any knowledge about the individual's faith, they can get it by inquiring from the client in order to stimulate the discussion in a helpful way.

In addition to restructuring distorted cognitions related to the client's mental health disorder, sometimes it is necessary to *restructure negative thoughts and beliefs related to their faith* (i.e. spiritual struggles, such as feeling that God is punishing them). Once this type of distortion has been identified, it is necessary to restructure these specific distorted spiritual beliefs because they can be sources of deep suffering. Also, therapists can encourage the use of spiritual positive coping strategies instead of negative ones (e.g. viewing God as punishing or abandoning them, being unable to forgive) (21, 25, 30). Index cards carrying positive spiritual coping statements can be used between sessions in order to better reassure the use of positive spiritual coping. One example is: 'No matter how bad it gets, I am never alone' (18).

Another approach involves religious imagery modification. This is an adaption of a less commonly used cognitive technique that combines cognitive restructuring with systematic desensitization techniques. In the spiritually adapted version, clients are invited to restructure their experiences using religiously based imagery (7, 31), in order to help change depressive images by using religious content. Clients are initially asked to recall depressive thoughts and feelings. Then they are given lists of religious coping statements and images using Beck's cognitive triad of depression (i.e. distorted and pessimistic concept of self, world, and future) and are invited to replace their negative thoughts and images with images such as visualizing Christ going with them into a difficult situation (31). Also, clients are encouraged to practise contemplative prayer or meditating on a specific religious passage in order to help them better manage negative thinking patterns (6, 17).

Conclusions

SIP involves the adaptation of secular psychotherapy in a culturally sensitive and *client-centred* way by addressing spiritual/religious life. In spiritually integrated CBT, clinicians adapt commonly used CBT methods by incorporating spiritual content into the treatment process. Of course, therapists must carefully avoid proselytism and recognize that treatment is first and foremost for the purposes of benefiting mental health—not spiritual growth. With that said, therapists must recognize that, for many patients, spiritual growth is an important catalyst for mental health. At a minimum, respecting the individual's spirituality, understanding in a non-judgemental way how their suffering may be related to their spirituality, or how their spirituality can help them deal with their suffering, is necessary. Furthermore, as is the case with all psychotherapy, we do not know which strategies are in fact the 'active ingredients' that improve symptoms. Therapists must therefore remain humble and open to spiritual as well as secular approaches to alleviate emotional pain.

References

1. **Kirmayer LJ, Ban L.** Cultural psychiatry: research strategies and future directions. *Adv Psychosomatic Medicine.* 2013;33:97–114.
2. **Moreira-Almeida A, Sharma A, van Rensburg BJ, Verhagen PJ, Cook CCH.** WPA position statement on spirituality and religion in psychiatry. *World Psychiatry.* 2016 Feb;15(1):87–8.
3. **Moreira-Almeida A, Koenig HG, Lucchetti G.** Clinical implications of spirituality to mental health: review of evidence and practical guidelines. *Revista Brasileira de Psiquiatria Sao Paulo, Brazil.* 2014 Jun;36(2):176–82.
4. **Lim C, Sim K, Renjan V, Sam HF, Quah SL.** Adapted cognitive-behavioral therapy for religious individuals with mental disorder: a systematic review. *Asian Journal of Psychiatry.* 2014 Jun;9:3–12.
5. **Anderson N, Heywood-Everett S, Siddiqi N, Wright J, Meredith J, McMillan D.** Faith-adapted psychological therapies for depression and anxiety: systematic review and meta-analysis. *Journal of Affective Disorders.* 2015 May;176:183–96.
6. **Koenig HG, Pearce MJ, Nelson B, Shaw SF, Robins CJ, Daher NS,** et al. Religious vs. conventional cognitive behavioral therapy for major depression in persons with chronic medical illness: a pilot randomized trial. *Journal of Nervous and Mental Disease.* 2015 Apr;203(4):243–51.
7. **Propst LR, Ostrom R, Watkins P, Dean T, Mashburn D.** Comparative efficacy of religious and nonreligious cognitive-behavioral therapy for the treatment of clinical depression in religious individuals. *Journal of Consulting and Clinical Psychology.* 1992 Feb;60(1):94–103.
8. **Pargament KI.** *Spiritually integrated psychotherapy: understanding and addressing the sacred.* New York and London: Guilford Press; 2011.

9. **Zimpel RR, Panzini RG, Bandeira DR, Heldt E, Manfro GG, Fleck MP,** et al. Can religious coping and depressive symptoms predict clinical outcome and quality of life in panic disorder? A Brazilian longitudinal study. *Journal of Nervous and Mental Disease.* 2018;**206**(7):544–8.

10. **Johnson CV, Hayes JA, Wade NG.** Psychotherapy with troubled spirits: a qualitative investigation. *Psychotherapy Research.* 2007 Jul;**17**(4):450–60.

11. **Martins, Moreira-Almeida A.** Terapia cognitivo comportamental— PROCOGNITIVA programa de atualização [Internet]. *Secad.* [cited 9 February 2018]. Available from: https://www.secad.com.br/produto/psicologia/ procognitiva-programa-de-atualizacao-em-terapia-cognitivo-comportamental/

12. **Baetz M, Griffin R, Bowen R, Marcoux G.** Spirituality and psychiatry in Canada: psychiatric practice compared with patient expectations. *Canadian Journal of Psychiatry.* 2004 Apr;**49**(4):265–71.

13. **Post BC, Wade NG.** Religion and spirituality in psychotherapy: a practice-friendly review of research. *Journal of Clinical Psychology.* 2009 Feb;**65**(2):131–46.

14. **Hook JN, Worthington EL, Davis DE, Jennings DJ, Gartner AL, Hook JP.** Empirically supported religious and spiritual therapies. *Journal of Clinical Psychology.* 2010 Jan;**66**(1):46–72.

15. **Worthington EL, Hook JN, Davis DE, McDaniel MA.** Religion and spirituality. *Journal of Clinical Psychology.* 2011 Feb;**67**(2):204–14.

16. **Gonçalves JPB, Lucchetti G, Menezes PR, Vallada H.** Religious and spiritual interventions in mental health care: a systematic review and meta-analysis of randomized controlled clinical trials. *Psychological Medicine.* 2015 Oct;**45**(14):2937–49.

17. **Pearce, M.J.** Cognitive behavioral therapy for christians with depression: a practical, tool-based primer. [Internet]. Templeton Press. 2016 [cited 9 February 2018]. Available from: https://www.templetonpress.org/books/cognitive-behavioral-therapy

18. **Rosmarin DH.** *Spirituality, religion, and cognitive-behavioral therapy: a guide for clinicians.* New York: Guilford Press; 2018.

19. **Beck JS.** *Cognitive behavior therapy: basics and beyond.* Second edition. New York: Guilford Press; 2011. 391 p.

20. **Armento MEA.** *behavioral activation of religious behaviors: treating depressed college students with a randomized controlled trial* (PhD dissertation) [Internet]. 2011 Aug 1; Available from: http://trace.tennessee.edu/utk_graddiss/1052

21. **Bowland S, Edmond T, Fallot RD.** Evaluation of a spiritually focused intervention with older trauma survivors. *Social Work.* 2012 Jan;**57**(1):73–82.

22. **Pecheur, D.** *A comparison of the efficacy of secular and religious cognitive behavior modification in the treatment of depressed Christian college students* (Doctoral dissertation). Rosemead School of Psychology. *Dissertation Abstracts International.* 1980; **41**, 1123B. Google Scholar.

23. **Pecheur DR, Edwards KJ.** A comparison of secular and religious versions of cognitive therapy with depressed christian college students. Biola University. 1984. https://doi. org/10.1177/009164718401200106

24. **Ebrahimi A, Neshatdoost HT, Mousavi SG, Asadollahi GA, Nasiri H.** Controlled randomized clinical trial of spirituality integrated psychotherapy, cognitive-behavioral therapy and medication intervention on depressive symptoms and dysfunctional attitudes in patients with dysthymic disorder. *Advanced Biomedical Research.* 2013;**2**:53.

25. **Razali SM, Aminah K, Khan UA.** Religious–cultural psychotherapy in the management of anxiety patients. *Transcultural Psychiatry.* 2002 Mar;**39**(1):130–6.

26. **VanderWeele TJ, Li S, Tsai AC, Kawachi I.** Association between religious service attendance and lower suicide rates among US women. *JAMA Psychiatry.* 2016;**73**(8):845–51.

27. **Johnson WB, Ridley CR.** Brief Christian and non-Christian rational-emotive therapy with depressed Christian clients: an exploratory study. *Counseling and Values.* 1992 Apr;**36**(3):220–9.

28. **VanderWeele TJ.** On the promotion of human flourishing. *Proceedings of the National Academy of Sciences of the USA.* 2017 Aug;**114**(31):8148–56.

29. **Hayes SC, Villatte M, Levin M, Hildebrandt M.** Open, aware, and active: contextual approaches as an emerging trend in the behavioral and cognitive therapies. *Annual Review of Clinical Psychology.* 2011;**7**:141–68.

30. **Zhang Y, Young D, Lee S, Zhang H, Xiao Z, Hao W,** et al. Chinese Taoist cognitive psychotherapy in the treatment of generalized anxiety disorder in contemporary China. *Transcultural Psychiatry.* 2002 Mar;**39**(1):115–29.

31. **Propst LR.** The comparative efficacy of religious and nonreligious imagery for the treatment of mild depression in religious individuals. *Cognotive Therapy and Research.* 1980 Jun;**4**(2):167–78.

Chapter 23

Religious and spiritual struggles and mental health: Implications for clinical practice

Kenneth I. Pargament and Julie J. Exline

Introduction

> I'm suffering, really suffering. My illness is tearing me down, and I'm
> angry at God for not rescuing me, I mean really setting me free from my
> mental bondage. I have been dealing with these issues for ten years now
> and I am only 24 years old. I don't understand why he keeps lifting me
> up, just to let me come crashing down again.
>
> *Personal communication, 2013, undergraduate with bipolar illness*

Psychiatric problems have an impact on people not only psychologically, socially, and physically, but spiritually as well, as we hear in the anguished words
of the undergraduate above. Life experiences, including physical and mental
illness, can shake and even shatter the individual's core spiritual beliefs, practices, values, and relationships. And, as a result, the individual may encounter
religious/spiritual (R/S) struggles that lead to further distress, disorientation,
and potential decline. We define R/S struggles as tensions, strains, and conflicts
with respect to sacred matters (1, 2). As we will see, these struggles, though
often overlooked in treatment, are not uncommon. Moreover, they have important implications for mental health, and need to be addressed in mental
health care.

This chapter will examine a growing literature on the relationship between
R/S struggles and mental health, and the implications of this literature for clinical practice. We will focus in detail on R/S struggles as they relate to the lives of
people with mental illness. Our chapter will begin with a conceptual overview
of R/S struggles. We will then briefly review the research literature showing the
prevalence of R/S struggles and their robust links with mental health. We will
see that R/S struggles represent an important topic for clinical practice, one that
should not be overlooked. The remainder of the chapter will offer pragmatic

recommendations for ways practitioners can assess and address R/S struggles in their clinical work.

Understanding religious and spiritual struggles

In the search for significant purpose and meaning in their lives, R/S offer people overarching orienting frameworks of belief, practice, experiences, relationships, and values (3). To put it another way, R/S are involved with both destinations and pathways for living that together define diverse life journeys. What these journeys have in common is a focus on the sacred however it is understood.

Empirical studies have shown that higher levels of R/S are generally associated with a number of mental health benefits (e.g. 4). At times, however, the individual's guiding R/S orientation to life may be shaken, as a result of exposure to major life stressors, the experience of developmental transitions, or vulnerabilities posed by temperamental factors such as neuroticism and emotional dysregulation (e.g. 5, 6, 7). These factors can set the stage for R/S struggles.

There are, in fact, a variety of specific but interrelated sub-types of R/S struggle. Conceptually, they can be grouped in terms of three general dimensions: supernatural struggles involving perceptions of higher powers (i.e. God or gods) or demonic or evil forces; intrapsychic struggles that involve tensions, conflicts, and strains about R/S beliefs, moral issues, and ultimate meaning; and interpersonal struggles that manifest as conflicts with other people about R/S matters. In support of this framework, factor analytic studies have identified six specific forms of R/S struggle: divine, demonic, doubt-related, moral, ultimate meaning, and interpersonal (8, 9). These studies indicate that R/S struggles can be analysed at the levels of both the specific six sub-types and the sum total of different R/S struggles. Box 23.1 defines each of the six sub-types of R/S struggle and presents illustrative items.

Research on religious and spiritual struggles and mental health

Prevalence of religious and spiritual struggles

R/s struggles are not rarities. According to surveys of community and college student samples, 33% reported experiencing an R/S struggle within the past few months (10). Within a community sample of military veterans, approximately one-third reported at least one R/S struggle (11). At least modest levels of R/S struggles have been shown across people of diverse age, gender, ethnicity, religious affiliation, and socio-economic status (12).

> ## Box 23.1 Six sub-types of religion and spirituality struggles, and illustrative items from the Religious and Spiritual Struggles Scale
>
> **Divine struggles**: anger or disappointment with God, and feeling punished, abandoned, or unloved by God. Sample item: Felt angry at God.
>
> **Demonic struggles**: worries that problems are caused by the devil or evil spirits, and feelings of being attacked or tormented by the devil. Sample item: Felt attacked by the devil or by evil spirits.
>
> **Doubt-related struggles**: feeling confused about R/S beliefs, and feeling troubled by doubts or questions about R/S. Sample item: Felt troubled by doubts or questions about R/S.
>
> **Moral struggles**: tensions and guilt about not living up to one's higher standards, and wrestling with attempts to follow moral principles. Sample item: Felt guilty for not living up to my moral standards.
>
> **Struggles of ultimate meaning**: concerns that life may not really matter, and questions about whether one's own life has deeper meaning. Sample item: Questioned whether my life will really make any difference in the world.
>
> **Interpersonal struggles**: conflicts with other people and institutions about sacred issues, anger at organized religion, and feeling hurt, mistreated, or offended by others in relation to R/S. Sample item: Felt as though others were looking down on me because of my R/S beliefs.

The prevalence of R/S struggles appears to be higher among people experiencing psychological problems. For example, among older adults with depression, 50% reported R/S struggles (13), as did 47% of outpatients being treated for a mood disorder (14). In a sample of people suffering from major depression and medical illness, 25%–35% indicated that they were experiencing some type of R/S struggle (15). Such issues are common among younger adults as well: one large-scale study of college students in campus counselling centres showed that one-third reported R/S struggles (16).

Links between religious and spiritual struggles and mental health

R/s struggles have been robustly associated with mental health status (see 8 for review). For example, in a nationally representative sample, R/S struggles were tied to higher levels of depressive symptoms and generalized anxiety

(12). Another study of a large US community sample showed significant links between R/S struggles and indicators of psychopathology, including anxiety, phobic anxiety, depression, paranoid ideation, obsessive-compulsiveness, and somatization (17). R/S struggles have also been strongly correlated with greater suicidality among veterans of the Iraq and/or Afghanistan wars (18). In addition, higher levels of R/S struggles increase the risk of symptoms of post-traumatic stress disorder (PTSD) among groups exposed to trauma, such as Muslims dealing with violence in London and the Middle East (19) and people near the Oklahoma City bombing (20).

Similar findings have been reported among people with various psychiatric problems. For instance, higher levels of R/S struggles were related to higher scores on a screening measure of psychiatric disorders within an outpatient psychotherapy centre serving economically disadvantaged individuals (21). R/S struggles were linked with suicidality among veterans in a PTSD residential rehabilitation programme (22), and patients in an anxiety and depression clinic (23). Among psychiatric patients in a partial hospitalization programme, R/S struggles were associated with higher levels of anxiety and depression prior to treatment (24). Stroppa and Moreira-Almeida (25) found that R/S struggles were linked with poorer quality of life within a sample of bipolar Brazilian out-patients. Finally, R/S struggles have also been associated with poorer medication adherence among Iranian psychiatric patients (26).

There are, in short, robust connections between R/S struggles and mental health status in the general population and among people with psychiatric problems. The findings reported thus far, however, are correlational in nature and cannot answer the question of whether R/S struggles are the cause or effect of psychological problems. This question has important implications for treatment. Fortunately, several studies have begun to address this question.

Primary versus secondary versus complex religious and spiritual struggles

Pargament and Lomax (27) have distinguished among three causal relations between R/S struggles and psychological problems: primary R/S struggles as a source of psychological problems, secondary R/S struggles as a consequence of psychological problems, and complex R/S struggles as both a cause and effect of psychological problems. This is not simply an academic distinction: it has implications for treatment. If R/S struggles are secondary to psychological problems, then treating the psychiatric issues might be sufficient to resolve the R/S struggles. However, if R/S struggles are primary to psychological problems, then treating the psychological problems without attending to the R/S struggles might not be effective. Finally, if R/S struggles are both a cause and consequence of psychological problems, then attending to the struggles or psychological problems alone might not be sufficient for effective treatment.

There is some evidence to support each of these three causal models. In support of a primary struggles model, several longitudinal studies of psychiatric patients have shown that R/S struggles are predictive of increased symptomatology over time, including symptoms of PTSD among military veterans (28), symptoms of manic depressive illness (29), frequency and intensity of suicidal ideation among patients with past or present psychosis (24), and symptoms of depression among Jews dealing with worry and stress (30). Another noteworthy study of medically ill elderly hospitalized patients revealed that R/S struggles at baseline increased the risk of mortality over the following two years, after controlling for initial medical and psychological status (31).

A smaller number of studies have also offered support for a secondary struggles model in which R/S struggles grow out of psychological problems, albeit in largely non-psychiatric samples. Reynolds et al. (32) measured R/S struggles and adjustment two years apart in a sample of adolescents with cystic fibrosis or diabetes. Depression predicted increases in R/S struggles over the two-year period for both medical groups. Neimeyer and Burke (33) conducted a six-month follow-up study of African-Americans who had lost a loved one to homicide. People who reported more complicated grief experienced more R/S struggles over time. And in a longitudinal study of a national sample of college students, R/S struggles among students in their junior year were predicted by the degree to which they felt depressed and emotionally overwhelmed at the time of their entry into college (34).

Only a few studies have addressed a complex model of R/S struggles. These studies have shown that R/S struggles appear to mediate the connection between exposure to trauma/stressors and psychopathology, including post-traumatic symptoms (35, 36) and depression and anxiety (37, 38).

Taken as a whole, these findings suggest that R/S struggles are potentially a cause of psychological problems, an effect of psychological problems, and, at times, both a cause and effect of these problems. Because these different models of R/S struggles have different implications for treatment, it is important to try to disentangle them, although the process may be challenging.

For example, Kao et al. (39) reported the case of a 55-year-old married father with a history of alcohol use disorder and major depressive disorder. He had been seen in a medical hospital following two self-inflicted gunshot wounds. He described terrible guilt over his history of drinking and extramarital affairs that had damaged his family. Interwoven into his depression were questions whether God could forgive him for his sins. To resolve his R/S struggle, he decided to 'gamble with God' by playing Russian roulette with a gun that he loaded with blanks and one live bullet. If God truly loved him, he believed, then he would be spared. The gun went off and the man sustained multiple facial injuries requiring several weeks of hospitalization. Upon discharge, his depression increased and, one year later, he tried to end his life by shooting himself in the chest, though he survived once again. Careful questioning in the process of treatment would be needed to disentangle the complex connections between this man's guilt, depression, and R/S struggles.

In sum, the research literature makes several points: R/S struggles are not at all unusual, especially among people with mental health problems; R/S struggles have been robustly tied to a variety of significant psychological concerns; and R/S struggles may be a cause and/or effect of psychological problems. It follows that, although R/S struggles are not typically addressed in treatment, they represent a potentially important concern. In the Kao et al. (39) case just described, it would be difficult to imagine how the patient could be treated effectively if his R/S struggles were ignored. And it is important to note here studies that show that chronic struggles, or struggles that remain unresolved over time, appear to be particularly problematic for mental health (e.g. 40, 41).

We have to be careful, however, not to equate R/S struggles with psychopathology. The process of wrestling with dilemmas and challenging questions, distressing and disorienting though it may be, has been viewed by key theorists (e.g. Piaget, Erikson, and Fowler) as a critical ingredient of growth. Many people—from exemplary religious figures in scriptures to modern-day figures—have described life-changing transformations that have followed periods of R/S struggle (e.g. 42). Among those who have experienced R/S struggles, a significant percentage indicate that they have grown through their experience (e.g. 43). A few studies also suggest that higher levels of R/S struggles are associated with greater perceptions of stress-related growth (e.g. 44).

Whether R/S struggles lead to psychological decline or growth may well depend on how they are understood and handled. Psychiatrists can play an important role here in fostering more productive efforts to come to terms with R/S struggles. The key question is 'how'?

Fortunately, we can look to a small but growing clinical and research literature on the topic for some guidance.

Addressing religious and spiritual struggles in clinical practice

Psychiatrists already find themselves tasked with understanding their patients at physical, psychological, and social levels. Attending to the R/S dimension of patients' lives may seem like a potentially overwhelming added responsibility. It does not have to be, however. Clinical work with R/S struggles does not call for a brand new form of treatment. Practitioners can draw on their general clinical skills when R/S issues arise. A foundational skill is the ability to form a strong therapeutic alliance, in part by creating a welcoming space for dialogue, particularly around sensitive issues, such as R/S.

Several factors can facilitate this welcoming space. First, it is important to show genuine curiosity about the patient's R/S life. Further conversation can be encouraged when mentions of R/S are met with a response of, 'That's really interesting. I'd like to hear more about that.' Second, practitioners should avoid assuming that they can know about the patient's R/S on the basis of their affiliation. Although people may have preconceived ideas about the beliefs and practices of a typical Christian, a typical Jew, or even a typical atheist, it is important to keep in mind that every patient has a distinctive story to tell and the therapist must be willing to learn about each special R/S narrative. Third, because R/S struggles often reflect profound questions about oneself, others, the world, and the sacred, they are not likely to be assuaged by a few words of comfort or advice. Thus, therapists should avoid the temptation of offering quick solutions, however well intended. Efforts at easy fixes may instead short-circuit conversation about the deeper meaning and value of R/S struggles. Moreover, practitioners must remember that they are not theologians or clergy and have no special authority when it comes to questions involving ontological truth. Fourth, R/S issues are often fraught with emotions for practitioners as well as patients. Self-awareness of therapists' own orientations and attitudes to R/S, be they positive, negative, or mixed, offers an important potential corrective to the R/S biases of all kinds that can interfere with treatment. Finally, a welcoming space for conversation grows out of respect for the patient's R/S—not that the practitioner must agree with the patient's R/S orientation. Rather, respect rests on the recognition that many patients find solace, strength, purpose, and identity from their R/S beliefs and practices, and attempts to proselytize or counter-convert patients toward or away from any R/S perspective are inconsistent with the ethics of clinical practice. Relevant here is research that shows that this kind of sensitivity to the R/S of patients predicts positive change in therapy more strongly than the level of R/S similarity between patients and therapists (45).

This welcoming space can be created in the context of one-to-one therapy or in a larger group milieu. For example, Phillips, Lakin, and Pargament (46) developed a seven-week spiritual discussion group for people with serious mental illness. The group covered diverse topics that focused on the relationship between their R/S and mental illness, including R/S struggles, R/S resources, hope, and forgiveness. Although participants had been involved in the mental health system for a number of years, the group was, for many, the first time R/S issues had been directly discussed in their treatment. Contrary to some concerns that had been raised by staff members before implementing the programme, the group did not trigger serious religious disturbances (e.g. delusions, hallucinations). Rather, participants appreciated the chance to share their feelings about R/S, both positive and negative within a non-judgemental context. Many felt relieved, supported, and informed by others who were also experiencing R/S struggles. Participants uniformly expressed a strong desire for continued dialogue on R/S in relation to their mental illness. In short, by creating a welcoming space for R/S dialogue, practitioners can help to build an effective working alliance, one that sets the stage for assessing and addressing R/S in treatment.

Assessing religious and spiritual struggles

A few questions about R/S are an appropriate part of the initial diagnostic interview (3). Particularly relevant to the possibility of R/S struggles is the question, 'How have your problems affected you religiously or spiritually?' This question can be raised when exploring other possible effects of the patient's problems.

The therapist should also be attentive to more implicit signs of R/S struggles. Language such as the following hints at the possibility of a deeper transcendent dimension to the patient's problems: 'Why is this happening to me?' 'I feel contaminated.' 'My world is falling apart.' 'Life is so unfair.' 'I'm feeling punished.' 'When will my suffering end?' Psychiatrists can also probe for R/S struggles through questions that make use of implicitly spiritual language, such as: 'What parts of your life are causing you great suffering or despair?' 'What are the questions that are most troubling to you?'

Responses to any of these initial or implicit queries may suggest that the patient is encountering R/S struggles and, if so, after normalizing R/S struggles, a more direct and explicit question can be posed: 'Have you been experiencing tensions, conflicts, questions, or struggles about religion or spirituality?'

It is important to keep in mind that R/S struggles can manifest themselves in the context of any psychiatric disorder (e.g. 47). Keep in mind also that patients may not express R/S struggles initially in treatment for a number of possible reasons: guilt and shame about their struggles, fear of a negative reaction from others including the psychiatrist, concerns about how God will react, or a lack of awareness. Thus, psychiatrists should remain alert to signs of struggle as treatment progresses, even if initial queries on the topic do not reveal obvious struggles. For example, Rosmarin (48) reports on his work with a 26-year-old single female who had been sexually assaulted by her father as a child. Although she initially described herself as completely secular, she later admitted feelings of anger toward God and her religious community for allowing the assaults to take place. She also noted that R/S stimuli, such as passing by a place of worship or seeing someone from her faith tradition, had triggered self-injury in the past. R/S struggles emerged as an important aspect of the clinical problem and subsequent treatment.

When R/S struggles arise in treatment, the practitioner should pursue more detailed questions about the particular kinds of struggles the patient is experiencing, whether the struggles are primary, secondary, or complex, the roots of these struggles, their clinical relevance, and the ways the patient has tried to cope with these conflicts. The patients' responses can help guide the direction of treatment.

Interventions with religious and spiritual struggles

There are several kinds of interventions that are appropriate to clinical work with people who are experiencing R/S struggles. Here, we briefly describe some of these interventions.

Name and normalize religious and spiritual struggles

As we have seen, R/S struggles can be distressing and disorienting. People going through these times of conflict may feel they are 'losing their minds', losing their spiritual foundation, or simply lacking a strong faith. Psychiatrists can reassure patients by giving a name to R/S struggles and educating them about these conflicts as normative life experiences, even among people who are deeply devout. In this vein, other illustrious R/S strugglers can be noted, from religious exemplars, such as Moses, Jesus, Buddha, and Muhammad, to more contemporary figures, including Gandhi, Mother Teresa, and Elie Wiesel. R/S struggles can also be reframed within a larger developmental context. Certainly, struggles are often a source of tension and turmoil, but they also carry the potential for positive transformation and growth. As Rupp (49) said, R/S struggles are a part of the larger cup of life, which has to be emptied out at times to pour something new in; the cup cannot always be full.

Facilitate acceptance and reflection

Empirical studies have shown that the effects of R/S struggles are exacerbated by attempts to suppress them (50). Psychiatrists can foster greater acceptance rather than avoidance of R/S struggles by encouraging patients to notice and observe the thoughts and feelings that accompany the struggles as they might other disturbing experiences. Kornfield (51) has developed a mindfulness exercise to facilitate the acceptance of R/S struggles:

> [After sitting quietly] cast your attention over all the battles that still exist in your life. Sense them inside yourself... If you have been fighting inner wars with your feelings... sense the struggle you have been waging. Notice the struggles in your thoughts as well.

> Be aware of how you have carried on the inner battles. Notice the inner armies, the inner dictators, the inner fortifications. Be aware of all that you have fought within yourself ... Gently, with openness, allow each of these experiences to be present. Simply notice each of them in turn with interest and kind attention. In each area of struggle, let your body, heart, and soul be soft. Open to whatever you experience without fighting. Let it be present just as it is. Let go of the battle. Breathe quietly and let yourself be at rest. Invite all parts of yourself to join you at the peace table in your heart (p. 30).

Greater acceptance of R/S struggles opens the door to greater self-reflection on their meaning (52). Because R/S struggles touch on core existential issues, greater insight into these struggles can illuminate areas of brokenness in the lives of patients, and lead to more intentional choices about their ultimate goals for living and the pathways they take to realize their dreams.

Martinez-Taboas (47) illustrates this point through the case of a 21-year-old Puerto Rican woman, Nancy, who was initially referred to a neurologist for constant seizures. However, she was not responsive to anticonvulsive medication and her electroencephalogram [EEG] was normal. Diagnosed with psychogenic non-epileptic seizures (PNES), a type of somatoform dissociation, Nancy was referred for psychotherapy where it was learned that she was experiencing conflicts about her pledge to become a nun. She had doubts about living the restricted life of a nun in the convent and giving up the possibility of sex, marriage, and family. At the same time, she feared that she would disappoint and anger family and friends if she were to retract her commitment. By identifying, accepting, and ultimately airing her conflicts about her ultimate purpose in life with family and friends, Nancy experienced a great deal of emotional relief and a reduction in the number of PNES episodes from 30 in a month to one or two in a month.

Access religious and spiritual resources

In the midst of their emotional problems, patients often lose touch with the resources that sustained them in the past. They may forget to eat regularly, get a good night's sleep, talk to family and friends, or get to work on time. This kind of dysregulation can extend to the R/S realm; patients may stop going to their religious institution, no longer pray or meditate, disconnect from their relationship with clergy, or discontinue practices that were once a source of spiritual solace and support. Encouraging patients to get back into the normal rhythm of their lives is a basic part of psychological treatment and the same kind of encouragement can be extended to the R/S sphere of life.

For example, McGee et al. (53) describe the case of Mrs A, a 58-year-old African-American woman diagnosed with early-stage Alzheimer's disease. Compounding her loss of cognitive functioning, Mrs A was encountering

R/S struggles that had been triggered by tensions and conflicts with members of her meditation group in the assisted living centre. As a result, Mrs A had become disengaged from her R/S resources. However, with the encouragement of her therapist, she was able to access several other sources of support, including reading inspirational books and scriptures, becoming involved in a Unitarian church, and engaging in regular spiritual practices such as walking the labyrinth that served as a reminder that she continued on a meaningful life path. Researchers have identified several R/S factors in mitigating the distressing effects of R/S struggles, including R/S coping activities, religious hope, religious commitment, and seeing life as sacred (54). Paradoxically, Abu-Raiya et al. note, R/S can be a significant part of the solution to the problems posed by R/S struggles.

In some instances, practitioners can help patients access R/S resources that have gone largely overlooked or untapped. For instance, Pargament (3) presents his clinical work with Rachel, a 35-year-old Roman Catholic woman, who was experiencing PTSD and suicidality following the trauma of being gang-raped. Rachel felt that the rapes represented a divine retribution for what she perceived as the unforgivable sin of an abortion she had had when she was a young adolescent. Unsure about whether her punitive judgement accurately represented the position of her church, the therapist consulted with a Roman Catholic priest who indicated that, although Rachel had committed a sin in the eyes of the Church, she could still experience forgiveness through the Sacrament of Reconciliation (i.e. confession and penance). With the therapist's encouragement, Rachel formed a relationship with the priest who guided her through this sacrament. By facilitating access to this ritual of purification, the therapist was able to help Rachel achieve significant relief from her symptoms and R/S struggles.

The effectiveness of interventions for religious and spiritual struggles

Empirical studies have shown that recently developed spiritually integrated treatments are as effective and, in some instances, more effective than standard mental health care (55). Interventions that target, at least in part, R/S struggles, have also been developed and evaluated with encouraging results. Changes in symptomatology and R/S struggles have been reported following clinical programmes designed for groups including traumatized military veterans (56, 57), HIV/AIDS patients (58), survivors of sexual abuse (59), medically ill people with major depressive disorder (15), and traumatized women with symptoms of PTSD (60).

To take one example, Dworsky et al. (61) developed a programme entitled *Winding Road* for college students dealing with R/S struggles in the process of transition from life-at-home to life-at-college. Winding Road is a 9-week group-based intervention unaffiliated with any particular religious tradition. It was designed to (a) facilitate understanding and acceptance of R/S struggles; (b) reduce stigma for struggles; and (enhance emotional, behavioural, and spiritual well-being. Over the course of the programme, participants made significant gains in terms of their R/S struggles, including lower levels of shame and stigma, improved affect, greater ability to regulate their emotions, and reductions in psychological distress. Many described a new perspective on their struggles. As one student put it: 'I had a lot of rash emotions coming into this experience ... [Now] I look at my struggles as more of a positive... I've matured in my view of the struggle—it doesn't have to be resolved right now ... Now it's not so much of a struggle as an evolution' (p. 328). Similar effects were reported in a replication of Winding Road among psychiatric inpatients (62).

Conclusions and future directions

Mental health professionals, including psychiatrists, have generally been reluctant to address R/S issues in treatment (63, 64), perhaps in part because they fear they may be overstepping their bounds and offending their patients. And yet patients themselves have voiced their interest in discussing R/S matters in therapy. For instance, in one study of 253 psychiatric patients, a majority expressed some desire to talk about R/S in treatment (48). Furthermore, 37% of patients without a religious affiliation showed interest in discussing R/S issues. Among clients encountering R/S struggles, the level of interest in discussing these topics in treatment may be even higher (65). Thus, many patients themselves would appear to welcome inclusion of R/S into the therapeutic conversation.

The reluctance of practitioners to broach the topic of R/S in treatment may have a more basic explanation—a lack of training. As a group, mental health professionals receive little education about how to understand and address R/S issues, including R/S struggles, in treatment (67, 67). Lacking training in this domain, practitioners may prefer to simply sidestep this area of a patient's life. In this chapter, we have tried to provide important information about R/S struggles—their definition, prevalence, and significant implications for health and well-being, with a focus on people with psychiatric problems.

All in all, the growing research literature underscores the importance of attending to R/S struggles in treatment. As we stressed, this process does not have to have to be overwhelming for practitioners. Nor does it require a brand new form of treatment. Psychiatrists can draw on basic clinical skills to integrate R/S into the diagnostic interview and assessment process, and address R/S struggles in treatment. Helping patients name and normalize their struggles, accept and reflect on these conflicts, and access R/S resources that offer potential resolutions to their struggles are all important elements of clinical care.

What psychotherapy with R/S struggles does require is an appreciation for the sensitive place R/S hold in the lives of many people. Matters of faith touch on some of the deepest of personal beliefs, emotions, values, connections, and commitments. So they must be approached with special care and sensitivity. Given the fact that mental health professionals as a whole are considerably less religious than those they see in treatment (e.g. 69), it is especially important for practitioners to be aware of their own orientation to R/S issues and guard against biases if they hope to address R/S struggles successively in treatment. There may be no faster way to close off potentially meaningful conversation than signs of R/S disinterest or discomfort from the therapist.

For practitioners interested in additional training in spiritually integrated therapy, a number of valuable texts have been written over the past 20 years. Some of these texts are geared to patients who come from diverse religious and spiritual backgrounds (e.g. 70; 3, 71). Other books focus on ways to integrate R/S into particular clinical orientations and/or work with specific religious groups (e.g. 72, 48, 73).

There is, of course, a great deal to be learned about how best to understand and address R/S in treatment. This point is particularly applicable to R/S struggles. We need to better understand the roots and consequences of R/S struggles, with particular attention to determining which model of struggles—primary, secondary, or complex—applies to specific clinical cases. Further studies are also needed that focus more closely on the implications of specific R/S struggles (divine, demonic, moral, ultimate meaning, doubt-related, and interpersonal) for psychological problems and their resolution. Additional studies are needed to clarify the ways people from diverse cultural and R/S backgrounds experience and express their struggles, and how they can be approached most effectively in treatment. Finally, there is a clear need for clinical case studies and evaluative studies that examine the impact of psychotropic medication, mainstream clinical psychotherapy, and spiritually integrated interventions on R/S struggles and psychiatric symptomatology.

Acknowledgements

We are grateful to the John Templeton Foundation (Grant # 36094) for its support of research cited in this chapter.

References

1. Exline JJ. Religious and spiritual struggles. In: KI Pargament, A Mahoney, EP Shafranske, (eds), *APA handbook of psychology, religion, and spirituality. Vol. 1: context, theory, and research.* Washington, DC: American Psychological Association; 2013, pp. 459–75.

2. Pargament KI, Murray-Swank NA, Magyar GM, Ano GG. Spiritual struggle: a phenomenon of interest to psychology and religion. In: WR Miller, H Delaney, (eds), *Judeo-Christian perspectives on psychology: human nature, motivation, and change.* Washington, DC: American Psychological Association; 2005, pp. 245–68.

3. Pargament KI. *Spiritually integrated psychotherapy: understanding and addressing the sacred.* New York: Guilford Press; 2011.

4. Koenig H, Koenig HG, King D, Carson VB. *Handbook of religion and health.* New York: Oxford University Press; 2012.

5. Krause N, Pargament KI, Hill PC, Wong S, Ironson G. Exploring the relationships among age, spiritual struggles, and health. *Journal of Religion, Spirituality & Aging.* 2017;**29**(4):266–85.

6. Stauner N, Exline JJ, Pargament KI, Wilt JA, Grubbs JB. Stressful life events and religiousness predict struggles about religion and spirituality. *Psychology of Religion and Spirituality.* 2018;**11**(3):291–96.

7. Wilt JA, Grubbs JB, Pargament KI, Exline JJ. Religious and spiritual struggles, past and present: relations to the big five and well-being. *International Journal for the Psychology of Religion.* 2017;**27**(1):51–64.

8. Exline JJ, Pargament KI, Grubbs JB, Yali AM. The religious and spiritual struggles scale: development and initial validation. *Psychology of Religion and Spirituality.* 2014;**6**(3):208–22.

9. Stauner N, Exline J, Grubbs J, Pargament K, Bradley D, Uzdavines A. Bifactor models of religious and spiritual struggles: distinct from religiousness and distress. *Religions.* 2016;**7**(6):68.

10. Wilt JA, Grubbs JB, Pargament KI, Exline JJ. Personality, religious and spiritual struggles, and well-being. *Psychology of Religion and Spirituality.* 2016;**8**(4):341–51.

11. Currier JM, McDermott RC, McCormick WH, Churchwell MC, Milkeris L. Exploring cross-lagged associations between spiritual struggles and risk for suicidal behavior in a community sample of military veterans. *Journal of Affective Disorders* 2018;**230**:93–100.

12. Abu-Raiya H, Pargament KI, Krause N, Ironson G. Robust links between religious/ spiritual struggles, psychological distress, and well-being in a national sample of American adults. *American Journal of Orthopsychiatry.* 2015;**85**(6):565–75.

13. Murphy PE, Fitchett G, Emery-Tiburcio EE. Religious and spiritual struggle: prevalence and correlates among older adults with depression in the BRIGHTEN Program. *Mental Health, Religion & Culture.* 2016;**19**(7):713–21.

14. Rosmarin DH, Malloy MC, Forester BP. Spiritual struggle and affective symptoms among geriatric mood disordered patients. *International Journal of Geriatric Psychiatry.* 2014;**29**(6):653–60.

15. Pearce M, Koenig, HG. Spiritual struggles and religious cognitive behavioral therapy: a randomized clinical trial in those with depression and chronic medical illness. *Journal of Psychology & Theology.* 2016;**44**(1):3–15.

16. **Johnson CV, Hayes JA.** Troubled spirits: prevalence and predictors of religious and spiritual concerns among university students and counseling center clients. *Journal of Counseling Psychology.* 2003;50(4):409–19.

17. **McConnell KM, Pargament KI, Ellison CG, Flannelly KJ.** Examining the links between spiritual struggles and symptoms of psychopathology in a national sample. *Journal of Clinical Psychology.* 2006;62(12):1469–84.

18. **Currier JM, Smith PN, Kuhlman S.** Assessing the unique role of religious coping in suicidal behavior among U.S. Iraq and Afghanistan veterans. *Psychology of Religion and Spirituality.* 2017;9(1):118–23.

19. **Berzengi A, Berzenji L, Kadim A, Mustafa F, Jobson L.** Role of Islamic appraisals, trauma-related appraisals, and religious coping in the posttraumatic adjustment of Muslim trauma survivors. *Psychological Trauma.* 2017;9(2):189–97.

20. **Pargament KI, Zinnbauer BJ, Scott AB, Butter EM, Zerowin J, Stanik P.** Red flags and religious coping: identifying some religious warning signs among people in crisis. *Journal of Clinical Psychology.* 1998;54(1):77–89.

21. **Olson MM, Trevino DB, Geske JA, Vanderpool H.** Religious coping and mental health outcomes: an exploratory study of socioeconomically disadvantaged patients. *Explore (NY).* 2012;8(3):172–6.

22. **Kopacz MS, Currier JM, Drescher KD, Pigeon WR.** Suicidal behavior and spiritual functioning in a sample of veterans diagnosed with PTSD. *Journal of Injury and Violence Research.* 2016;8(1):6.

23. **Exline JJ, Yali AM, Sanderson WC.** Guilt, discord, and alienation: the role of religious strain in depression and suicidality. *Journal of Clinical Psychology.* 2000;56(12):1481–96.

24. **Rosmarin DH, Bigda-Peyton JS, Öngur D, Pargament KI, Björgvinsson T.** Religious coping among psychotic patients: Relevance to suicidality and treatment outcomes. *Psychiatry Research.* 2013;210(1):182–7.

25. **Stroppa A, Moreira-Almeida A.** Religiosity, mood symptoms, and quality of life in bipolar disorder. *Bipolar Disorder.* 2013;15(4):385–93.

26. **Movahedizadeh M, Sheikhi MR, Shahsavari S, Chen H.** The association between religious belief and drug adherence mediated by religious coping in patients with mental disorders. *Social Health and Behavior.* 2019 Jul 1;2(3):77.

27. **Pargament KI, Lomax JW.** Understanding and addressing religion among people with mental illness. *World Psychiatry.* 2013;12(1):26–32.

28. **Currier JM, Holland JM, Drescher KD.** Spirituality factors in the prediction of outcomes of PTSD treatment for U.S. military veterans. *Journal of Traumatic Stress.* 2015;28(1):57–64.

29. **Currier JM, Foster JD, vanOyen Witvliet C, Abernethy AD, Luna LM, Schnitker SA,** et al. Spiritual struggles and mental health outcomes in a spiritually integrated inpatient program. *Journal of Affective Disorders.* 2019;249:127–35.

30. **Pirutinsky S, Rosmarin DH, Pargament KI, Midlarsky E.** Does negative religious coping accompany, precede, or follow depression among Orthodox Jews? *Journal of Affective Disorders.* 2011;132(3):401–5.

31. **Pargament KI, Koenig HG, Tarakeshwar N, Hahn J.** Religious struggle as a predictor of mortality among medically ill elderly patients: a 2-year longitudinal study. *Archives of Internal Medicine.* 2001;161(15):1881–5.

32. **Reynolds N, Mrug S, Hensler M, Guion K, Madan-Swain A.** Spiritual coping and adjustment in adolescents with chronic illness: a 2-year prospective study. *Journal of Pediatric Psychology* 2014;**39**(5):542–51.

33. **Neimeyer RA, Burke LA.** Complicated grief in the aftermath of homicide: spiritual crisis and distress in an African American sample. *Religions.* 2011;**2**(2):145–64.

34. **Bryant AN, Astin HS.** The correlates of spiritual struggle during the college years. *Journal of Higher Education.* 2008;**79**(1):1–27.

35. **Harris JI, Erbes CR, Engdahl BE, Ogden H, Olson RH, Winskowski AM,** et al. Religious distress and coping with stressful life events: a longitudinal study. *Journal of Clinical Psychology.* 2012;**68**(12):1276–86.

36. **Wortmann JH, Park CL, Edmondson D.** Trauma and PTSD symptoms: does spiritual struggle mediate the link?. *Psychological Trauma.* 2011;**3**(4):442–52.

37. **Krumrei EJ, Mahoney A, Pargament KI.** Spiritual stress and coping model of divorce: a longitudinal study. *Journal of Family Psychology* 2011;**25**(6):973–85.

38. **Pomerleau JM, Pargament KI, Krause N, Ironson G, Hill P.** Religious and spiritual struggles as a mediator of the link between stressful life events and psychological adjustment in a nationwide sample. *Psychology of Religion and Spirituality.* 2020;**12**(4):451–9.

39. **Kao LE, Shah SB, Pargament KI, Griffith JL, Peteet JR.** 'Gambling with God': a self-inflicted gunshot wound with religious motivation in the context of a mixed-mood episode. *Harvard Review of Psychiatry.* 2019;**27**(1):65–72.

40. **Pargament KI, Koenig HG, Tarakeshwar N, Hahn J.** Religious coping methods as predictors of psychological, physical and spiritual outcomes among medically ill elderly patients: a two-year longitudinal study. *Journal of Health Psychology.* 2004;**9**(6):713–30.

41. **Park CL, Holt CL, Le D, Christie J, Williams BR.** Positive and negative religious coping styles as prospective predictors of well-being in African Americans. *Psychology of Religion and Spirituality.* 2018;**10**(4):318–26.

42. **Chittister J.** *Scarred by struggle, transformed by hope.* Grand Rapids (MI): Wm. B. Eerdmans Publishing; 2003.

43. **Desai KM, Pargament KI.** Predictors of growth and decline following spiritual struggles. *International Journal for the Psychology of Religion.* 2015;**25**(1):42–56.

44. **Gall TL, Charbonneau C, Florack P.** The relationship between religious/spiritual factors and perceived growth following a diagnosis of breast cancer. *Psychology & Health.* 2011;**26**(3):287–305.

45. **Wade NG, Worthington Jr EL, Vogel DL.** Effectiveness of religiously tailored interventions in Christian therapy. *Psychotherapy Research.* 2007;**17**(1):91–105.

46. **Phillips III RE, Lakin R, Pargament KI.** Development and implementation of a spiritual issues psychoeducational group for those with serious mental illness. *Community Mental Health Journal.* 2002;**38**(6):487–95.

47. **Martinez-Taboas AL.** The case of the shaking legs: somatoform dissociation and spiritual struggles. *Frontiers in the Psychotherapy of Trauma & Dissociation.* 2018;**1**:124–34.

48. **Rosmarin DH.** *Spirituality, religion, and cognitive-behavioral therapy: a guide for clinicians.* New York: Guilford Press; 2018.

49. **Rupp J.** *The cup of our life: a guide to spiritual growth.* Notre Dame, IN: Ave Maria Press; 2012.

50. **Dworsky CKO, Pargament KI, Wong S, Exline JJ.** Suppressing spiritual struggles: the role of experiential avoidance in mental health. *Journal of Contextual Behavioral Science.* 2016;5(4):258–65.

51. **Kornfield J.** *A path with heart: a guide through the perils and promises of spiritual life.* New York: Bantam; 2009.

52. **Murray-Swank NA, Murray-Swank AB.** Navigating the storm: Helping clients in the midst of spiritual struggles. In: **Aten J, O'Grady, K, Worthington Jr. E** (eds), *The Psychology of Religion and Spirituality for Clinicians.* New York (NY): Routledge; 2013, pp. 231–58.

53. **McGee JS, Zhao HC, Myers DR, Seela Eaton H.** Spiritual diversity and living with early-stage dementia. *Clinical Gerontologist.* 2017:**24**;1–7.

54. **Abu-Raiya H, Pargament KI, Krause N.** Religion as problem, religion as solution: religious buffers of the links between religious/spiritual struggles and well-being/mental health. *Quality of Life Research.* 2016;**25**(5):1265–74.

55. **Captari LE, Hook JN, Hoyt W, Davis DE, McElroy-Heltzel SE, Worthington EL.** Integrating clients' religion and spirituality within psychotherapy: a comprehensive meta-analysis: *Journal of Clinical Psychology.* 2018;**74**(11):1938–51.

56. **Harris JI, Erbes CR, Engdahl BE, Thuras P, Murray-Swank N, Grace D,** et al. The effectiveness of a trauma focused spiritually integrated intervention for veterans exposed to trauma. *Journal of Clinical Psychology.* 2011;**67**(4):425–38.

57. **Starnino VR, Angel CT, Sullivan JE, Lazarick DL, Jaimes LD, Cocco JP, Davis LW.** Preliminary report on a spiritually-based PTSD intervention for military veterans. *Community Mental Health Journal.* 2019;**55**:1–6.

58. **Tarakeshwar N, Pearce MJ, Sikkema KJ.** Development and implementation of a spiritual coping group intervention for adults living with HIV/AIDS: A pilot study. *Mental Health, Religion & Culture.* 2005;**8**(3):179–90.

59. **Murray-Swank NA, Pargament KI.** God, where are you?: Evaluating a spiritually-integrated intervention for sexual abuse. *Mental Health, Religion & Culture* 2005;**8**(3):191–203.

60. **Loewenthal KM.** EMDR—eye movement desensitization and reprocessing therapy and religious faith among orthodox Jewish (hareidi) women. *Israel Journal of Psychiatry and Related Sciences.* 2019;**56**(2):20–7. 61. **Dworsky CKO, Pargament KI, Gibbel MR, Faigin CA, Haugen MR, Desai KM,** et al. Winding road: preliminary support for a spiritually integrated intervention addressing college students' spiritual struggles. *Research in the Social Scientific Study of Religion.* 2013;**24**:309–39.

62. **Gibbel MR, Regueiro V, Pargament KI.** A spiritually integrated intervention for spiritual struggles among adults with mental illness: Results of an initial evaluation. *Spiritual Clin Pract.* 2019;**6**(4):240–55.63. **Huguelet P, Mohr S, Borras L, Gillieron C, Brandt PY.** Spirituality and religious practices among outpatients with schizophrenia and their clinicians. *Psychiatric Services.* 2006;**57**(3):366–72.

64. **Verbeck EG, Arzoumanian MA, Estrellado JE, Delorme JI, Dahlin KR, Hennrich EM,** et al. Religion, spirituality, and the working alliance with trauma survivors. In: **DR Walker, CA Courtois, JD Aten,** (eds), *Spiritually oriented psychotherapy for trauma.* Washington, DC: American Psychological Association; 2015, pp. 103–26.

65. **Exline JJ, Yali AM, Sanderson WC.** Guilt, discord, and alienation: the role of religious strain in depression and suicidality. *Journal of Clinical Psychology*. 2000;**56**(12):1481–96.

66. **Oxhandler HK, Parrish DE, Torres LR, Achenbaum WA.** The integration of clients' religion and spirituality in social work practice: a national survey. *Social Work*. 2015;**60**(3):228–37.

67. **Schafer RM, Handal PJ, Brawer PA, Ubinger M.** Training and education in religion/ spirituality within APA-accredited clinical psychology programs: 8 years later. *Journal of Religion & Health*. 2011;**50**(2):232–9.

68. **Shafranske EP, Cummings JP.** Religious and spiritual beliefs, affiliations, and practices of psychologists. In: **Pargament KI, Mahoney A, Shafranske EP,** (eds), *APA handbook of psychology, religion, and spirituality (Vol. 2): an applied psychology of religion and spirituality*. Washington, DC: American Psychological Association; 2013, pp. 23–41.

69. **Griffith JL.** *Religion that heals, religion that harms: a guide for clinical practice*. New York: Guilford Press; 2010.

70. **Vieten C, Scammell S.** *Spiritual and religious competencies in clinical practice: guidelines for psychotherapists and mental health professionals*. Oakland, CA: New Harbinger Publications; 2015.

71. **Pearce M.** *Cognitive behavioral therapy for Christians with depression: a practical tool-based primer*. West Conshohocken, PA: Templeton Foundation Press; 2016.

72. **Schreurs A.** *Psychotherapy and spirituality: integrating the spiritual dimension into therapeutic practice*. London: Jessica Kingsley Publishers; 2001.

Chapter 24

Spirituality and end-of-life experiences: Meeting the spiritual needs of the dying

Peter Fenwick and Bruno Paz Mosqueiro

Introduction

Until quite recently, medical treatment of the dying has been focused almost entirely on pain control and easing the end of life. And yet health care should not simply be caring for a patient's physical needs. It should also be about providing spiritual care to help people (especially older folk) to search for hope, and understand the mental and spiritual experiences of the dying.

A recent study shows that the greatest fear among Britons is that of dying alone: a worrying factor because more than half the complaints received by the UK National Health Service (NHS) concern end-of-life care, with an emphasis on spiritual matters. Much has been written on the spiritual needs of the dying, but many health professionals still find this area difficult to approach with the dying. They lack the confidence and/or training to recognize or talk about spiritual aspects of death and dying, and to enter a discussion that affirms the spiritual need of a dying person to be able to see beyond their present situation and die at peace.

Perhaps this is because of the assumption that death is simply the shutting down of the brain and so is of little interest to the medical profession, who feel that at this point they cannot control the process and are no longer involved. Very little is known about, and little research has been done, on the mental states during the dying process. And yet it is these experiences that research has shown to have a profound and positive effect on the dying themselves, and which suggest that death need not be the fearful process we may have imagined, but can indeed be something that is positive, indeed joyful.

When we conducted our own studies, from 2006 to 2010, our data came from interviews with carers in one palliative care team, one nursing home, two hospices in England, and three hospices in Holland, and with data collected in an

Irish hospice study by Dr. Una McColville. We found that, although almost all the carers we interviewed were aware of and interested in the phenomena they had observed, very few understood their significance. Only the Dutch carers had received proper training in this area: the British were poorly trained and the Irish training was abysmal. There is, unsurprisingly, no mention at all of the strange, inexplicable, but essentially comforting phenomena that so many of the dying report. When we started our own research study, we quickly found that medical practitioners have been slow to recognize them—indeed, the doctors we talked to were quite confident that we would find nothing like this ever happened to their patients. The prevailing culture of the institutions was such that these experiences were something of a taboo topic and not generally acknowledged or discussed. Carers received no training in how to respond if their patients had such experiences and wanted to talk about them.

So the training of carers—doctors, nurses, palliative care, and auxiliary staff—is a priority, though ideally education about the dying process should begin in schools and be made available to every adult. So far, though, it seems that very little has changed. In 2019, I asked a medical student who had just completed his first four years of medical training whether his palliative care training had been based entirely on pain control, or whether he had been given any advice about alleviating any mental distress the patient might have. This was his reply.

In my four years I've had a very limited amount of experience with dying/palliative patients. I don't think I had any training, either lectures, small group sessions or practical experience with palliative patients until my fourth year of medical school.

We had 3 weeks of placement in various hospices and with community palliative teams. The majority of the teaching however was focused around breaking the initial bad news of a terminal diagnosis, and then some basic symptom management such as pain relief but we didn't really go into much detail on that.

Death is one of the very few universal experiences. We know how to deal with death. It has its own rituals to help the bereaved acknowledge and come to terms with death—the wake, the condolences, the funeral service, and the burial. But these rituals do nothing to help prepare the dying themselves. Many people would say they are frightened of death but, when questioned more closely, what most of us fear is not death itself—is there much point in fearing the inevitable?—but the process of dying, the anticipation of annihilation. Most healthcare professionals frequently encounter grief among their patients after the death of a family member or close friend but few have been trained in the healing potential of end-of-life experiences (ELEs).

And yet, it is these experiences that research has shown to have a profound and positive effect on the dying themselves. Our ELE research suggests that these experiences, such as deathbed visions and deathbed coincidences, are not uncommon, and imply that the dying process appears to involve an instinctive need for spiritual connection and meaning.

Dr Robin Youngson's report (1), 'Compassion in healthcare: the missing dimension of healthcare reform' outlines how a lack of compassion can negatively affect the welfare of patients. Nurses and doctors, he says, cannot spend as much time as they should with patients because targets are driven by the need to satisfy budgets rather than by care and quality. This follows a study by Dignity in Dying (2) suggesting that the greatest fear for 32% of Britons is to die alone. Dignity in Dying also highlights that the current average budgetary spend for dying patients from 31 primary care trusts across London is less than 0.5%. Fifty-six per cent of us die in hospital (3) where more than half of the complaints received relate to end-of-life care for the dying and demonstrate the lack of empathetic understanding from medical staff that led to relatives being unprepared to face the death of their loved one, or being given no time to arrange for other family members to be present at the time of death (4). This issue is discussed by Curtis et al. (5) who express concern that most physicians do not discuss how long patients have to live, what dying might be like, or the patient's spiritual needs as they approach death. Rousseau (6) also draws attention to the fact that innumerable patients endure considerable anguish during the dying process, partly due to a lack of understanding or acknowledgement of their spiritual needs.

What do the dying tell us?

Anecdotal accounts of apparitions of dead relatives seen by the dying, or of 'visits' the dying themselves make to someone to whom they are emotionally close, at or around the time of death, have been current for over 300 years, and the first serious scientific study of the phenomena, Sir William Barrett's *Deathbed Visions*, was published in 1926 (7).

The first comprehensive and objective study of such visions was made by Karl Osis and Erlendur Haraldsson (8). In 1961, Osis conducted a questionnaire survey of 5,000 physicians and 5,000 nurses, asking about the hallucinations they had observed in terminally ill patients under their care. He analysed the 640 replies and categorized two types of hallucination: non-human visions of nature or landscapes, and apparitions of people, usually dead relatives or friends who were perceived to have come to help the dying in their transition to the next life. Together with Professor Erlendur Haraldsson, Osis carried out two further surveys, in the United States and India, and found an interesting cultural bias in these 'take-away' visions. In the United States survey, the most common apparitions were of dead relatives and friends, while religious escorts were much less frequent. However, in the Indian experiences, the reverse was true;:it was religious figures such as the 'yamdoot'—the messenger sent by the God of death—who were the most frequent take-away companions, while apparitions of dead relatives or friends appeared far less often (9).

Wholihan (10) points out that these experiences are under-recognized and cannot easily be explained within a traditional medical model, but that the most consistent caregivers, nurses, assess, recognize, and validate such experiences. And Melvin Morse, a paediatrician and researcher found 'deathbed phenomena to be an integral aspect of the dying process', which, he says, ' … should be interpreted as being part of the spectrum of spiritual events that happens to the dying, their families and their caretakers' (11).

My own interest in these ELEs was sparked off by an account sent to me by a patient, describing the day before her mother died:

> Suddenly she looked up at the window and seemed to stare intently up at it … She suddenly turned to me and said 'Please Pauline, don't ever be afraid of dying. I have seen a beautiful light and I was going towards it … it was so peaceful I really had to fight to come back'. The next day when it was time for me to go home I said 'Bye mum, see you tomorrow'. She looked straight at me and said 'I'm not worried about tomorrow and you mustn't be, promise me'. 'Sadly she died the next morning … but I knew she had seen something that day which gave her comfort and peace when she knew she had only hours to live.

The account intrigued me. First, because it contained so many elements of the near death experience—the experience of light, the feeling of peace; and, second, because the glimpse of another reality that Pauline's mother had been shown and from which she was reluctant to return seemed to have abolished any fear of death. This made me think that we should perhaps not look at any of these experiences in isolation as something that occurs only as life is almost extinguished, but as part of a continuum—a single process, the process of dying, and that part of this process might be a preparation beginning in the hours or even days before death.

Our first pilot study, during which we interviewed members of a palliative care team, indicated that this was an area well worth further investigation. The carers and palliative care workers we interviewed—the people who actually spent time with their patients and talked to them—assured us not only that these ELEs occurred, but that they were relatively common and seemed to be an intrinsic, transitional, and important part of the dying process, comforting for both the patient and their family. The dying person felt that the purpose of their 'visitors' was to give them help and support through the dying process. Even though it was hard to find an acceptable scientific explanation for them, all our interviewees agreed that these experiences were not pathological but a valuable, intensely personal, and often spiritual experience that helped the patient to become reconciled with events in their life, and therefore to come to terms with their death (12).

Further studies in hospices and nursing homes in the UK and Holland confirmed that most of the carers we talked to were well aware of these phenomena, said that they were not unusual, and believed that they gave hope and comfort to the dying (13, 14).

An overview of recent ELE indexed publications retrieved from a PubMed search database reinforces the renewed interest in ELE experiences in scientific literature (see Tables 24.1 and 24.2). Different studies report the prevalence of ELE across different cultures (United States, Switzerland, Japan, Brazil, Moldova, England), within diverse clinical settings, especially among patients with cancer and in palliative care settings (cancer care hospitals, nursing homes, hospices and community settings). Reports of ELE are provided by healthcare professionals in 57% of studies (8/14), some of them with prospective daily deathbed observations and records (2/8). Other experiences are retrieved by patients' self-reports in structured or opened interviews (3/14) and by family members' records of ELE in close relatives (3/14). Table 24.2 shows a clinical overview of the main ELEs reported in quantitative studies.

Deathbed visions

The best known of the phenomena reported around the time of death is the occurrence of visions, occasionally of unknown or spiritual presences, but usually of dead relatives. Reported incidences of deathbed visions in quantitative studies are estimated as 36%–87% in family members' retrospective surveys and as 48%–88% of health professional records in cancer care and hospice settings (view Table 24.2). Interestingly, in survey responses, most health professionals who witness these experiences reported by their patients in healthcare settings consider ELE different from drug, fever-induced hallucinations or delirium (45%–69%) and accept the hypothesis that ELE might represent a sort of transpersonal experience (70%–89%). So absolutely real do these apparitions seem that the dying person is often witnessed interacting with them, and expecting others to do so too. Many nurses told us about deathbed visions they had witnessed when caring for dying patients. One said:

> I was attending a patient with a fellow nurse—again around 4 in the morning. The patient asked us to stand one on each side of him because he wanted to thank us for looking after him. He then looked over my shoulder towards the window and said 'Hang on I will be with you in a minute, I just want to thank these nurses for looking after me'. The patient repeated himself a couple of times then died!

Table 24.1 End-of-Life Experiences Study Characteristics (PubMed**)

Author	Year	Country	Type	Respondents	Setting	Sample	Age	Female	Assessments	Design	Methods
Renz, M.	2018	Switzerland	Qualitative Quantitative	Patients Observation	Cancer palliative care patients	80	62	50%	O-Protocol. Semi-structured questionnaire	Prospective	Descriptive analysis Mixed method analysis Interpretative Phenomenological Analysis (IPA)
Santos, C.	2016	Brazil	Quantitative	Professionals Report	Nursing homes, a Palliative Care Unit, a Cancer Center	133	41	78.9%	ELE questionnaire, DUREL, Depression, Anxiety and Stress Scale	Retrospective	Descriptive analysis Chi-Square and ANOVA tests
Morita, T.	2016	Japan	Quantitative	Family Report	Nationwide survey of bereaved family cancer patients	2221	72.9*	42%*	Protocol with Questions, Good Death Inventory, PHQ-9	Retrospective	Descriptive analysis T-test and Logistic Regression
Renz, M.	2015	Switzerland	Qualitative	Patients Observation	Advanced cancer hospitalized patients	251	–	–	O-Protocol. Semi-structured questionnaire	Prospective	Mixed method analysis Interpretative Phenomenological Analysis

Author	Year	Country									
Nosek, C.	2015	USA	Qualitative	Patients Self-Report	Hospice Unit inpatients	63	75	65.1%	Protocol with questions	Transversal	Mixed method analysis Concurrent triangulation approach
Kerr, C.	2014	USA	Quantitative	Patients Self-Report	Hospice Unit inpatients	59	74.9	67.8%	Protocol with questions	Prospective	Descriptive analysis Univariate analysis
Arnold, B.	2014	USA	Qualitative	Patients Self-Report	San Diego Hospice and The Institute for Palliative Medicine patient's	85	74	46%	Unstructured interviews	Transversal	Multimodal perceptual analysis strategy
Moore, L.	2013	USA	Quantitative	Professionals Report	Nursing faculty National League of Nursing	571	52.9	94%	Near-Death Phenomena Knowledge and Attitudes Questionnaire (NDPKAQ)	Retrospective	Descriptive analysis T-test and Regression
Lawrence, M.	2013	USA	Quantitative Qualitative	Professionals Report	Patients from a local hospice and hospice nurses across the USA	60 (Patients) 75 (Nurses)	–	–	Protocol with questions and a Chart	Prospective (Patients) Retrospective (Nurses)	Descriptive analysis
Kellehear, A.	2012	Moldova	Quantitative Qualitative	Family Report	Carers of dying Community Sample	102	68*	55%*	Protocol with questions	Retrospective	Descriptive analysis Content analysis

(continued)

Table 24.1 Continued

Author	Year	Country	Type	Respondents	Setting	Sample	Age	Female	Assessments	Design	Methods
Fenwick, P.	2011	UK	Qualitative	Family and Community Report	Bereaved relatives and friends	300	–	–	E-mail letters	Retrospective	Content analysis and descriptive analysis of reports
Fenwick, P.	2010	UK	Quantitative Qualitative	Professionals Report	Palliative care and Hospice teams	38	48	–	Validated Protocol with questions and tape-record	Retrospective Prospective	Content descriptive analysis
Brayne, S.	2008	UK	Quantitative Qualitative	Professionals Report	Nurses and Assistants from a Nursing Home	10	40.1	100%	Validated Protocol with questions and tape-record	Retrospective and Prospective	Observational, Descriptive analysis
Brayne, S.	2006	UK	Qualitative	Professionals Report	Palliative Care Team nurses, doctors, support worker	9	30-40	66%	Validated Protocol with questions and tape-record	Retrospective	Qualitative content analysis of tape-records interview

* Age and gender of patients reported by family members.

** The Pubmed Database search terms include a combination of words identified in literature regarding *end-of-life experiences, deathbed experiences, deathbed phenomena, deathbed visions, deathbed coincidences, deathbed communications, terminal lucidity, near-death experiences, anomalous experiences and near-death awareness* from inception to October 2019. Selected studies include: 1. Adult participants (aged 18 or over). 2. Peer-Reviewed Journals only. 3. Meeting the definition of end-of-life experiences (ELE) or deathbed phenomena (DBP), which includes visions, dreams, apparitions, coincidences or spiritual experiences associated with approaching death, that could provide comfort, meaning, to the dying person, or prepare him or her spirituality to death.

Table 24.2 Frequency of End-of-Life Experiences Reported in Quantitative Studies

Types of End-of-Life Experiences	Santos, 2017	Morita, 2016	Kerr, 2014	Moore, 2013	Lawrence, 2013	Lawrence, 2013	Kellehear, 2012	Fenwick, 2010	Fenwick, 2010	Brayne, 2008
Study design	Retrospective	Retrospective	Prospective	Retrospective	Retrospective	Prospective	Retrospective	Retrospective	Prospective	Retrospective
Sample	133	2221	59	571	75	70	102	38	29	10
Country	Brazil	Japan	USA	USA	USA	USA	Moldova	UK	UK	UK
Responders	Professionals	Family	Patients	Professionals	Professionals	Patients	Family	Professionals	Professionals	Professionals
Setting	Cancer Center, Hospices	Community family of cancer patients	Hospice Inpatient Unit	Nursing faculty	Hospice nurses across the USA	Hospice patients	Community carers of dying and Hospice patients	Palliative care and Hospice teams	Palliative care and Hospice teams	Nurses and Assistants Nursing Home
Any ELE reported by patients	79.8%	21%	88%	46%	48%	16.6%	40%	62%	43%	–
Visions	88.2%	87%	–	–	–	–	36%	62%	48%	50%
Reports of a different reality or afterlife	52.7%	54%	–	–	–	–	–	33%	48%	–
Dying end-of-life dreams	68.8%	–	–	–	–	–	18.5%	62%	50%	60%

(continued)

Table 24.2 Continued

Types of End-of-Life Experiences	Santos, 2017	Morita, 2016	Kerr, 2014	Moore, 2013	Lawrence, 2013	Lawrence, 2013	Kellehear, 2012	Fenwick, 2010	Fenwick, 2010	Brayne, 2008
Consider that ELE different from drug, fever-induced hallucinations or delirium	69.3%	45%	–	–	–	–	–	67%	65%	–
Consider ELE a transpersonal experience	78.5%	38%	–	–	–	–	–	70%	89%	–

*Any spiritual experience approaching death

We found, too, that the cultural differences noted by Osis and Haraldsson held true in our own investigations. Hospices and nursing homes in the UK, Ireland, and Holland showed that here deathbed visitors are most likely to be dead friends or family members—at any rate, someone the dying person has had a close emotional relationship with. While angels were common in the US 'Bible belt' in the UK survey, we found that out of 118 visions only 3% were of angels—the most common visitors (25%) were close relatives, while 17% were spiritual beings, though not angels.

Travelling companions

These visitors seem to come with a definite purpose, to help the person through the dying process. They draw closer as death draws nearer and, intriguingly, often sit on the person's bed, as a parent might do to comfort a sick child, and promise to return and accompany them on their journey when the time comes. In many instances, these experiences were remembered for many years by relatives who had been present and had also found them helpful and supportive. The following fascinating and detailed account we were given by a woman describing the last days of her 90-year-old mother who was in hospital, dying of pneumonia, shows very clearly the parallel worlds the dying seem able simultaneously to inhabit. As the various members of her family visited her, she was able to talk to them 'very calmly and clearly'. During all this time, her heart and oxygen levels were being monitored and were steady:

> She occasionally mentioned that she was aware that people were watching over her, and that they were in the gardens surrounding the hospital. She couldn't describe them, as they were behind the bushes, but she knew that they were there to help her 'if her head fell forward'. She said to my son that she also saw 'Dad' in the hospital room (as she used to call my father), and wasn't bothered by this. My son looked at her medical attachments and saw no fluctuation in the readings of the medical instrumentation. She would then continue talking normally to him.
>
> When my daughter arrived, shortly afterwards, she too had a really good visit. Her medical responses were calm and steady, and when she referred to, and saw, 'these people' her heart and oxygen levels didn't move. At this time 'the people' were in the ward, but near the inside of the windows. She was very calm and explained that she knew my daughter couldn't see them—but would understand when 'her time comes'. She calmly waved and spoke to 'these people' and introduced them to my daughter—as if they were talking to her. She would then carry on discussing Christmas and other aspects of normal life. I joined my daughter, after an hour, at the hospital and we both sat chatting to my mother. She spoke to me about my life—remembering vividly situations and many memories. She spoke to me about my future—all interspersed with references to 'these people' who were now at the end of her bed. She told us that she wouldn't be there the next day as 'these people' would 'pick her up when she fell and take her on a journey'. We were slightly spooked at her comments, but she was totally at ease.

By about 5 p.m. that afternoon, 'these people' were sitting on her bed next to her granddaughter, and she was having a three-way conversation with them. She died peacefully later that day.

It seems that occasionally these visitors can even be negotiated with to postpone the final time of departure. One man described how his car broke down on his way to visit his dying father. His sister broke the news to their father that he had been delayed. Then:

> My sister heard Dad talking very crossly to someone in his room. Fearing that one of her children had gone in and upset him she went in to see what was going on. Only Dad was there in his bed. My sister asked him who he was talking to. He replied 'I was telling the angels that I was not ready to go yet!' He knew I was coming and was determined to stay alive until I had seen him.
>
> All the people concerned (and myself) are and were practising Catholics, though this sort of phenomenon has nothing to do with our Faith. We were all as surprised as anyone of any faith or no faith would be.

It is interesting that these experiences seem to depend on neither expectation nor religious faith—they seem to bewilder and amaze believers and non-believers alike. Another of our correspondents told us about the death of his elderly aunt, a woman with a lifelong and deeply held conviction that death was the end of everything. They had had many discussions about this, as he himself had always doubted death's absolute finality. As she lay dying, she asked if she could speak to her nephew alone for a moment. She called him by his name and told him, 'You were right after all.'

By far the most common reaction is to feel the visitor as a comforting presence, there to help with the dying process and escort the person over the borders of death. The apparitions are nearly always seen as welcoming, and the dying person responds with interest or joy"

> Suddenly my Gran sat up in bed and smiled. She said 'I'm going now and here's Dad and John come to meet me.' She then died still with this big smile on her face. My mother never forgot it.

This kind of description recurs again and again:

> My mother's face lit up with joy.
>
> She smiled the most marvellous smile. She seemed to come alive.
>
> She suddenly sat up in bed her arms out towards someone with a great look of happiness and then after a pause sank back on the pillow and died not long after.

Quite often the visitor comes as a surprise, though usually a pleasant one. A district nurse told us this very typical story of an 80-year-old woman she used to visit once a week, to help and supervise the family who were giving her care.

She eventually became weaker and was semi-conscious, only reacting to painful stimuli. She died and I visited the next day to help. Her daughter said that she was lying peacefully and suddenly sat bolt upright with a beaming smile on her face and said 'Bobby how nice of you to come and see me.' Bobby was her deceased husband; then she lay back down again and died soon after. The daughter was very sensible and practical and really believed that her father had visited.

The third-party testimony of the nurse who told us this story indicates how compelling the daughter, in her opinion a thoroughly down-to-earth and credible witness, found the whole episode. It was also one of the many cases when a patient who has been comatose or unconscious has a sudden lucid interval just before death. From being someone who only reacted to painful stimuli, this woman suddenly rallied, sat bolt upright, and recognized and welcomed her visitor. There are cases of Alzheimer patients who have not recognized their family for some considerable time, who shortly before death sit up, greet their relatives by name and say goodbye.

Transiting to a new reality

As death approaches, some of the dying report that they go in and in out of another reality similar to that of the near-death experience, which they perceive as being more real than the real world, and interpenetrated by light, love, and compassion. Within this area, they experience a widening of their spiritual vision (15):

My father was at his (my grandfather's) bedside, deeply distressed. My grandfather quietly said to my father 'Don't worry Brady, I'm all right. I can see and hear the most beautiful things and you must not worry.' He quietly died, lucid to the end.

Visions of both relatives and strangers may be seen, and nearly always they are experienced as a comforting presence, there to help with the dying process and holding out a promise of the possibility of a continuation of consciousness.

The mother of a 32-year-old woman dying of breast cancer described to me what happened in the last two to three days of her daughter's life:

She was conscious of a dark roof over her head and a bright light. She moved into a waiting place where beings, her grandfather amongst them, were there to help her and told her everything would be ok. She moved into and out of this area, and was adamant that it was not a dream.
  We were comforted by her calmness—and her awareness of her forthcoming death—and the thought that she was totally at peace with it all.

It is very difficult to find a unitary mechanistic cause for these experiences. Carers who are familiar with both end-of-life and drug-induced experiences are clear that they are not drug induced, and are quite different in both form and quality. Neither can they be attributed to an organic confusional state—they mainly occur in clear consciousness. Are they contextual? Yes, they seem to be a part of the dying experience, but this does not help explain their mechanism. Are they simply a comfort experience? This is certainly their effect, but again it does not explain the mechanism. They do not seem to be due to expectation, and occur irrespective of any previous religion or belief, although belief may certainly colour them.

It is not only the dying themselves who have inexplicable experiences that seem to help them through the dying process. Relatives too often have experiences at the time someone they love dies, which they find enormously comforting. The perception of something leaving the body around the time of death is a little discussed phenomenon, reported consistently by professional carers and, most importantly, relatives, but usually only when they are directly asked about it. Light may be seen in the room or around the body, and 'something' often described as smoke or mist, or a form or shape seen leaving the body. Clocks are often reported to stop at the time of death, pets to behave strangely (16).

Deathbed coincidences

Some of the most interesting experiences are the reports by people who were close to someone who died, but were not with them at the time and may not even have known they were ill. And yet they may have some intimation of their friend or relative's death at the time it actually occurred. Such experiences are brief and may take the form of a 'visit' from the dead person, or simply be a sudden strong conviction that the person has died, often with the feeling that they have come to say goodbye. Or it may just be that they have an inexplicable and overwhelming feeling of unease or burst of grief, which they later discover occurred at the time of death. A woman described what happened 20 years ago when her brother was killed in a car crash.

> I had been at work, intending to work till 5 o'clock. At 4.20 p.m. I was uneasy and began getting cross with myself. I just packed up and went home despite really needing to stay at work. I found out at 2.30 a.m. the next morning that my brother had been killed instantly by a drunk driver at 4.20 p.m.

More detailed accounts make it clearer that coincidence is usually a pretty unsatisfactory explanation. This is another woman's account of what happened on the day her husband's grandfather died. He had lived with them for three years and had developed cancer of the oesophagus:

> One night my husband—a musician—was working and another grandson was visiting him. I asked Grandad if he would like a cup of tea and he said 'yes please' so I went into the kitchen and put the kettle on. As I waited for it to boil, the phone rang and my husband said 'Is Grandad alright?' so I said that yes he was alright and I was just making

him a cup of tea. He went on to say that he had been playing his guitar at work and a very strong feeling came over him that his grandad was there and he just had to get off the stage and phone me. I reassured him that Grandad was definitely OK and put the phone down. I made the tea and just as I was about to take it in, my brother in law came out and said 'he's gone'. He had just closed his eyes and died.

Although her husband knew that his grandfather was terminally ill, the fact that his feeling of unease was so intense that he was compelled to leave the stage and phone home, and the precise timing of his call at the moment his grandfather died does suggest strongly that this was more than just coincidence. To maintain that both these factors are due simply to chance seems far more improbable than the alternative explanation—that this man had in fact somehow reached out to make contact with his grandson as he was dying.

About two-thirds of the experiences we were told about occurred in the form of a dream and were more explicit. Always the person seems to indicate that they are dying, have come to say goodbye, and that they are all right. Distance is no object—the farewell visit can cross continents, and we were even told of someone who was 'visited' by their dying grandfather when they were in a submarine deep in the ocean. In October 1987, a man was serving in the Royal Navy as a submariner on-board HMS Revenge and had sailed for an 8-week patrol:

Two days after diving I was asleep in bed and had a very real dream that my grandfather had 'died'. The dream was very strange in that all of our family was waiting in the place where our grandparents had lived and that I was the last one to arrive. When I arrived and my grandfather saw that we were all there, he picked up my nephew's bike and said 'that's it, I'm off' and pedalled off over a walk way and disappeared. I woke up the next morning and told my best friend 'I had a really weird dream that my grandad had died'. My friend reassured me that it was only a dream and not to worry.

Whilst on patrol submariners are never told of any bad news. This was a problem for the Royal Navy as our next of kin were only allowed 40 words a week to inform us of any news (family-grams)—the Navy duly vetted such messages. My mother insisted that my wife put in the 'family-gram' that she was 'sorry about grandad'. On receipt of my wife's message the Royal Navy withheld all family-grams for me for 3 weeks—so I knew something was wrong! The Captain then decided to tell me that the reason for my messages being withheld was because my paternal grandfather had passed away, at approximately 3.00am on the 18th October 1987, I had no idea that he had been ill. At the time of his death I was fast asleep 200 feet under the Atlantic ocean. Very spooky . . .

This again highlights the fact that space is no bar for these communications, and even being underwater cannot stop them. It is certainly not uncommon for people who are away from their families to have anxiety dreams about them, but here again the timings are so precise that communication rather than co-incidence is much the most likely explanation. There is no ambiguity about either the message or the messenger—the people who have this experience are never in any doubt about who is contacting them, and what they are saying. And, however they occur, these visits, with their very specific farewell message, are almost always described as comforting and reassuring. The relatives are left with the strong impression that all is well and many say that they themselves subsequently lose any fear of death.

Perhaps not surprisingly, these experiences have not been taken seriously by the medical profession. Visions are usually attributed to medication, the pathological process of dying, or to expectation based on religious belief. But their nature and clarity, and the fact that many of those who experience them have no particular religious belief and certainly no expectation of a visit, makes none of these explanations tenable. The sense of somehow knowing, at the actual time of their death, that someone you love is dying is dismissed as coincidence. But there are enough accounts of these deathbed coincidences, in which the timing is so accurate and the emotional impact on the person who has the experience so intense, to suggest that, although some may indeed be simple coincidences, they cannot all be easily dismissed in this way.

Whether these phenomena are 'true' in a literal sense is unimportant. The fear of death is one of the most fundamental and universal human fears, and what these experiences seem to do is to extinguish this fear, not only for the dying themselves, but often for the family who may witness or be told about them, and on whom they have a profound and lasting impact (17,18).

What to say, and how to say it

Death isn't easy to talk about at the best of times and, for someone who is having to come to terms with the end of their own life, it can be harder still. Hard too, for those who are caring for them. But, if someone has had one of the experiences just described, they may want to talk about it, and it will probably make it easier for you to talk to them about what is happening. Watch their body language and look them in the eye. Be ready to listen to them, encourage them to describe who or what they have seen and, above all, don't question or belittle their experience, whatever you believe yourself. Ask them open questions (such as how, who, when, where). If you seem interested and curious, rather than incredulous or dismissive, it will help them to feel that talking about what happened is a normal—and very positive—part of the dying process.

Dying a good death

What exactly do we mean by a 'good death'? It should simply mean that the person has died as they wanted to die. For some, this might mean at home surrounded by their family; for others, it might mean a hospice with professional carers. I was impressed by the head of a hospice in Canada whom I once talked with at a conference. Often her patients lived in isolated places and might be some way away from home and relatives. But, she told me, 'No one ever dies alone in my hospice.' She described how she would wait until the dying person had a deathbed vision and then told them that, the next time they were 'visited', they should take their hand and leave with them.

Some people wait to die until they are on their own, others seem able to hold onto life until someone they particularly want to say farewell to has arrived at their bedside. But, for most people a 'good death' probably means dying with an untroubled mind, with conflicts and misunderstandings resolved. The Maoris in New Zealand say that one should always approach death 'walking backwards'. This way you can look back over your life, see what conflicts, differences, difficulties there have been, and do what you can to resolve them for your own peace of mind.

Reconciliation

One of the most impenetrable barriers to a 'good death' is unfinished business, and one of the most essential facilitators is reconciliation. If we are to die in peace, we need to forgive others, seek their forgiveness, and forgive ourselves for any wrongs or misunderstandings. If you are caring for the dying, the most valuable thing you can do for them is to make sure they have the opportunity, however late in the day, to try to mend broken or troubled relationships. This is not only so that the dying person can let go in peace, but so that the people left behind can have a peaceful and guilt-free parting. How important this is can be seen from the following account by a man of something that happened to him 40 years ago, when he was just 21 years old:

> My father and I had never got on and thus I left home 6 months after leaving school at the age of 16 years. I managed to find work and get myself stabilized in the south of England where I worked in the transport industry. I never visited home in the following 5 years nor did I think about the family I had left behind in Yorkshire.
>
> However, one morning at 7.30 am I was on my way to work as I had done for quite a few years when suddenly I turned right where I always turn left for my workplace, and started heading for London and the North. I could not reason with this, other than I found a sudden urge to visit my home in Yorkshire. I just felt a sudden need to do this.
>
> When I arrived at my parents front door my Mum came rushing out in tears and threw her arms around me saying 'Thank God you're here … we hadn't a clue where to get in touch, but your Dad is dying of cancer and you're the only one left to see him.'
>
> I went upstairs and made my peace with my dad who said that now he had seen all his family he was ready to go, and, next morning, when my elder brother called to see him he was dead in his bed.
>
> I could not explain this phenomenon and it has troubled me ever since.

This account was given to me by a close friend who had helped her mother take care of her dying brother:

> My brother developed cancer of the oesophagus about two years after his wife left him, and my mother always felt his illness was somehow 'her fault' even though he had been a heavy smoker and liked a drink or two. By the time he became ill he had met another lovely woman, and she and I helped my mother look after him at home during his last weeks. Although I knew in my heart that he should be given the chance to say goodbye to her last wife my mother still felt so antagonistic to her that I felt I couldn't ask her to come over. But in the last hour or so before he died, he was restless and the only word I heard him say was her name. I know now that there was unfinished business there that he should have been given the chance to resolve, and I will always regret that I didn't somehow find an opportunity for him to have this final meeting.

Many of the carers who were interviewed in our study said that the death process itself may somehow create the conditions that make the resolution of personal conflicts easier. They say that in the two or three days before death the room becomes extremely peaceful and dominated by feelings of love, and it is within this setting that families find it is easier for conflicts to be resolved and for reconciliation to be achieved. This isn't always possible, but it is always worth making the attempt. The nursing-home staff interviewed in our survey who had managed to effect reconciliation between estranged family members felt a sense of completion, as if the resident could rest. And the following account shows how profoundly such reconciliations can help the grieving process of family members.

Peter Beresford and his family had always had a difficult relationship with his mother and, because she would always refuse to talk through any differences or disagreements, their problems were always left unresolved. As he says, it is the most troubled relationships that are the most difficult to resolve after death, and he was given the chance to escape all that through the kindness of a hospice nurse who had been with his mother on the night she died and who wrote to him describing the conversation they had had that night. His mother had been anxious to talk about her past, and about things she wished she had done differently. He described the effect the nurse's letter had had in an article in *the Guardian* (19):

> What was so wonderful about the nurse's letter was that here truly was a voice from the grave, a kind of deathbed confession, where you knew the messenger had no ulterior motive, had no interest other than to try and help as an unbiased outsider. Just as we felt we were not judged, so we knew that neither was my mother, so what had rarely ever happened before for once did. We heard an authentic warm voice from my mother . . . in what she said, there was appreciation, there was recognition, there was apology, above all there was warmth to Suzy . . . Over the years I have been able to develop an honest picture of my mother and mourn that. And that is greatly due to the nurse's simple, diligent and generous action.

Dying as transition

The recent research carried out by Dr Monika Renz, a Swiss palliative care theologian who has studied a large number of dying patients in hospices, has taken our knowledge of the dying process a step further in her recent and most comprehensive and interesting research into what happens to consciousness as we die (20).

Dr Renz showed that there seem to be three stages in the death process that mark the alterations that consciousness undergoes. These she calls pre-transition, transition, and post-transition. In the pre-transitional state, the person realizes that dying is inevitable. They may fear losing control, and realize that they will have to give up everything they are attached to. It is in this state that the dying person may suffer from the anxiety and struggle that are called 'terminal restlessness'. Inability to accept this will hold them in the pre-transitional state and lead to further suffering.

If you feel that a patient is restless or anxious, it may be that they want to resolve some unresolved issue. Someone to listen to them may be all they need, but they may ask for your help. Even if they do not, it is worth asking them if anything particular is worrying them, or if they would like you to contact a friend or relative for them. It is important to take any final requests they may make seriously—they may make all the difference between a restless and a peaceful death.

But, once they have acknowledged and accepted the inevitable, they will pass into the next stage: transition. Now there is a loosening of ego consciousness. Old traumas may be reactivated but on the whole the person becomes quieter and may simply lie quietly and stare.

In this final, post-transitional state, the sense of ego is no longer dominant and the patient enters a new state of consciousness, which is known as 'non-duality'. They become serene, in a state beyond anxiety, pain, or powerlessness, and, although they may be unable to speak, they can still hear and communicate by gestures or single words. Such transformative experiences are comparable to a spiritual awakening: the patient has completed their journey. This is an important state to recognize because it shows an expansion of consciousness with love and light, rather than its cessation.

The progress from pre- to post-transition is not essentially linear: the patient may pass back and forth from level to level during the days preceding death. But the real significance of these findings is that death need not be a fearful process. We can die happy and should not be afraid. Dr. Renz has noted that there seem to be various protective factors that make it easier to reach this final peaceful state. The people who seemed to suffer least during the dying process, to pass most easily to the post-transitional state, were the ones who had been medita-tors, or prayed regularly, or had had a previous near-death experience, or who were simply curious about the death process. Any of these factors seemed to make a person less likely to be afraid when they met it face to face.

We may never find a logical scientific explanation that would fully explain the experiences described in this chapter and, even if we did, something within us might not be satisfied with the explanation. We do not like to believe that something that makes such a powerful emotional impact might be essentially either mechanical or meaningless. Most people want to believe that they have meaning in a wider sense—that they are more than brain function, more than just a speck in creation, and that, finally, personal consciousness will continue in some form or other. And the knowledge we have now about the whole pro-cess of dying suggests that this may indeed be an expansion of consciousness rather than the diminution and extinction of consciousness, which is the more traditional way of regarding death. It is incumbent upon all teachers to make certain that, when they teach palliative care and dying, they make certain that the dying person is fully aware of the dying process and that all carers are aware of the phenomena discussed in this chapter.

References

1. **Youngson R.** Compassion in healthcare: the missing dimension of healthcare reform? London: The HNS Confederation, 17 August 2009. Available from: https://www.nhsconfed.org/resources/2009/08/compassion-in-healthcare

2. **Campaign for Dignity in Dying.** Survey finds that being alone is Britain's biggest fear about death. 22 April, 2008. Available from: http://www.dignityindying.org.uk/uploadedFiles/About_Us/Dying%20Alone.pdf.

3. **Higginson I.** Priorities for end-of-life care in England, Wales and Scotland National Council. Powerpoint presentation by Department of Health: What is the End-of-life Care Programme. [Online] 2003. [Cited: 12 June 2008.] https://uk.search.yahoo.com/yhs/search?hspart=trp&hsimp=yhs-001&type=Y143_F163_201897_020721&p=www.endoflifecare.nhs.uk+.&rdr=1

4. **Mayor, S.** Care of dying patients and safety dominate report by NHS complaints. *BMJ News*, 10 February 2007, **334**: 278. Available from: https://www.ncbi.nlm.nih.gov/pmc/articles/PMC1796720/

5. **Curtis JR, Engelberg RA, Nielsen EL, Au DH, Patrick DL.** Patient-physician communication about end-of-life care for patients with severe COPD. *European Respiratory Journal*. 2004;24:200–5.

6. **Rousseau P.** Spirituality and the dying patient. *Journal of Clinical Oncology*. 2000;18(9, May):2000–2.

7. **Barrett W.** *Deathbed visions*. 1926 republised White Crow books 2011.

8. **Osis K, Haraldsson E.** *At the hour of death*. New York: Hastings House; 1986, orig. 1977.

9. **Osis K.** Deathbed observations by physicians and nurses: a cross-cultural survey. *Journal for the American Society for Psychical Research.* 1961;71(3):237–59.

10. **Wholihan D.** Seeing the light: end of life experiences—visions, energy surges and other deathbed phenomena. *Nursing Clinics of North America.* 2016;51(3, Sep):489–500.

11. **Brayne S, Lovelace H, Fenwick P.** An understanding of the occurrence of deathbed phenomena and their effects on palliative care physicians. *American Journal of Hospice and Palliative Medicine.* 2006;23(1):17–24.

12. **Brayne S, Lovelace H, Fenwick P.** Perceptions of nursing home carers on the spiritual experiences of residents at the end of life. *European Journal of Palliative Care,* 2008;15(3).

13. **Brayne S, Lovelace H, Fenwick P.** (2008). End of life experiences and the dying process in a Gloucestershire nursing home as reported by nurses and care assistants. *American Journal of Hospice and Palliative Medicine.* 2008;25(3):195–206. doi:10.1177/1040090108315302

14. **Fenwick P, Fenwick E.** *The art of dying.* London: Bloomsbury Continuum. 2008.

15. Fenwick P, Fenwick E. *The Truth in The Ligh 2012.* White Crowe Books.

16. **Barbato M.** Parapsychological phenomena near the time of death. *Journal of Palliative Care.* 1999;15(2):30–7.

17. **Kellaher A.** *The inner life of the dying person.* New York: Columbia University Press; 2014.

18. **Betty LS.** Are they hallucinations or are they real? The spirituality of deathbed and near death visions. *Omega.* 2006;53(1–2):37–49.

19. *Guardian Newspaper,* Family section p.2. 18.08.07

20. **Renz M. Reichmuth O, Bueche D, Traichel B, Schuett MM, Cerny T, Strasser F.** Fear, pain, denial, and spiritual experiences in dying processes. *American Journal of Hospice and Palliative Medicine.* 2017. PMID:28823175 PMCID:PMC5794111. doi:10.1177/1049909117725271

Chapter 25

Fruitful collaborations with religious and spiritual communities to foster mental health in general society: An international perspective

Wai Lun Alan Fung, Victor A. Shepherd, King Yee Agatha Chong, Sujatha D. Sharma, and Avdesh Sharma

Section 1: overview

Wai Lun Alan Fung

Interprofessional Collaborations and Education has been widely recognized (by the World Health Organization and various other national organizations) as instrumental for improving the quality of health care. In the World Psychiatric Association (WPA)'s position statement on spirituality and religion in psychiatry (1), one of the seven recommendations is that 'Psychiatrists, whatever their personal beliefs, should be willing to work with leaders/members of faith communities, chaplains and pastoral workers, and others in the community, in support of the well-being of their patients, and should encourage their multi-disciplinary colleagues to do likewise.' A similar recommendation was made in the Royal College of Psychiatrists (UK) Position Statement PS03/2013 titled 'Recommendations for psychiatrists on spirituality and religion' (2).

In the United States, the American Psychiatric Association (APA)—partnering with the APA Foundation and the Interfaith Disability Advocacy Coalition—formed the Mental Health and Faith Community Partnership (of which this writer has served on the Steering Committee) in 2014—'a collaboration between psychiatrists and clergy aimed at fostering a dialogue between two fields, reducing stigma, and accounting for medical and spiritual dimensions as people seek care' (3). The partnership was aimed at 1) providing an

All authors contributed to this chapter equally.

opportunity for psychiatrists and the mental health community to learn from spiritual leaders, to whom people often turn in times of mental distress; and 2) providing an opportunity to improve understanding of the best science and evidence-based treatment for psychiatric illnesses among faith leaders and those in the faith community. In 2015, the partnership had published *Mental Health: A Guide for Faith Leaders*, as well as an accompanying *Quick Reference Guide*—both freely available for downloading (3). These resources have been utilized by thousands in North America and beyond.

The relevance of such partnerships has recently been illustrated by a cluster randomized controlled trial reporting that a collaborative shared care model delivered by traditional and faith healers (TFHs) and conventional healthcare providers for people with psychosis in Nigeria and Ghana was effective and cost-effective (4). The authors have noted that this model may be especially promising for resource-constrained settings. Nonetheless, there have also been concerns about harmful practices and absence of evidence on safety and effectiveness of TFH care, and such collaborative models with TFHs have thus far been uncommon (5, 6). Of note, these studies have grouped faith healers together with traditional healers and these faith healers may be quite different from other spiritual care professionals—say, those belonging to a major organized religion or a newer religious movement.

Regardless of the scope of spiritual care provider or community under discussion, one should always be cognizant of not just the potential benefits of such collaborations but also the potential harms. More generally, such collaborations must be ethical (7). Indeed, these issues have been explicitly addressed by recommendations 4 and 7 of the WPA position statement (1). Similarly, the Royal Australian and New Zealand College of Psychiatrists position statement 96 recommends that psychiatrists 'be willing to work with members of religious/spiritual communities in support of the well-being of individuals, and their families and communities, *only ever with the valid consent of the individual*' (8).

While the APA Mental Health and Faith Community Partnership has presented one such model—at the national level—such collaborations may take various forms at different levels (from local to global), and in different cultural and geographical contexts—as will be illustrated in the following sections. In Section 2, Reverend Victor Shepherd, a Canadian Christian pastor and theology professor, describes his perspectives on such collaborations from the religious/spiritual side, filled with practical examples at a local level and tips that anyone from the faith community could quite readily implement. In Section 3, Dr Agatha Chong, a psychiatrist in Hong Kong, describes various examples (at the local/regional levels) of partnerships between mental health and faith communities in Hong Kong—which has a predominant Chinese culture but also strong Western influence from being a former British colony. In Section 4, Dr Avdesh Sharma, a psychiatrist from India, and his wife, Dr Sujatha Sharma, a clinical psychologist, describe their decades-long collaborations with the spiritual organization, Brahmakumaris, with numerous examples at the local, national (India) and international levels (e.g. through collaborations with the WPA). In Section 5, I discuss some implications from these sections.

Section 2: a Canadian Christian pastoral response to mental health needs

Victor A. Shepherd

Acquire the capacity to discriminate

In my final year of theology studies (1970), University of Toronto, I enrolled on a course whose instructor was a psychiatrist connected with Toronto's Centre for Addiction and Mental Health. Months later, I emerged from the course not merely with medical information I had heretofore lacked: I emerged with a world I hadn't known to exist.

The 'world' that I was to indwell for the rest of my ministry was the irreducible complexity of the human person, together with the multidimensionality, pervasiveness, and relentlessness of human suffering. This 'world' was the constellation of the stresses, frequently swelling to distresses—intra-psychic, social, biological, historical, religious—that bear upon people, together with the configuration of responses—individual and societal—to such stresses. Indwelling this world spared me a shallow, unrealistically simplistic approach to the people I would see every day for the next 40 years in my work as pastor.

One month after the course had concluded, I was ordained, and then appointed to one of the poorest regions in Canada. Immediately I found myself face to face with people whose difficulties were the 'common cold' of the psychiatric world: for example, mood disorders, anxiety disorders, schizophrenia. I also witnessed suffering less frequently seen in the twentieth century: hysterical limb paralysis and even hysterical blindness when someone without neural or ocular deficits was 'put on the spot' in a troubling social situation only to find her vision fading and returning repeatedly. In addition, I saw factitious disorders (under-employment found some people adeptly avoiding the employment they could have had), impairment born of organic brain disorders (lumberjacks are especially prone to forest mishaps entailing major head injuries), children emotionally warped in families beset with addiction (the rate of alcoholism in my region was three times the North American average.) Aware of their pain, I eschewed the approach of fellow pastors who naively and unhelpfully counselled mentally ill congregants to pray more, trust more, repent and repudiate more—thereby compounding a medical problem with religiously induced neurotic guilt, anxiety, and self-rejection.

Recognize the mental health need

Most elementally, pastors and church counsellors must acquire *the capacity to recognize the mental health need*. Even moderate sophistication here will enable church workers to discern what is at issue regardless of how sufferers assess their problem. (Mentally ill people who belong to faith communities tend to fault themselves spiritually for their illness. Church workers must be able to move sufferers beyond their spiritual misdiagnosis rather than confirm them in it.)

Rudimentary skills in this regard can be acquired readily.

a. In addition to emotional floridness, for instance, one of the first signs of mania is irresponsible use of money: someone with limited resources gathers up magazines in a variety store and in one hour adds $2,000 to their credit card tally.

b. While depression is often associated exclusively with persistent feelings of sadness or worthlessness, some depressed people chiefly exhibit not sadness but psycho-motor retardation: inability to 'get going', stalling when confronted with tasks they normally performed and dismissed routinely. The businessperson who daily makes a dozen decisions worth $100,000 each now finds himself unable to make any. And if he adds, 'By the way, I also feel there's something gnawing at my innards', his nihilistic self-delusion only confirms his depression.

c. Since 1% of the world's population is schizophrenic, it is crucial that church workers be able to recognize the affliction: withdrawal or isolation, accompanied by 'pillar-to-post' thinking, inability to concentrate, inability to think in shades of grey, and inappropriate mood responses—laughing when nothing funny has been said, or weeping when nothing unhappy is occurring. (The 'split' in the schizophrenic person is not a Jekyll-and-Hyde split in character: it's a split between situation and affect.)

d. Addictions are legion. While substance misuse, such as that of alcohol, tobacco, or drugs, is readily understood (supposedly) as addictive, few people understand non-substance addictions—for example, gambling. Here, it must be grasped that addiction has a neurophysiological component, a psychological element, and, of course, the ever-present spiritual dimension.

What is frequently overlooked is the suffering of addicts: the alcohol-habituated, for instance, are often deemed devious or vulgar or obnoxious or weak or stupid. What is not grasped is that, underneath their bravado (usually deployed to mask pathetically diminished self-esteem), they are suffering atrociously and should be approached in terms of their pain.

Have a ready-to-hand means of referral

Any pastor can direct an ill person to a psychotherapist, while only a physician or nurse practitioner can refer to a psychiatrist. For this reason, much awkwardness can be avoided if pastor or church-counsellor has a friend, physician, or nurse-practitioner, who will see a congregant on short notice and make the appropriate referral.

A woman in my congregation, a mathematics teacher by profession, phoned me at midnight. She was in distress. She and her husband had attended a symphony concert, and had returned home late in the evening, when she decided the kitchen floor needed to be washed; not washed once, but washed three times. She had phoned me, dismayed that her obsession had clung to her for years, had impaired her marriage, and now threatened to collapse it. She had hidden her difficulty so very well that prior to her call I had had no idea of her problem. Next day I phoned my psychiatrist instructor from the course I had taken 15 years earlier. He recommended a psychiatrist in another neighbourhood who specialized in obsessive–compulsive disorder in women. My congregant had her family doctor refer her to this latter psychiatrist. The bottom line was that the suffering woman was treated pharmaceutically, was relieved of her torment, and went on to have the two children she never thought she could, as well as live in a manner she had never dreamed she would be able to.

In one of my seminary classes whose topic was suicide, a quiet student spoke in a barely audible whisper, 'I've been down to the subway tracks several times, planning to leap in front of an oncoming train, only to step back at the last moment.' The class fell silent. Gently I told her that it was inappropriate for me to discuss her predicament in front of others; she should see me after class. I contacted a colleague on the seminary faculty who was also a family doctor. He treated her (family doctors treat more mentally ill people than psychiatrists do), and she remains fine— as long as she continues to take her prescribed medication.

Be ready to respond

It is important to distinguish between 'How to respond' and 'How to treat' (let alone 'How to cure'). Only professionals treat; anyone else may respond.

A major aspect of our response is the ministry to the family of the ill person. While it is difficult to overlook the suffering of the ill person, it is too easy to overlook the suffering of the ill person's family. If we have spent even a few hours with a psychotic person who talks past our world because our world has little to do with his, then we should try to imagine the frustration of family members who live with this situation every day.

Recently, I decided to treat a paranoid, psychotic person I have long looked out for to a restaurant meal. We were about to sit down when my friend shouted, 'There's a tape recorder under my seat!' The waitress, frightened and frozen at once, looked at me pleadingly. Quietly, I asked her to find us a seat devoid of tape recorders. I reassured her that my friend was unusual and I would see that no harm befell fellow diners. Quickly she found us another seat and our meal together unfolded without incident.

The paranoid fellow lives with his unmarried sister. Her anguish, different from his to be sure, is anguish nonetheless. In ministering to him, we must never fail to minister to her.

If we have spent even a few hours with someone whose major depression can lower the mood of a room, we have insight enough into what burden is sustained by family members who live with her. If we have spent any time with a substance-addicted person who is a public embarrassment, we have insight enough into the embarrassment that person is to those who live with him.

Earlier, I mentioned that the addicts, plus their families, are suffering extraordinarily. One day I called on a man whose alcoholism was unrelieved. People in the congregation avoided him: they found his addiction repugnant and diminished impulse control disgusting. While I was speaking with him, late one afternoon, his wife returned home from work. She was humiliated that the pastor had found her husband intoxicated and dirty. Gently I said to her, 'Your husband is suffering terribly; and you are suffering no less.' She wept—and then asked, 'Will you join us for supper?'

How badly is this fellow suffering? As a child, he was beaten repeatedly by his father; as an adult, he lost his business in a store fire. How badly is his wife suffering? Her first husband was shot and killed on the steps of a downtown hotel in a case of mistaken identity.

The ill person and family members may not be suffering in the same way, but all are suffering *alike*. There is a ministry to be rendered to all because all are afflicted with loneliness. While much is said today about guilt and shame, in my first congregation, I discovered loneliness to be the miasma whose noxious vapour distorts life. A physician friend with whom I raised this issue (he had graduated at the top of his medical school class, had married a well-to-do woman, and lacked nothing with respect to wealth and social advantage); when I had voiced my opinion concerning loneliness, he added soberly, 'The whole world is lonely'—meaning, of course, that *he* was lonely.

Loneliness drives people to behave uncharacteristically. For this reason, loneliness renders people at risk: we are most at risk spiritually when we are most needy emotionally. Wise pastoral friendship always fosters spiritual vigilance in the face of uncommon loneliness.

Loneliness is exacerbated by stigma, the stigma sticking like flypaper to ill people and to their families simultaneously. Stigma assumes various expressions: someone is deemed morally defective, intellectually deficient, socially unacceptable.

'Stigma' is a Greek word meaning 'brand, scar, mark'. In the ancient Greek world, slaves were branded indelibly. In the ancient Roman world, a runaway slave, upon being caught, was branded with the letter 'F'—for *fugitivus*, 'fugitive', escapee. Such a person was marked for life, readily identified, and forever despised.

Much can be done to denature stigma. Simple friendship is a good place to start. Charlie Brown, was rendered famous by Charles Shulz's comic strip, *Peanuts*; Charlie plays on a baseball team that loses every game by 40 runs. Snoopy exclaims, 'It must be terrible to play on a team that loses every game by 40 runs.' 'No,' rejoins Charlie, 'losing isn't what hurts; what hurts is that no one comes to see us play. And therefore the agony of defeat we must bear alone.' Simple hospitality is a step towards overcoming the isolation of the chronic sufferer.

Simple hospitality must be emphasized. Too often people are held off exercising hospitality because they fear their homes are insufficiently grand, their furniture insufficiently elegant, and their food insufficiently cordon bleu. Sufferers are aware of none of this. What matters to these people is human company in a context of warmth, sharing, generosity, and undisguised acknowledgement that everyone is lacking (for now) the wholeness and holiness for which we were created. Everyone needs to reflect to everyone else the truth that our suffering does not define us: that a day has been appointed when our restoration will be complete and no one will be impaired, rejected, or stigmatized.

We are told, 'Do not neglect to show hospitality to strangers, for by doing that some have entertained angels without knowing it' (Hebrews 13:8, New Revised Standard Version). According to rabbinic texts, Abraham planted a tamarisk tree at Beersheba (Genesis 21:33) and then called on the name of El Holam, the Everlasting God. The medieval rabbis maintained that Abraham did this so that all who passed that way and were refreshed might name God's name; that is, in according the sufferer hospitality *we* become an *icon of God for* the person in pain. According to 1st Timothy 3:2 and Titus 1:8, Christian leaders must be given to hospitality.

Not only is there a response individuals, or individuals plus their families, can make: there is also a response congregations can make. In a group home adjacent to the church I pastored for 21 year, we came upon a dozen residents who were seriously ill and could not be left unattended. They were adequately cared for materially, but otherwise lived a relatively bleak existence. The congregation recognized the need on its doorstep and drew up a schedule for taking these people to a local restaurant to give them an outing they would otherwise not have. We made sure to have two congregants for every resident, just in case someone decompensated. And then together we shared a meal that gloriously anticipated the messianic banquet.

Were the residents in the group home the congregation's neighbours? In the parable of the Good Samaritan, the question is posed, 'Who is my neighbour?'—and is never answered. At the conclusion of the parable, the questioners are interrogated, 'Who *proved* to be neighbour?' (Luke 10:35, English Standard Version) The neighbour is neither someone we have nor someone we are: the neighbour is someone we *prove* ourselves to be.

Because the communities of the Abrahamic traditions maintain, for instance, that there is no human being, anywhere, in even the most distressing predicament, who is ever God-forsaken, the community that upholds this truth must embody it. Because God doesn't abandon, despise, or reject (regardless of how God-forsaken many might feel), there must be a community that does not abandon, despise, or reject.

Our concrete embodiment of this truth takes at least two forms.

1. Most simply, the community shares its material resources with those who are especially needy. Everyone is aware, of course, that there is a government-enforced, non-voluntary sharing of our material resources with the needy. This enforced, non-voluntary assistance is found in the combination of graduated income tax and social assistance and health care. Unquestionably, this provision is the indirect illumination arising from scripture-steeped communities. We ought never to sell it short, and we should continue to ask ourselves what the social texture of our society might be if secularism extinguishes the indirect illumination of the gospel.

   The Mississauga congregation I pastored for 21 years did much to develop two affordable housing projects (value: $35 million CND). This housing accommodated needy people, among whom were many psychiatrically troubled. We discovered that not a few of the people we housed were undernourished—whereupon we developed Mississauga's first food bank. Next, we noticed that many children were so poorly fed that they were underachieving at school—whereupon we fashioned a 'breakfast club' in order to give them a nutritious start to the school-day. At one point, there were 44 people from my own congregation serving in the 'breakfast club'.

The most elemental level of community is serving the neighbour's material scarcity through our material abundance.

2. The second expression of community is sharing the neighbour's suffering. To share the neighbour's suffering, where mental illness is concerned, is at least to befriend that person and thereby at least reduce their isolation and loneliness.

The mentally ill person suffers what every human suffers in terms of frailty, disease, and bodily breakdown through accident, sickness, and aging. In addition, the mentally ill person suffers from her particular psychiatric problem, indeed *lives*, lives out that problem, as the non-psychiatrically afflicted do not live *that* problem, at least. And in the third place, the mentally ill person suffers the social stigma visited upon the psychiatrically troubled. The community must be aware of all three levels of such suffering, and remain aware that such suffering, cumulatively, is an appalling burden.

When I was a pastor in Mississauga, my wife and I invited back to lunch each Sunday a different family from the congregation. Several matters need to be noted here.

1. The unmarried person is still a family, and should not be overlooked in a society almost exclusively couple oriented.

2. In a congregation of 400 families, there are always several people who have been diagnosed with assorted psychiatric problems.

3. As already discussed at length, the entire family of the mentally ill person is suffering.

4. While these people are invited to lunch, many linger as late as 5 p.m., and this on account of the invisible loneliness discussed above.

In the course of our simple hospitality, we welcomed to our home and table those whose suffering beggared description, including the 'dual diagnosed'— for example, the mentally ill person who is also blind or in trouble with the law.

Concluding remarks

The role of the community of faith is not to mimic the mental health professional; and certainly it is not to suggest that medical intervention is superfluous. The role of the community of faith is to render concrete its conviction that ill people matter and should not be ignored. Not least, the role of the community of faith is to hold up—for the sufferer herself but also for the wider society—the truth that the troubled of this earth have been appointed to a future release and recovery more glorious than their pain allows them to glimpse at this time.

Section 3: partnership between mental health and faith communities in enhancing mental health— the Chinese context

King Yee Agatha Chong

Religion and spirituality (R/S) has been playing an important role in the Chinese culture for five millennia, long before the era of modern psychology. These religions demonstrate ritual, ethical, social, and doctrinal dimensions—through which the mental health of Chinese people is enhanced through developing acceptance, gratitude, commitments, ethics, and virtues, as well as positive relationships. While the majority of Chinese people (more than 1.4 billion) reside in the Greater China Area—a term usually referring to mainland China, Taiwan, Hong Kong, and Macau—there are also more than 50 million ethnic Chinese residing outside the Greater China Area.

This essay focuses on Hong Kong—officially the Hong Kong Special Administrative Region of the People's Republic of China—with a population of around 7.25 million, 92% of whom are ethnic Chinese (9). It was a British colony between 1841 and 1997.

According to 2016 estimates, 27.9% of the population of Hong Kong believe in Buddhism or Taoism; 6.7% in Protestantism; 5.3% in Roman Catholicism; 4.2% in Islam; 1.4% in Hinduism; and 0.2% in Sikhism (9). Over half (54.3%) of the population of Hong Kong have reported either no religion, or beliefs in other religions—the majority in the form of Chinese folk religious practices like worshipping ancestors and local Gods like Guanyin, Wong Tai Sin, and Che Kung. Of note, many people practise Confucianism, regardless of their religion or not having a religious affiliation (9).

The role of religion/spirituality and faith communities on enhancing mental well-being and addressing mental distress

While sense of hopelessness is one of the diagnostic criteria of depressive disorder, a hopeful person has better mental health and less likely to have depression or suicidal idea. There are local studies showing higher prevalence of mood disorder in patients with chronic or terminal illnesses. For those who have illness, their hope for afterlife or eternal life can ameliorate their fear of death.

Early Western medical services in Hong Kong were mostly carried out by overseas missionary organizations. Missionaries provided people with medical services and at the same time preached the gospel to them. In olden days, hospital staff always talked to outpatients and every ward had a morning prayer session. They recited the Bible and gave sermons to patients. They often quoted Bible sayings to encourage patients, whether they were inpatients or outpatients.

Nowadays, chaplaincy service is readily available in all hospitals of Hong Kong. Psychiatrists can readily refer a patient with a spiritual need to a chaplain. Chaplaincy services include counselling, psycho-spiritual support to patients, relatives or hospital staff, referring patients to appropriate support groups, arranging funerals, as well as organizing religious activities for patients and hospital staff. Chaplains also recruit volunteers and provide training, including clinical pastoral education for voluntary workers in a systemic approach. Chaplaincy services can be tailored to individuals' religious faiths.

Under the grief theory of Elisabeth Kübler-Ross, there are five stages of grief: denial, anger, bargaining, depression, and, finally, acceptance (10). Denial, anger, and bargaining commonly occur in a clinical setting, causing tension and even conflict among patient and relatives as well as medical professionals. Not only are emotional health and relationships jeopardized, medical decisions can be affected when people are overwhelmed by numerous changes and emotions. The chaplaincy service plays an important role here to support patients and relatives through all these stages, finally reaching the stage of acceptance of the loss.

End-of-life care should be individualized according to the patient's and/or relatives' religious belief. It is not uncommon for people who are atheist all along to finally commit to one religion at the end of their lives. Most funerals in Hong Kong have religious themes—and most often a Taoist, Buddhist, or Christian approach. If the deceased did not have any religious belief, the Taoist approach is often adopted because Taoism is not only a religion but also a major part of Chinese tradition and culture. According to the Buddhist conception of equality for all, people normally would go through four stages of life (birth, aging, sickness and death). These four stages are equal in nature—which means that we need not fear one or the other, or death over life—for they are both part of a life cycle (11). Dying is a natural and unavoidable process, just like living.

Religious rituals are grief-healing and able to facilitate the smooth transition of stages of grief. People who are vulnerable to mood disorder or pathological grief are encouraged to attend a funeral with support, rather than avoiding mourning, so that they are able to reconcile their grief and find continued or new meaning in life, knowing that they are not alone in their grief.

Collaborations among different religions for enhancing mental health and addressing mental ill health

To enhance collaboration among Chinese religions for the betterment of mental and spiritual health, the 'Colloquium of Six Religious Leaders of Hong Kong' was established in June 1978. It is composed of representatives of six associations of major religions among Hong Kong Chinese: the Hong Kong Taoist Association, Hong Kong Buddhist Association, Catholic Diocese of

Hong Kong, Hong Kong Christian Council, Confucian Academy, and Chinese Muslim Cultural and Fraternal Association. The Colloquium enhances friendship through regular dialogues and joint activities in order to establish a model of social harmony. It also emphasizes the importance of respecting different religions through understanding, and the member associations have been collaborating in various social aspects related to the mental well-being of the population.

The leaders of the six religions make a joint New Year statement to Hong Kong people every year, which responds to major social phenomena or events in the previous year. In the face of any social instability, they emphasize the importance of peace and the role of religious people in turning conflict into cooperation, turning bad feelings into good will, and raising the level of spiritual life. The Colloquium also organizes conferences and other inter-religious activities every year for exchanging ideas about social, economical livelihood, and religious problems through inter-religious dialogues.

During the period of social unrest in Hong Kong in 2019 against the Anti-Extradition Law Amendment Bill, the Colloquium issued appeals on different occasions throughout months of social conflict, during which many Hong Kong people suffered from stress-related mental disorders. Also, the theme of the bi-annual conference held during that time was about how faith could help people deal with emotional distress (12).

Different religious perspectives were introduced to the audience. Buddhism encourages people to understand their own 'heart' (mind), be still in mind, to let go of their 'attachments' and 'ego-grasping', and to be altruistic. Taoist followers can have their mind stay calm through Taoism rituals, physical practices of 'Qi', and prayer. The doctrines of Islam also uphold 'forgiveness' and 'love (for) one another'. From the Confucianism point of view, people develop emotional distress because of the lack of 'cultivation' of thoughts, mind, and noble personal character towards benevolence, righteousness, propriety, wisdom, and faith (13). For Christianity, Jesus Christ is the model for His believers when they are in times of adversity. The suffering of Jesus Christ and His sacrifice on the cross is a major theme of the spiritual exercise for Christians. These religious teachings helped the general public to cope with emotional distress.

Collaborations between mental health professional and faith community in addressing mental ill health—a case report

Identifying data and personal history: Miss C was a 36-year-old single woman. She was born into a lower-middle-class family and she lived in a public housing estate with her parents. She did not dare to lose her job and therefore would never say no to any of her colleagues, despite the requests sometimes being unreasonable. Her parents had a poor marital relationship and the atmosphere of her family was always tense. She described herself as the 'bridge' for communication between her parents because they were always in a 'cold war' and did not talk to each other. After completing high school, she worked as a clerk in an office. Having been attending church regularly for more than 10 years, she was a devoted Christian.

History of present illness: One month before she was first seen by a psychiatrist, her job demand had been increasing and her communication with her parents had been getting poorer. In view of stress from both her work and her family, she developed depressive symptoms including insomnia, tearfulness, poor appetite, and low energy level. She lost her motivation to join any church activity. She had a sense of uselessness, feeling that it was useless to go to church and that she herself was useless too. She also felt no hope in getting better and she could not find the meaning of life. She believed that she was 'unlovable', 'worthless', and she could not feel the 'love of God'. She was socially withdrawn and refused to go back to her church.

Diagnosis: She was diagnosed to have major depressive disorder without psychotic features.

Recommended management: The psychiatrist recommended the initiation of a selective serotonin re-uptake inhibitor (SSRI) to help with her biological and mood symptoms, as well as cognitive behavioural therapy (CBT) to address her negative cognitions.

Barriers: Miss C was reluctant to accept the treatment recommendations, because she felt that there would be no hope for her to get better and she had the idea that she was depressed because of 'lack of faith'.

Addressing the treatment barriers through collaborations between her church community and mental health professionals: Miss C's church sisters and pastor continued to visit her from time to time. She was first advised to rely on prayers, talk to church friends, or 'leave her burden to the Lord' in order to relieve her emotional distress, but was unsuccessful. She also struggled about whether she was really loved by God and whether her depressive symptoms were caused by 'lack of faith'. Eventually, Miss C decided to stop all her church activities. Fortunately, the pastor did not criticize her and took a supportive attitude to understand her mental condition and to acknowledge her emotional turmoil. Given her persisting insomnia and other depressive features, the pastor helped her find a Christian psychiatrist, and a church sister accompanied her for psychiatric consultation and follow-up appointments. Miss C was prescribed an antidepressant with good recovery. The Christian psychiatrist also recommended a Christian psychotherapist, with whom Miss C had 12 sessions of CBT addressing her cognitive distortions—including some concerning her distress related to her faith. Her mood eventually improved, and she went back to church after nine months of professional treatments. Her negative cognitions had also subsided, and she managed to enjoy her church activities, spiritual exercises, and reading scriptures again.

Learning Points

1. Evidence-based pharmacological treatments, such as SSRI antidepressants, biochemically improve the brain function of emotion processing. A biologically healthy brain enables an individual to develop a healthy mind.

2. Spiritual experience is subjective and a positive spiritual experience would be diminished by the believer's depressive state.

3. Depressive cognitions such as hopelessness, self-blaming, self-perceived uselessness, unlovable and worthlessness are more readily observed in depressive patients in a religious context.

4. Somatic symptoms like anhedonia, day-time malaise, and insomnia would affect patients' participation in religious activities. These can be the result rather than the cause of depression.

5. Because symptoms of mood disorders may be subtle and mood deterioration occur so gradually that patients themselves may not be aware of it, longitudinal observation from peers of religious groups, who may have known the patient for years or decades, may provide useful information for the mental health professional.

6. Religious groups can provide psychosocial support and relevant resources to facilitate mental recovery. Some churches in Hong Kong even sponsor their congregants for psychiatric consultation or have in-house counsellors to provide psychotherapy.

7. Spiritual recovery usually occurs sometime later, and may take months to years after physical and mental recovery because cognitive recovery often occurs later.

8. Pastors and religious leaders should consider the possibility of a mood disorder or other mental health issues when a believer reports a negative spiritual/religious experience. If in doubt, it would be advisable to consult a psychiatrist for assessment.

Section 4: interface of mental health with spiritual organizations—illustrated by the example with Brahmakumaris

Avdesh Sharma and Sujatha D. Sharma

We need to realize as mental health professionals, and the society at large, that disease, health, and well-being form a continuum. The perceived causation for disease and its proposed management not only depends on science but also resources, especially human resources. It also needs to be kept in mind that application of research may differ from culture to culture or religion/spiritual perceptions about health and disease. 'Modern medicine', as we know it, is suited for disease or illness management to an extent (there are many other ways of medical management and other forms of treatment). In India, the (Ayurveda, Yoga, Unani, Siddha and Homeopathy [AYUSH)] systems of medicine), which have philosophical underpinnings about health are well established. They constitute part of the government's recognized forms of disease management, apart from 'modern medicine'.

The prevention of disease and promotion of health and well-being have been largely left out by modern medicine, especially psychiatry. The reasons have been not only inadequate resources but also the lack of acknowledgement of their importance accorded by the professionals themselves. The R/S organizations have usually provided culturally accepted ways of dealing with these preventive and promotive aspects of health. These may include cultural, social, philosophical, and anthropological perspectives including texts, scriptures, and stories about life and emotional well-being as a narrative, for handling mind, moods, relationships, crisis situations, and purpose of life.

Our collaborations with the spiritual organization 'Brahmakumaris' as mental health professionals

These started as a personal experience about 30 years back when I (Avdesh Sharma) participated in an international spiritual retreat at Mount Abu, Rajasthan, India. The retreat with about 90 participants from about 30 countries had intense discussions, workshops, and experiences of meditation from 4 a.m. to 10 p.m. I started experiencing parapsychological phenomenon such as of out-of-body experiences, pre-cognition, telepathy, complete sense of calm, peace and happiness, and high levels of energy and déjà vu from the second day onwards, and these lasted for about five days. At a party that I soon attended after returning to Delhi, I realized that I could neither drink even a few sips of beer nor even tolerate its smell as I started vomiting! (I used to be a social drinker then.) Even today, I cannot smell or drink alcohol because it causes nausea. That to me was the personal experience of a shift in consciousness causing changes in the body–mind axis. I pursued the knowledge of spiritual principles, meditative experience, and also how they could have an impact on mental health. My wife, Dr Sujatha Sharma, a clinical psychologist by profession has also since then been pursuing the spiritual practices of Brahmakumaris (a worldwide non-profit organization that does not charge for any activities, programmes, or conferences) and, over a period of time, we have carried out programmes integrating spirituality and mental health.

The spiritual beliefs and practices of Brahmakumaris have a presence in 138 countries through 8,500 centres. Its teachings are in all major languages of the world. In essence, the principles are that we are all essentially soul(s) (consciousness), which—through the mind—plays its assigned part (role) as an actor; that we should try to realize our highest self by letting go of all in the physical/ mental/social, and spiritual planes that interfere with our spiritual growth; that we should try to create positivity around ourselves and in our interactions; that we should consciously avoid hurting another person, species, or nature; that we should serve others unselfishly; and that meditative lifestyle makes us become better human being by a constant connection with The Supreme Soul, God. This is carried out by not renouncing the world or denying oneself a worldly life or necessary treatment of physical or mental disorders.

Below are some of the programmes carried out with Brahmakumaris and its affiliated non-profit organization, the Rajyoga Education and Research Foundation (RERF) in addressing the interface of spirituality and mental health:

1. Psychiatric conferences and workshops in the premises of Brahmakumaris with integrated programmes having both technical (psychological) and spiritual sessions.

2. Audiovisual programmes, television and web series.
   - Mindwatch (1995–2000), a 26-episode, documentary series on mental health was shot partially in the headquarters of Brahmakumaris at Mount Abu, India, and had inputs from spiritualists for the well-being section in each episode of mental health. This series, made for Indian National Television, Doordarshan, by Dr Avdesh Sharma and Dr Sujatha Sharma, was run 10 times on national television with a reach of 350 million people. It has been dubbed in seven Indian regional languages (English being the original) and has been the longest running mental health documentary series in the world.
   - Mind Matters (2009), 32-part television series in Hindi on psychospiritual health, having Dr Avdesh Sharma and Sister BK Shivani (an internationally acclaimed spiritual motivational speaker) as guest experts, was run on three television channels dedicated to spirituality.

- Zindagi Bane Aasan (2016–18) (Hindi, translating as 'Making life easy'), 52 episodes of half an hour each with Dr Avdesh Sharma as a guest expert giving psychospiritual perspectives on dealing with life situations and psychological issues. The telecast has been on a spiritual channel (Peace of Mind) with more than one million viewers.
- Khushian Khede Sadhe Vehre (2017–19) (Punjabi, regional language), 22 episodes of half an hour each with Dr Avdesh Sharma as guest expert, telecast on the Peace of Mind television channel with a viewership of more than a million.
- Mysteries of the Mind and Mann Ke Raaz (Hindi) (2018–20), 70 10-minute long episodes on various aspects of mental health followed by reflections, having Dr Avdesh Sharma as an expert for Awakening Television, Awakening App and the Awakening YouTube channel.

3. Joint webinars in 2020 on spirituality and mental health, healing the earth, building emotional resilience, etc. by Drs Avdesh and Sujatha Sharma with spiritual leaders of Brahmakumaris for healthcare professionals, psychiatrists, and the general public during and before the lockdown due to coronavirus.

4. Messages by spiritual leaders on mental health from a spiritual perspective but reiterating the message of being aware of mental health problems, seeking help and treatment, for the YouTube channel, Mind Specialists. This is a non-profit organization having mental health awareness and education as a focus and is managed by Drs Avdesh and Sujatha Sharma as Ffunders.

5. Medical conferences in Mount Abu, Rajasthan, India, and other major cities, and retreat centres in India, usually about two big events (1,500–5,000 health professionals) where the programme is a mix of technical sessions on health/mental health and spiritual teachings. This has been an ongoing programme for more than 20 years in which Drs. Avdesh and Sujatha Sharma are regular faculty members in these conferences.

6. Training in counselling skills to the staff of Global Hospital and Research Centre, a 140-bedded hospital in Mount Abu, Rajasthan, India, run by the RERF and Brahmakumaris. It provides an integrated approach to treatment through modern medicine, the Indian system of medicine, and spiritual lifestyle practices. This has been carried out by Dr Sujatha Sharma, regularly from time to time for the past 10 years.

7. Dr. Avdesh Sharma has done workshops and symposiums on 'Psychospiritual management' at various forums including the Indian Psychiatric Society and Indian Association of Private Psychiatry Conferences, Annual Conference of Royal College of Psychiatry, American Psychiatric Association, and RERF.

8. *Spirituality and Mental Health: Reflections of the Past, Applications in the Present and Projections for the Future*, 2009, a 608-page book with 39 chapters, edited by Dr, Avdesh Sharma, is a joint publication of the Indian Psychiatric Society and the RERF. It has contributions from renowned mental health and other professionals of international repute, including Professor Dinesh Bhugra, Past President of the WPA and senior spiritual teachers on various faiths. It was freely distributed to all the members (about 5,000 copies) of the Indian Psychiatric Society in hard copy, and is also freely available as an E-book now.

9. Publications in peer-reviewed journals, such as 'Effect of Raj Yogi Lifestyle on Tobacco De Addiction in India' by Dr Avdesh Sharma et al. (Indian Journal of Private Psychiatry, Vol. 9, Issue 2, November 2015).

10. Brahmakumaris has a presence in 138 countries through more than 8,500 centers. Dr Avdesh Sharma and Dr Sujatha Sharma have made public appearances, lectures, television and radio programmes on more than 200 forums in India, the USA, Canada, the UK, France, Spain, Israel, Australia, South Africa, Malaysia, Nepal, the UAE, etc.

11. In collaborations with the WPA:

    a. At the 2016 WPA International Congress in Cape Town, South Africa, a round-table discussion with Faith leaders was organized by Brahmakumaris on 20 November, 2016. Faith leaders from 12 organizations and 15 mental health professionals held a day-long deliberation leading to a white paper. On the same date, public programmes for interfaith leaders and mental health professionals were held at the Nelson Mandela Auditorium, Cape Town, organized by Brahmakumaris in association with the WPA section on R/S and psychiatry.

    b. The International Congress on Spirituality and Mental Health, 1–4 December 2019, Jerusalem, Israel, organized by the WPA section on R/S and psychiatry with other co-organizers, had among the plenary speakers: Brahmakumari Sister Gayatri, United Nations Representative of Brahmakumaris on 'Compassion Fatigue'; Dr Avdesh Sharma on 'Integrating spirituality and mental health; and Dr Sujatha Sharma on 'Integrating principles of Rajyoga in psychotherapy'. The Congress drew participants from 35 countries.

    c. Sister BK Shivani, an immensely popular international motivational speaker of Brahmakumaris, has been the Goodwill Ambassador of WPA and has been promoting mental health through various forums in conferences, videos, and lecture tours.

Some concluding thoughts on our collaborations with Brahmakumaris

The programmes carried out have been mutually beneficial. They have led to our own growth as individuals and mental health professionals, helped us integrate culturally acceptable spiritual principles in our therapeutic work, and improved therapeutic alliance with clients. It has helped the spiritual organization, Brahmakumaris, to be able to help those with mental health issues and also create awareness about handling mental health problems through integrated psychospiritual principles. It is hoped that other health/mental health professionals may also explore opportunities to collaborate with spiritual/faith-based organizations around them in attaining quality, holistic, cost-effective, culturally acceptable care that is also humane.

Section 5: commentaries and conclusions

Summary

Wai Lun Alan Fung

The authors of Sections 2, 3, and 4 have vividly illustrated the diverse range of possible collaborations between mental health and faith communities in promoting mental health, across different cultural and geographical contexts, and all the way from the local to international levels.

With Reverend Shepherd and other mental health and spiritual care professionals, this writer had co-founded the Working Group for the Promotion of Mental Health in Faith Communities (mentalhealthandfaith.org) in Canada—which has been involved in the organization of conferences, seminars, and other activities to promote mental health among Christian and other faith communities. These activities were well received based on quantitative and qualitative feedback. In another project that this writer had co-led in Toronto, Canada, a series of low-cost psychoeducational intervention in collaborations with local mosques and Islamic organizations—aiming at improving mental health literacy—resulted in statistically significant improvements in knowledge, behaviour, attitudes towards mental health service utilization, and stigma related to mental ill health (14). This writer had also initiated and co-organized other half- to one-day conferences addressing the interface between mental health and spirituality in publicly funded, secular settings in Canada, such as the North York General Hospital (2012) and the University of Toronto (2014)—which in both cases had resulted in significantly increased participants' self-rated knowledge level about the interface between mental health and spiritual care, competence levels in caring for patients with spiritual concerns and mental illness, and likelihood of collaboration with the other professions (i.e. between mental health and spiritual care). Together, these suggest that endeavours addressing the interface between mental health and spirituality—with the goal of enhancing mental health—may not necessarily be resource-intensive, and thus may be quite feasibly implemented even in resource-constrained settings, and something with global implications.

Indeed, to enhance the global reach of the WPA position statement on spirituality and religion in psychiatry (1)—originally written in English—the position statement has been translated into multiple other languages, available from religionandpsychiatry.org/main/wpa-position-statement-on-spirituality-and religion-in-psychiatry. In particular, Dr Agatha Chong (莊勁怡醫生) and Dr Alan Fung (馮偉麟醫生) were in charge of the Chinese (traditional and simplified characters) translations of the Position Statement (世界精神醫學會的靈性及宗教與精神醫學立場聲明). The full texts of these Chinese versions are available in the aforementioned website.

An additional layer of complexity of the role of culture in the interface of spirituality and mental health is migrant populations—for instance, visible minorities in the Western world. The case of Miss C in Section 3 has illustrated how collaborations between faith communities and mental health professionals may help address the challenges involved in treating a Chinese woman in Hong Kong with major depressive disorder. Nonetheless, mental health issues and service provisions for Chinese migrants in the Western world are often even more complicated (15, 16) and such collaborations between mental health professionals and faith leaders may be especially valuable (17).

Assuming that one is convinced about the importance of collaborations between mental health professionals and faith communities, what are some guiding principles for such endeavours? As discussed in Section 4, at the 2016 WPA International Congress in Cape Town, South Africa, a round-table discussion was held among mental health professionals and leaders of various faith-based organizations to consider such collaborations. Chaired by Dr Avdesh Sharma, Dr Sujatha Sharma and this writer were among the participants. Subsequently, Dr Sujatha Sharma prepared the Round Table meeting proceedings. Based on the Round Table discussions and proceedings, this writer had formulated some suggested principles of interprofessional collaborations between mental health and spiritual care professionals—as listed in Box 25.1.

The aforementioned discussions also have significant implications for the training of mental health professionals. In a 2012 survey (led by this writer) on the self-rated attitudes, behaviours, and competencies of psychiatry residents at the University of Toronto (which has one of the largest psychiatry residency programmes in North America) on spirituality in clinical care, two-thirds of

Box 25.1 Some suggested principles of interprofessional collaborations between mental health and spiritual care professionals

1. Spirituality/religion plays an important role in mental health, for coping with human sufferings, as well as for facilitating the pursuit and attainment of purpose and meaning of life.

2. Both spiritual care and mental health professions have long been working towards similar goals in caregiving, mitigating human suffering and enhancing human well-being.

3. The different paradigms and parlance used in the two professions have at times led to conflicts.

4. It would be important for the two professions to collaborate in order to address the mental health needs of the general population.

5. Steps of establishing and enhancing collaborations between the two professions may include:
    i. building trust between the two professions by establishing common parlance as well as identifying common goals in terms of helping those with mental health issues and/or distress;
    ii. identifying further facilitators and barriers to collaborations between the two professions;
    iii. identifying and/or establishing best practice models of integrative/collaborative care between spiritual care and mental health professionals;
    iv. identifying core competencies and establishing 'best practices' for training:
        a. in mental health, for spiritual care professionals and trainees;
        b. in spirituality/religion, for mental health professionals and trainees.

6. The general principle of interprofessional collaborations between the two professions should be advocated globally, but should also take local factors into consideration to ensure relevance (i.e. glo-cal)—for instance, indigenous perspectives.

Note: The implications of such collaborations for the younger generation should be further explored—given the growing existential crises of the younger generation as well as their growing mistrusts in religious groups due to perceived associations of religious groups with injustice and conflicts. The younger generation—including those in the two professions—should be involved in shaping this discussion.

respondents agreed that there would be a need for training in how to address R/S issues in psychiatric practice, and 89% agreed that there would be clinical situations in psychiatry where it would be important to consider R/S-related issues. Nonetheless, only one-quarter endorsed often taking a spiritual history or discussing spiritual issues with patients; one-quarter having enough experience and/or training to take a spiritual history/discuss spiritual issues; and one-fifth understanding when to use the diagnosis of religious and spiritual problems. The most often reported barriers included lack of time in clinical work (70%) and lack of training (61%). A recent systematic and scoping review of educational endeavours on teaching spiritual/religious competencies to psychiatry residents (co-led by this writer) has revealed that such training endeavours, while only available in a minority of psychiatric programmes worldwide, have generally been well tolerated and appreciated by both psychiatry trainees and patients (18). Indeed, a proposed core curriculum for R/S in psychiatry residency programmes has recently been published (19).

In conclusion, interdisciplinary collaborations and partnerships have been advocated for global well-being (20). Authors of this chapter have illustrated different ways of how mental health professionals and faith communities could collaborate in enhancing mental health as well as mental health service provision. We now appeal to YOU—readers of this chapter and our newest collaborators—to act NOW in contributing to these efforts.

References

1. **Moreira-Almeida A, Sharma A, Janse van Rensburg B, Verhagen PJ, Cook CCH.** WPA position statement on spirituality and religion in psychiatry. *World Psychiatry.* 2016;**15**(1):87–88. Available from: religionandpsychiatry.org/main/wpa-position-statement-on-spirituality-and religion-in-psychiatry

2. **Cook, CCH.** *Recommendations for psychiatrists on spirituality and religion. Position statement PS03/2013.* London: Royal College of Psychiatrists; 2013.

3. **American Psychiatric Association (APA).** Mental health and faith community partnership. United States: APA; 2018 [cited 1 June 2020]. Available from: https://www.psychiatry.org/psychiatrists/cultural-competency/engagement-opportunities/mental-health-and-faith-community-partnership

4. **Gureje O, Appiah-Poku J, Bello T, et al.** Effect of collaborative care between traditional and faith healers and primary health-care workers on psychosis outcomes in Nigeria and Ghana (COSIMPO): a cluster randomised controlled trial. *Lancet.* 2020 Aug 29;**396**(10251):612–22.

5. **Hanlon C, Alem A.** A leap of faith for more effective mental health care. *Lancet.* 2020 Aug 29;**396**(10251):584–5.

6. **Nortje G, Oladeji B, Gureje O, Seedat S.** Effectiveness of traditional healers in treating mental disorders: a systematic review. *Lancet Psychiatry.* 2016 Feb;**3**(2):154–70.

7. **Peteet JR, Dell ML, Fung WLA** (eds). *Ethical considerations at the intersection of psychiatry and religion*. Oxford: Oxford University Press; 2018.

8. **The Royal Australian and New Zealand College of Psychiatrists Section of History, Philosophy and Ethics of Psychiatry.** *Position statement 96: the relevance of religion and spirituality to psychiatric practice*. Melbourne: The Royal Australian and New Zealand College of Psychiatrists; 2018.

9. **Central Intelligence Agency** [Internet]. The world factbook: Hong Kong. Washington, DC: Central Intelligence Agency; 2020. [cited 1 June 2020]. Available from: https://www.cia.gov/library/publications/the-world-factbook/geos/hk.html

10. **Kübler-Ross E.** *On death and dying*. New York: Macmillan Publishing Co.; 1969.

11. **Lee KH.** *A Buddhist theory and method of end of life care: equality, compassion, enlightenment and conversion* (dissertation). Taiwan: National Central University; 2016 (cited 14 June 2020]). Available from: http://ir.lib.ncu.edu.tw:88/thesis/view_etd.asp?URN=971404004

12. **Hong Kong Sheng Kung Hui** [Internet]. Hong Kong: Hong Kong Sheng Kung Hui. Colloquium of six religious leaders discusses emotional distress. 23 December 2019. [cited 14 June 2020]. Available from: www.hkskh.org/article.aspx?lang=1&id=14118&cID=95

13. **Zhao D.** Research on Confucius cultivation thought into the personal morality education of college students [dissertation on the Internet]. China: Hebei University of Technology; 2015. [cited 14 June 2020]. Available from: http://www.cdmd.cnki.com.cn/Article/CDMD-10080-1017873869.htm

14. **Ali-Mohammed S, Malick A, Islam F, Kutuadu A, Qasim K, Fung WLA.** *Increasing mental health literacy among Muslim Canadians through a spiritually and culturally integrative psychoeducation workshop program*. Manuscript under review.

15. **Ahmad F, Maule C, Wang J, Fung WLA.** Symptoms and Experience of Depression Among Chinese Communities in the West: A Scoping Review. *Harvard Review of Psychiatry*. 2018 Nov/Dec; 26(6):340–351. doi: 10.1097/HRP.0000000000000202.

16. **Ahmad F, Wang J, Wong B, Fung WLA.** Interactive mental health assessments for Chinese Canadians: A pilot randomized controlled trial in nurse practitioner-led primary care clinic. *Asia-Pacific Psychiatry*. 2020 Jun 30:e12400. doi: 10.1111/appy.12400. Online ahead of print.

17. **Fung WLA.** [Internet]. Canada: The Globe and Mail. Culture's role in mental health is overlooked. 31 May 2011. [cited 14 June 2020]. Available from: https://www.theglobeandmail.com/opinion/cultures-role-in-mental-health-is-overlooked/article581457/

18. **Hathaway DB, de Oliveira E Oliveira FHA, Mirhom M, Moreira-Almeida A, Fung WLA, Peteet JR.** Teaching spiritual and religious competencies to psychiatry residents: A scoping and systematic review. *Academic Medicine*. 2021 May 18. doi: 10.1097/ACM.0000000000004167. Online ahead of print.

19. **de Oliveira e Oliveira FHA, Peteet JR, Moreira-Almeida A.** Religiosity and spirituality in psychiatry residency programs: why, what, and how to teach? *Brazilian Journal of Psychiatry*. 2020 Oct 23:S1516–44462020005035204. doi: 10.1590/1516-4446-2020-1106. Online ahead of print.

20. **Halbreich U, Schulze T, Botbol M,** et al. Partnerships for interdisciplinary collaborative global well-being. *Asia-Pacific Psychiatry*. 2019 Jun;11(2):e12366.

Index

For the benefit of digital users, indexed terms that span two pages (e.g., 52–53) may, on occasion, appear on only one of those pages.

Notes

As this work concerns religion and spirituality, entries under these headings are kept to a minimum. Users are advised that all entries related to these two terms. *vs.* indicates a comparison

Tables, figures and boxes are indicated by *t*, *f* and *b* following the page number